Social determinants of health

Social determinants of health

Edited by

Michael Marmot

International Centre for Health and Society, University College London, UK

and Richard G. Wilkinson

Trafford Centre for Medical Research, University of Sussex, UK, and
International Centre for Health and Society, University College London, UK

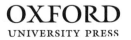

OXFORD

UNIVERSITY PRESS

OXFORD
UNIVERSITY PRESS

Great Clarendon Street, Oxford OX2 6DP

Oxford University Press is a department of the University of Oxford.
It furthers the University's objective of excellence in research, scholarship,
and education by publishing worldwide in

Oxford New York

Auckland Bangkok Buenos Aires Cape Town Chennai
Dar es Salaam Delhi Hong Kong Istanbul Karachi Kolkata
Kuala Lumpur Madrid Melbourne Mexico City Mumbai Nairobi
São Paulo Shanghai Taipei Tokyo Toronto

Oxford is a registered trade mark of Oxford University Press
in the UK and in certain other countries

Published in the United States
by Oxford University Press Inc., New York

© Oxford University Press, 1999

The moral rights of the author have been asserted

Database right Oxford University Press (maker)

First published 1999
Reprinted 2000 (three times), 2001 (twice), 2002, 2003 (twice), 2004

British Library Cataloguing in Publication Data
Data available

Library of Congress Cataloging in Publication Data
Social determinants of health/edited by Michael Marmot and
Richard G. Wilkinson.
Includes bibliographical references and index.
1. Public Health – Social aspects. 2. Social medicine. 3. Medical policy
– Social aspects.   I. Marmot, M.G. II. Wilkinson, Richard G.
RA418.S4225   1999   362.1—dc21   99–22942

10

ISBN 0 19 263069 5

Printed in Great Britain
on acid-free paper by
Biddles Ltd, King's Lynn, Norfolk

Contents

Contributors

Mel Bartley Department of Epidemiology and Public Health, University College London, 1–19 Torrington Place, London WC1E 6BT, UK. e-mail: m.bartley@ public-health.ucl.ac.uk

David Blane Division of Neuroscience, Imperial College of Science, Technology and Medicine; at Department of Behavioural and Cognitive Science, ICSTM Charing Cross, St Dunstan's Road, London W6 8RP, UK. e-mail: d.blane@ic.ac.uk

Eric Brunner International Centre for Health and Society, University College London, 1–19 Torrington Place, London WC1E 6BT, UK. e-mail: e.brunner@ucl.ac.uk

George Davey Smith Department of Social Medicine, University of Bristol, Canynge Hall, Whiteladies Road, Bristol BS8 2PR, UK. email: zetkin@bristol.ac.uk

Danny Dorling School of Geographical Sciences, University of Bristol, University Road, Bristol BS8 1SS, UK. e-mail: d.dorling@geography.leeds.ac.uk

Jill L. Farrington WHO Centre for Urban Health, WHO Regional Office for Europe, Scherfigsvej 8, DK 2100 Copenhagen Ø, Denmark. e-mail: jfa@who.dk

Amanda Feeney Department of Epidemiology and Public Health, University College London, 1–19 Torrington Place, London WC1E 6BT, UK. email: m.feeney@public-health.ucl.ac.uk

Jane Ferrie Department of Epidemiology and Public Health, University College London, 1–19 Torrington Place, London WC1E 6BT, UK. email: j.ferrie@public-health.ucl.ac.uk

Martin J. Jarvis ICRF Health Behaviour Unit, Department of Epidemiology and Public Health, University College London, 1–19 Torrington Place, London WC1E 6BT, UK. email: martin.jarvis@ucl.ac.uk

Mark McCarthy Department of Epidemiology and Public Health, University College London, 1–19 Torrington Place, London WC1E 6BT, UK. e-mail: m.mcarthy@ucl.ac.uk

Michael Marmot   International Centre for Health and Society, University College London, 1–19 Torrington Place, London WC1E 6BT, UK. e-mail: m.marmot@public-health.ucl.ac.uk

Scott M. Montgomery   Department of Medicine, Royal Free and University College Medical School, Rowland Hill, London NW3 2PF, UK. email: smm@rfhsm.ac.uk

Aileen Robertson   WHO Regional Office for Europe, Scherfigsvej 8, Copenhagen, Denmark. e-mail: aro@who.dk

Mary Shaw   School of Geographical Sciences, University of Bristol, University Road, Bristol BS8 1SS, UK. e-mail: mary.shaw@bristol.ac.uk

Aubrey Sheiham   International Centre for Health and Society, University College London, 1–19 Torrington Place, London WC1E 6BT, UK. e-mail: a.sheiham@ucl.ac.uk

Johannes Siegrist   Department of Medical Sociology, Medical Faculty, University of Duesseldorf, Moorenstrasse 5, D-40225 Duesseldorf, Germany. e-mail: siegrist@uni-duesseldorf.de

Stephen A. Stansfeld   International Centre for Health and Society, University College London, 1–19 Torrington Place, London WC1E 6BT, UK. e-mail: s.a.stansfeld@qmw.ac.uk

Tores Theorell   National Institute for Psychosocial Factors and Health, Box 230, S-17177 Stockholm, Sweden. e-mail: tores.theorell@ipm.ki.se

Agis D. Tsouros   WHO Centre for Urban Health, WHO Regional Office for Europe, Scherfigsvej 8, DK 2100 Copenhagen Ø, Denmark. e-mail: ats@-who.dk

Michael Wadsworth   MRC National Survey of Health and Development, University College London, Department of Epidemiology and Public Health, 1–19 Torrington Place, London WC1E 6BT, UK. e-mail: m.wadsworth@ucl.ac.uk

Jane Wardle   ICRF Health Behaviour Unit, Department of Epidemiology and Public Health, University College London, 1–19 Torrington Place, London WC1E 6BT, UK. e-mail: j.wardle@ucl.ac.uk

Richard G. Wilkinson   Trafford Centre for Medical Research, University of Sussex, Brighton BN1 9RY, UK. e-mail: r.g.wilkinson@sussex.ac.uk

Foreword

The health of populations is related to features of society and its social and economic organization. This crucial fact provides the basis for effective policy making to improve population health. While there is, understandably, much concern with appropriate provision and financing of health services and with ensuring that the nature of the services provided should be based on the best evidence of effectiveness, health is a matter that goes beyond the provision of health services. Policies pursued by many branches of government and by the private sector, both nationally and locally, exert a powerful influence on health – and this book shows the direction in which we should be going. Just as decisions about health services should be based on the best evidence available, so should policies related to the social determinants of health.

Researchers associated with the International Centre for Health and Society at University College London have accumulated a wealth of knowledge on the social determinants of health. The World Health Organization Regional Office for Europe's Centre for Urban Health was concerned to package that knowledge in a way that is useful to policy-makers. The result was *Social Determinants of Health – The Solid Facts* (Wilkinson and Marmot 1998). This accumulation of evidence was also fundamental to the *Independent Inquiry into Inequalities in Health* which I was commissioned to chair by the Government in Britain (Acheson 1998). Indeed, many of the authors of this book were closely involved in the presentation of evidence that underpinned the formulation of recommendations for policy development that resulted from that Inquiry.

This book results from the welcome efforts of members of the International Centre for Health and Society and their collaborators to summarize their research evidence around themes useful to policy-makers. Policy making will always involve a multiplicity of influences. The research summarized here shows that important among those influences must be the evidence on the social determinants of health.

Sir Donald Acheson
Chairman
International Centre for Health & Society
University College London

References

Wilkinson, R. and Marmot M., eds 'Social Determinants of Health – The Solid Facts', World Health Organization, 1998

Acheson, Sir Donald. Independent Inquiry into Health Inequalities Report. London: The Stationery Office 1998

Acknowledgements

Without the essential provision of research funds, much of this work would not be possible. Funding organizations have been acknowledged by individual authors at the end of each chapter.

A special word of thanks is due to Patricia Crowley, ICHS Centre Administrator, who has co-ordinated the efforts of all those involved in providing the scientific material for this book and who was the main point of contact for the editors, authors, staff from the WHO Regional Office for Europe's Centre for Urban Health, and Oxford University Press.

1 Introduction

Michael Marmot

1.1 Introduction

The distinction between pure and applied research is, appropriately, blurred. Research that increases knowledge and understanding is of social value whether or not its practical implications are followed through in the short term. Curiosity-driven research might turn out to have greater application than research directed at an immediate practical problem. Knowledge and understanding might well have been the main social justification that most of the authors of this book would have given for their research. Those of us involved in research on social inequalities in health feel particularly vulnerable on the 'so what?' question. Time and again, we have been confronted by the question of whether research on social inequalities in health has any practical application. The hard form of this argument asserts that there are no societies without social inequalities, hence the research has little relevance.

Even an area with such obviously practical implications for public health as the research on smoking as a cause of premature mortality was initially greeted with some scepticism. If individuals will not change their behaviour, so the argument ran, what use is it to show that smoking increases risk of illness? The smoking example perhaps has some relevance. Indeed, it was the case that 'simply' showing the smoking disease link was insufficient to benefit the public health. There have been a number of important contributors to policies to reduce the burden of smoking-related diseases. Important among these have been summaries of the evidence in a form amenable to policy makers, and widespread public information about the links between smoking and health. Both of these have been important in developing policies which relate to taxation, advertising and sponsoring, health education, labelling, and restriction in public places. What concerns us here is not the details of smoking control policies but how to promote a discourse among policy makers and the public about relevant research findings. In this example we might note that we are interested not only in smoking as a cause of disease but in the determinants of smoking: the causes of the causes.

This seemed to be the right analogy when the Centre for Urban Health, WHO Regional Office for Europe, approached us at the International Centre for Health and Society at University College, London to inquire if we could summarize work on the social determinants of health in 10 messages. The aim was that these messages should be relevant both to policy makers and the public. An important consideration was that each message should be supported by evidence. This book grows directly out of that process. Members of the International Centre for Health and Society and colleagues, represented in this book, developed 10 messages that were brought together in a booklet *Social determinants of health – the solid facts*, distributed widely by WHO to policy makers, researchers, and practitioners (Wilkinson and Marmot 1998). The ten messages form the topics for Chapters 2–11 of this book. Each of these chapters presents a summary of relevant research, giving the evidence under-lying the message. A description of the WHO campaign, of which the Solid Facts is a part, and for which this book provides the evidence is given in the Epilogue.

Two key assumptions underlie the approach we took in producing messages for WHO and the chapters in this book. First, the impact of the social environment on health, as represented by social inequalities in health, is not a 'given'. By understanding how the social environment affects health, its specific features and pathways, it is potentially possibly to affect these with consequent impact on health. The second assumption follows from the first, namely that the social environment is not inchoate and amorphous, but that specific social determi-nants of health can be characterized and their separate effects on health studied.

1.2   Social and economic environment and health

1.2.1   Medical care?

For many commentators there is the untested assumption that inequalities in health arise from inequalities in health care. In one sense, it would be quite easy to see how this conflation of two disparate ideas could happen. In the industrialized world, countries spend between about 6 per cent and 14 per cent of gross domestic product on health care. It therefore looms large in health policy dis-cussions. The logic might be characterized as follows: countries would not spend this much money on health care, actually medical care, if it were not effective; there are undoubted inequalities in access to medical care; therefore inequalities in health must result from inequalities in access to and delivery of medical care.

There is, of course, a gap in this logic. Because there are inequalities in access, it does not follow that these are the causes of inequalities in health. On the contrary, there are inequalities in the onset of new disease, which is not a medical care issue, and there are inequalities in mortality from diseases not amenable to medical intervention (Mackenbach et al. 1989).

The purpose of this book, however, is not to examine the effectiveness and limits of medical care. Universal access to high-quality and effective medical care (if it were not effective it could not be high quality) should be part of an advanced civilized society. Lack of access to effective medical care is likely to lead to unnecessary morbidity and suffering. For the purposes of this book we take this as unproblematic and not requiring further elaboration. Medical care is only relevant to this book's discussions of the social determinants of health if we have somehow got it wrong. In other words, are we mistaken in concluding that childhood environment, the work environment, unemployment, patterns of social relationships, social exclusion, food, addictive behaviour, and transport are related to causation of ill health when, in fact, these apparent relationships could all be accounted for by lack of access to good-quality medical care? Clearly, we judge that these relationships are causal and are determinants of differences in disease rates within and between societies. They create problems with which the medical care system must cope. Defects in the medical care system are not the cause of the problems.

1.2.2 Constitution or individual risk?

There is much interest in the genetic basis of human disease. Researchers in this tradition look for the interaction of genetic predisposition with individual exposures to account for individual differences in disease. Thus, for example, smoking causes lung cancer; most smokers do not die of lung cancer; there must therefore be some genetic or other factor determining which smokers succumb and which do not. We do not question such a formulation, but point out that it is only part of the picture. It is important to ask whether it can account for differences in risk of disease between *populations*.

Two of the clearest types of evidence demonstrating the importance of the environment come from migrant studies and time trends. When people change environment their patterns of disease risk changes. In my earliest work on epidemiology, I was part of a collaborative group studying heart disease and stroke in men of Japanese ancestry living in Japan, Hawaii, and California (Marmot et al. 1975; Syme et al. 1975; Worth et al. 1975; Winkelstein et al. 1975; Nichaman et al. 1975). The further the Japanese migrated across the Pacific, the higher their incidence of coronary heart disease and the lower the rate of stroke. One might be tempted to argue that this is not a demonstration of the importance of the environment in changing risk of disease, but that the Japanese who were genetically more likely to develop heart disease were more likely to leave Japan. If there were such selective migration, this genetic predisposition would have to determine not only the fact of leaving Japan but the distance travelled. Japanese in Hawaii have rates of heart disease intermediate between those in Japan and those in California. A simpler interpretation of the facts is that environment and life style affected disease rates. In California, we had evidence that the rate of heart disease went up with degree of acculturation (Marmot and Syme 1976). Whatever the importance of genetic predisposition, the environment in which these people lived played an important role in determining their disease risk.

Over short periods of time, genetic predisposition to disease of individuals and populations cannot change materially but disease rates can change markedly. Figure 1.1 shows the changing pattern of suicide mortality by socio-economic status (Registrar General's Social Class) in England and Wales. Over the 20 year period, the social gradient increased dramatically in a way that could not be accounted for by a shift of predisposed individuals between social classes (Drever et al. 1996).

It is also worth making a distinction between individual risk factors and environmental causes of disease. Syme has pointed to two limitations of the individual risk-factor approach. First, individual risk factors explain only a part of variations in the occurrence of disease. Secondly, it has proved difficult to modify individual risk factors by trying to persuade individuals to change their behaviour (Syme 1996). There has been success in modifying individual risk in people at especially high risk, such as drug treatment of high cholesterol and high blood pressure. As Rose has pointed out, while this has benefit for the individuals concerned, it makes a limited contribution to reducing disease rates in the whole population (Rose 1992). Rose goes further and suggests that the causes of individual differences in disease may be different from the causes of differences between populations. It is these population determinants that are the focus of this book.

1.2.3   Social and economic environment – non-infectious disease

The overall relation between economic fortunes and health is shown in Fig. 1.2, taken from the World Development Report (World Bank 1993). It

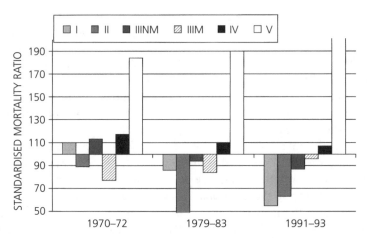

Fig. 1.1 Suicide by social class in England and Wales, males, 1970–93. 1970–72 does not include undetermined injury, Professional; II, employers and managers; IIINM, intermediate and junior non-manual; IIIM, skilled manual and non-professional; IV, semi-skilled manual and personal service; V, unskilled manual. (From Drever et al. 1996.)

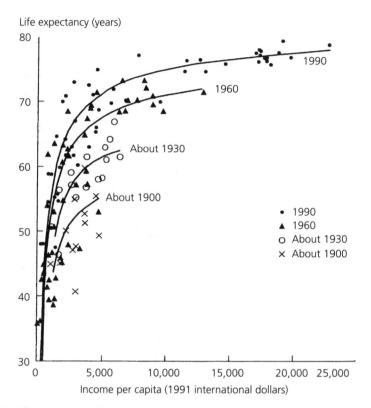

Fig. 1.2 Life expectancy and income for selected countries and periods (World Bank 1993).

shows that, for the poor countries of the world there is a clear relation between gross national product (GNP) per capita and life expectancy. At the lower end of the range of GNP, the relationship is quite steep: small increases in per capita GNP are related to relatively large increases in life expectancy. This causes little surprise. Malnutrition and infectious diseases that result in a high burden of maternal, infant, and childhood deaths are related to poverty. Improvement in living conditions that goes along with increases in GNP in poor countries will result in improvements in life expectancy. This is well understood.

What is perhaps less well understood is that the major causes of morbidity and mortality in developed countries, non-infectious diseases and external causes of death, are also related to the social environment. Increasingly, these are also the major health problems for the developing world. Figure 1.3 (a and b) is taken from the WHO Global Burden of Disease study (Murray and Lopez 1996). By looking at probability of death between 15 and 60 years of age, it removes the contribution of deaths in infancy, childhood, and old age. It shows that by 2020, for every region of the world, chronic diseases, including cardiovascular disease, cancer, and respiratory disease will be more important causes of death

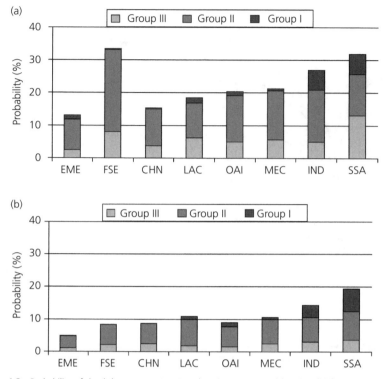

Fig. 1.3 Probability of death between ages 15 and 60 in year 2020: (a) males; (b) females. Group I, infections, perinatal, nutritional, maternal; Group II, cardiovascular disease, cancer, respiratory, other; Group III, external causes. EME, Established market economies; FSE, formerly socialist economies of Europe; CHN, China; LAC, Latin America and the Caribbean; OAI, other Asia and islands; MEC, Middle Eastern crescent; IND, India; SSA, sub-Saharan Africa. (From Murray and Lopez 1996.)

than the group including infections, perinatal, nutritional, and maternal deaths. Figure 1.3b shows the probability of death between 15 and 60 to be considerably lower in women than men. The death rate due to external causes is lower and, once again, the chronic diseases including cardiovascular disease emerge as the major cause of death.

Figure 1.3 shows the high mortality in middle-age in the former socialist economies of central and eastern Europe. In men, mortality rates were actually higher in these countries than in any other region of the world. This is a new development. Figure 1.4 (a and b) shows that around 1970 life expectancy in the countries of central and eastern Europe was similar to that in the European Union (Marmot and Bobak 1997). Over the subsequent two and a half decades life expectancy continued to improve steadily in the EU and Nordic countries and declined in the countries of central and eastern Europe. In women there was not a decline in life expectancy but the gap between 'west' and 'east' increased. The former Soviet Union, and then

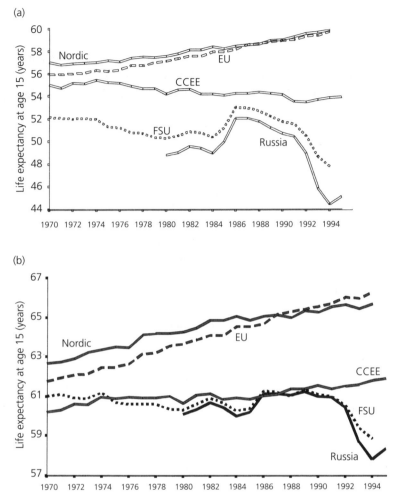

Fig. 1.4 Life expectancy at age 15 in Europe: (a) men; (b) women. CCEE; Countries of Central and Eastern Europe. EU, European Union; FSU, former Soviet Union. (From Marmot and Bobak 1997.)

Russia, shows even more marked divergence from the 'west'. The apparent increase in life expectancy in Russia around 1985 has been attributed by some to the Gorbachov reforms designed to reduce alcohol consumption (Leon et al. 1997). Similarly, it has been argued that alcohol has made a major contribution to the marked decline in life expectancy in more recent years (Leon et al. 1997), although the magnitude of this contribution has been questioned (Bobak and Marmot 1996).

More than half of the east/west difference in mortality is due to cardiovascular disease and a further 20 per cent per cent to external causes of death (Marmot and Bobak 1997).

1.3 Accounting for the global burden of disease

Figure 1.5 is adapted from the work of Murray and Lopez (Murray and Lopez 1996). It shows their best estimates of how much of the global burden of deaths could be attributed to different risk factors. In their analyses the largest single contributor is malnutrition, accounting for nearly 12 per cent of deaths. This, and all the other major risk factors that they consider account for about 40 per cent of the global burden of deaths. How are we to think about these figures? One obvious response is to assume that measurement error or other data analytical problems has led to an under-estimate of the contribution of risk factors. Possibly, but it seems unlikely that this would change the conclusion that about half of the global burden of deaths remains unexplained by major risk factors. Certainly the figures fit well with analyses of cardiovascular disease that suggest a similar conclusion in relation to international differences (Tunstall-Pedoe et al. 1994).

It also seems unlikely that Murray and Lopez (1996) have 'forgotten' a major risk factor. Better specification of 'malnutrition' could perhaps encompass the nutritional causes of cardiovascular disease and cancer, and thereby account for a larger proportion of deaths. Be that as it may, there are other reasons for believing that something important is not included in this analysis of risk factors. There is a developing research base that relates disease patterns to the organization of society and the way society invests in its human capital (for example, Amick et al. 1995; Blane et al. 1996; Wilkinson, 1996). Not only may these social determinants of health start to fill in the 'other' category in Fig. 1.5, but several of the risk factors in Fig. 1.5 themselves have social determinants.

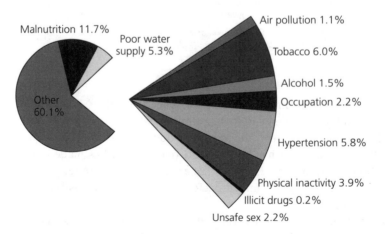

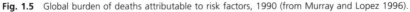

Fig. 1.5 Global burden of deaths attributable to risk factors, 1990 (from Murray and Lopez 1996).

1.3.1 Sustainable development and chronic disease

One formulation of sustainable development is:

> 'development that meets the needs of the present without compromising the ability of future generations to meet their own needs' (Interdepartmental Working Group on UK's Sustainable Development Strategy of 1994).

One way of thinking about it is the developing of goods and services which meet people's needs but involve the use of fewer natural resources. This implies managing and protecting the natural environment and resources. To take one example, Fig. 1.6 shows projected global energy use up to the year 2010. Although beyond the present purpose, we may note the inequities here: in that the projected increase in energy use of non-OECD countries still does not bring them up to the level of use in the OECD (Organization of Economic Co-operation and Development) countries (Joint publication by World Resources Institute, United Nations Development Programme, 1998). We may point to two problems relevant to our current concern. First, this increasing use of energy will lead to increasing levels of air pollution, not to mention global warming due to emission of greenhouse gases. Murray and Lopez (1996) estimate that about 5 per cent of deaths in the former socialist economies could be attributed to air pollution. The second problem relates to transport. A significant proportion of this global energy use will be from the automobile. The downside to the convenience afforded by the car is decreasing use of walking and cycling as modes of transport. These have the advantage to individuals of being readily accessible to all and, in the richer countries, reducing the burden of obesity and of cardiovascular disease.

1.3.2 The natural environment and the social environment

There is now active work enlarging the concept of sustainable development to include the building of sustainable communities for people to live and work in.

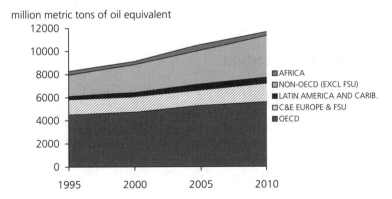

Fig. 1.6 Projected global energy use 1995–2010. FSU, former Soviet Union; OECD, Organization of Economic Co-operation and Development. (From World Resources Institute and United Nations Development Programme 1998).

Although the major focus of this work is not the improvement of health, the areas it covers are relevant to the social determinants of health. In the broadest terms, the relevance of social determinants was illustrated above in Fig. 1.2, which showed the association between GNP and life expectancy.

There are three further observations to be made about Fig. 1.2. First, for a given level of income (standardized to $1991), life expectancy has been increasing over the four time periods shown. This could be attributed to improvements in public health and medical care. But it could also be related to the causes underlying the other two observations. Second, there is a scatter of life expectancy around a given GNP level. This is illustrated further in Fig. 1.7 (a, b and c). It compares countries with equivalent levels of GNP and shows that adult mortality is inversely related to levels of adult literacy. The suggestion here is not necessarily that adults who are literate will have better health than those who are not, although that is plausible. Rather, one should view adult literacy as an indicator of investment in human capital. Even poor countries who invest in human capital will have better health than those who do not.

The third observation relates to the flattening of the curve in Fig. 1.2. Above a GNP per capita of about $5000, the relationship between GNP and life expectancy is weak. Wilkinson shows that, for these richer countries, there is a strong relation between income inequality of a country and life expectancy (Wilkinson 1996).

In the final chapter of this book Wilkinson develops the argument that income inequality reflects the social environment. His thesis is that a more fragmented society goes along with wider income inequalities. Income inequalities may be a driver of the system. It is possible, however, that fragmentation of the social system may have profound adverse effects on health, whatever is happening to income inequalities. This may be relevant to the trends in central and eastern Europe illustrated in Fig. 1.4 (Walberg et al. 1998). They may be a reflection of a decline in the degree to which these countries provide suitable circumstances for people to live and work in. This may be thought of as erosion of social capital, or unsustainable development.

1.4 Social inequalities

If the social environment is an important cause of ill health, this is likely to be manifested as social inequalities in health. For three decades we have been following the health of British civil servants in the Whitehall studies. This may, at first, seem to be an unlikely choice of population to use in order to study social inequalities in health. These people all live in a relatively affluent part of a relatively affluent country. They are office based, non-industrial employees in stable jobs, and, in the first Whitehall study, they were all white males. The results of 25 year follow-up of the first Whitehall study are shown in Fig. 1.8 (Marmot and Shipley 1996). At the

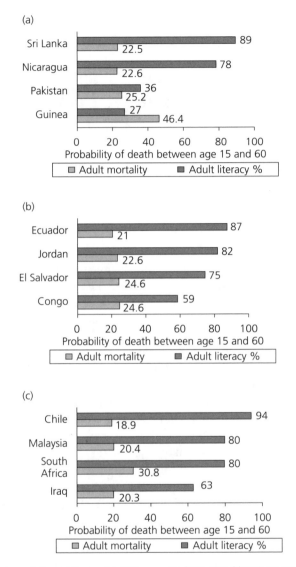

Fig. 1.7 Male mortality and literacy: (a) GNP per capita $400–500; (b) GNP per capita $1000–1100; (c) GNP per capita $2300–2600. (From Human Development Report 1994.)

younger ages, men in the lowest, office support, employment grades have a four times higher mortality rate than men in the highest administrative grade. Just as striking as the difference between top and bottom is the gradient. Position in the hierarchy shows a strong correlation with mortality risk. Men second from the top have higher mortality than top-grade civil servants; clerical officers have higher mortality rates than the men above them in the hierarchy.

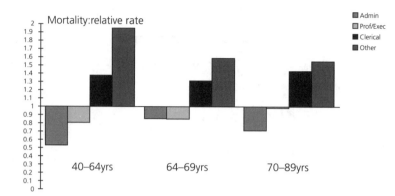

Fig. 1.8 All-cause mortality by grade of employment; Whitehall men, 25 year follow-up. (From Marmot and Shipley 1996.)

There are abundant data showing a link between poverty and ill health. These results from Whitehall have influenced us in coming to the view that inequality is also important. The problem of inequality in health is not confined to the poorest members of society but runs right across the social spectrum. In Whitehall the social gradient was seen not only for total mortality, but for all the major causes of death, including coronary heart disease and stroke (Marmot et al. 1984).

In several of the countries of central and eastern Europe, all-cause mortality and heart disease mortality are higher in people with less education. As mortality has increased in those countries between the early 1980s and early 1990s, the mortality disadvantage in those of lower status has increased (Blazek and Dzurova 1997; Shkolnikov et al. 1998).

1.5 Social determinants: selection or causation?

As David Blane explains in chapter 4, the causal direction may be two-way: health may determine socio-economic position as well as social circumstances affecting health. Where the link is between individual social status and health outcome, this has superficial plausibility. Health could be a major determinant of life chances. This has been termed health selection. The implication being that health 'selects' people into different social strata.

Perhaps one way of judging the social causation hypothesis is to consider the merits of the alternate, health selection hypothesis. For the purpose of argument, let us consider the extreme case to see whether *all* the observed relations could be the result of health selection. This would lead to the argument that ill health led to: lower position in the social hierarchy, social exclusion, having a job that offered less opportunities for control and imbalance between efforts and rewards, increased risk of unemployment and job insecurity, living in a deprived neighbourhood, having less participation in social networks, eating worse food, indulging in addictive behaviour, and breathing in polluted air, as well as being sedentary.

These have varying degrees of plausibility. Plausibility, however, is no guarantee that selection is actually operating. Apart from judging the relative plausibility of the causation and selection arguments, there have been a number of other research strategies, of which two are worth highlighting. The first deals with the question head on. Longitudinal studies allow a judgement to be made as to which came first, health or social circumstances. This has been examined in considerable depth by a number of studies (Goldblatt 1990). Perhaps the clearest answers come from the birth cohort studies referred to by Wadsworth (Chapter 3) and studied also in the 1958 birth cohort (Power et al. 1991). In the 1946 birth cohort, children who showed evidence of illness were less likely to be upwardly mobile than healthy children and more likely to be downwardly mobile (Wadsworth 1986). The effect was small however and could not account for the relation between social position and ill health in adulthood (Blane et al. 1993).

The second approach to dealing with selection is to examine the effect of social circumstances that could not have plausibly been affected by health status of individuals. For example, it is plausible that sick individuals may be more likely to lose their jobs and remain unemployed than healthy people. Where unemployment is imposed from the outside, as in large-scale factory closures, individual illness is unlikely to be a determinant of unemployment status. This evidence is reviewed in the chapter by Bartley (Chapter 5). Similarly, geographic and population differences in disease rates could not all be attributed to selective migration of healthy people to 'good' areas or of unhealthy people to 'bad' areas. More plausibly, as elaborated in the chapters by Shaw et al. (Chapter 10) and Wilkinson (Chapter 12), these area differences in disease rates relate to characteristics of the social environment. The causal direction, therefore, is likely to be from social environment to illness, not the other way.

1.6   How does the social environment affect health?

As stated above, in the discussion of Fig. 1.2, for the poor countries of the world an increase in living standards that reduces malnutrition and infectious disease will make a major contribution to improving health. These are the most obvious ways that the social environment can affect health. This book is concerned primarily with the health problems of the developed world, although, as the Global Burden of Disease study shows, these will increasingly become the problems of the developing world.

This book attempts to unpick the social environment in a way that is susceptible to scientific inquiry and relevant to policy. It focuses on the environment rather than on individual psychology and behaviour, although these may be influenced by the environment. The categories in the chapters may overlap, because the more we attempt to unpick the environment in which people live and work and separate it into discrete analytical categories, the further we retreat from reality. Nevertheless, the attempt to be specific is potentially important for the development of policy. We have not recommended specific policies but areas where our judgement of the scientific evidence suggests that policies should be developed. Our hope is that we may rouse awareness of these important issues and contribute to informed debate.

References

Amick, B., Levine, S., Tarlov, A. and Walsh, D. (eds.) (1995). *Society and Health*, Oxford University Press, New York.

Blane, D., Davey Smith, G. and Bartley, M. (1993). Social selection: what does it contribute to social class differences in health? *Sociol. Hlth Illness*, **15**, 1–15.

Blane, D., Brunner, E.J. and Wilkinson, R.G. (eds.) (1996). *Health and Social Organization*, Routledge, London.

Blazek, J. and Dzurova, D. (1997). The case of the Czech Republic. Part of the WIDER Project 'Economic shocks, social stress and the demographic impact'. United Nations University, Helsinki.

Bobak, M. and Marmot, M.G. (1996). East–West mortality divide and its potential explanations: proposed research agenda. *BMJ* **312**, 421–5.

Drever, F., Whitehead, M. and Roden, M. (1996). Current patterns and trends in male mortality by social class (based on occupation). *Popn Trends* **86**, 15–20.

Goldblatt, P. (1990). Mortality and alternative social classifications. In: *Longitudinal Study: Mortality and Social Organisation* (ed. P. Goldblatt) pp. 163–92. HMSO, London.

Interdepartmental Working Group on UK's Sustainable Development Strategy of 1994 (1998). Indicators of sustainable development for the United Kingdom. HMSO, London.

Leon, D., Chenet, L. and Shkolnikov, V. (1997). Huge variation in Russian mortality rates 1984–94: artefact, alcohol, or what? *Lancet* **350**, 383–8.

Mackenbach, J.P., Stronks, K. and Kunst, A.E. (1989). The contribution of medical care to inequalities in health: differences between socio-economic groups in decline of mortality from conditions amenable to medical intervention. *Soc. Sci. Med.*, **29**, 369–76.

Marmot, M.G., Syme, S.L., Kagan, A., Kato, H., Cohen, J.B. and Belsky, J. (1975). Epidemiologic studies of coronary heart disease and stroke in

Japanese men living in Japan, Hawaii and California: Prevalence of coronary and hypertensive heart disease and associated risk factors. *Am. J. Epidemiol.* **102**, 514–25.

Marmot, M.G. and Syme, S.L. (1976). Acculturation and coronary heart disease in Japanese Americans. *Am. J. of Epidemiol.* **104**, 225–47.

Marmot, M.G., Shipley, M.J. and Rose, G. (1984). Inequalities in death – specific explanations of a general pattern. *Lancet* i, 1003–6.

Marmot, M.G. and Shipley, M.J. (1996). Do socioeconomic differences in mortality persist after retirement? 25 year follow up of civil servants from the first Whitehall study. *BMJ* **313**, 1177–80.

Marmot, M. and Bobak, M. (1997). Psychosocial and biological mechanisms behind the recent mortality crisis in central and eastern Europe. In: Cornia, A.G. and Panicci R., eds *The Mortality Crisis in Transitional Economies* in press.

Murray, C. and Lopez, A. (1996). *The global burden of disease*, Harvard University Press.

Nichaman, M.Z., Hamilton, H.B., Kagan, A., Sacks, S., Greer, T. and Syme, S.L. (1975). Epidemiologic studies of coronary heart disease and stroke in Japanese men living in Japan, Hawaii and California: distribution of biochemical risk factors. *Am. J. Epidemiol.* **102**, 491–501.

Power, C., Manor, O. and Fox, J. (1991). *Health and class: the early years.* Chapman & Hall, London.

Rose, G. (1992). *The strategy of preventive medicine*, Oxford University Press, Oxford.

Shkolnikov, V., Leon, D., Adamets, S., Andreev, E. and Deev, A. (1998). Educational level and adult mortality in Russia: an analysis of routine data 1979–94. *Soc. Sci. Med.* **47**, 357–69.

Syme, S.L., Marmot, M.G., Kagan, A., Kato, H. and Rhoads, G.G. (1975). Epidemiologic studies of coronary heart disease and stroke in Japanese men living in Japan, Hawaii and California: introduction. *Am. J. Epidemiol.* **102**, 477–80.

Syme, S.L. (1996). To prevent disease: the need for a new approach. In: *Health and Social Organisation* (ed. D. Blane, E. Brunner, and R. Wilkinson) pp. 21–31. Routledge, London.

Tunstall-Pedoe, H., Kuulasmaa, K., Amouyel, P., Arveiler, D., Rajakangas, A.M. and Pajak, A. (1994). Myocardial infarction and coronary deaths in the World Health Organization MONICA project. Registration procedures, event rates, and case-fatality rates in 38 populations from 21 countries in four continents. *Circulation* **90**, 583–612.

United Nations Development Programme (1994). *Human Development Report (1994)*. Oxford University Press, New York.

Wadsworth, M.E.J. (1986). Serious illness in childhood and its association with later-life achievement. In: *Class and health* (ed. R.G. Wilkinson) pp. 50–74. Tavistock Publications Ltd, London.

Walberg, P., McKee, M., Shkolnikov, V., Chenet, L. and Leon, D. (1998). Economic change, crime and mortality crisis in Russia: regional analysis. *BMJ* **317**, 312–8.

Wilkinson, R.G. (1996). *Unhealthy societies: the afflictions of inequality*, Routledge, London.

Winkelstein, W., Kagan, A., Kato, H. and Sacks, S. (1975). Epidemiologic studies of coronary heart disease and stroke in Japanese men living in Japan, Hawaii and California: blood pressure distributions. *Am. J. Epidemiol.* **102**, 502–13.

World Bank (1993). *World Development Report 1993*, Oxford University Press, New York.

World Resources Institute and United Nations Development Programme (1998). *World Resources 1998–99. A guide to the global environment.* Oxford University Press, New York.

Worth, R.M., Rhoads, G., Kagan, A., Kato, H. and Syme, S.L. (1975). Epidemiologic studies of coronary heart disease and stroke in Japanese men living in Japan, Hawaii and California: mortality. *Am. J. Epidemiol.* **102**, 481–90.

Acknowledgements

Professor Marmot's research is supported by by an MRC Research Professorship.

2 Social organization, stress, and health

Eric Brunner and Michael Marmot

2.1 Introduction

Two major health problems have been described in this book that illustrate the social determinants of health: the social gradient in disease, and the striking differences in life expectancy between the countries of western Europe and those of central and eastern Europe that have emerged over the last 25 years. In relation to the social gradient, observed in the Whitehall studies of British civil servants (Marmot et al. 1984, 1991), we argued that it is significant that it runs right across the social hierarchy from the top employment grades to the bottom. The fact that civil servants in the second grade from the top have worse health than those at the top shows that we are not dealing only with the effects of absolute deprivation. Rather, position in the hierarchy is important. This suggests some concept of relative rather than absolute deprivation. This is a psychosocial concept. What this might mean is discussed in other chapters of this book, for example chapters 6 and 8. Is it plausible that circumstances in which people live and work, which differ according to where they are in the hierarchy, could powerfully influence health by acting through psychological pathways?

Similarly, when we review the evidence from central and eastern Europe (Bobak and Marmot 1996), we come up with the hypothesis that psychosocial factors play an important role in accounting for the worse health of those countries compared to the more favoured countries of the 'West' Fig. 2.1. Is it again plausible that these factors might be crucial and, if so, how do they operate to cause disease?

This chapter takes up the issue of biological plausibility (Brunner 1997). There are, in fact, two broad issues here. First, is it plausible that the organization of work, degree of social isolation, and sense of control over life, could affect the likelihood of developing and dying from chronic diseases such as diabetes and cardiovascular disease? The answer is an emphatic 'yes'. As we shall discuss, a variety of biological pathways can plausibly change the risk of developing major disease. The second issue is more complicated: do any of the

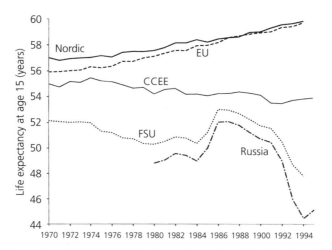

Fig. 2.1 Life expectancy trends in the EU, Nordic countries, and countries of the former USSR and central and eastern Europe, 1970–95. The powerful impact of social organization on health is seen over the period of transition from the centrally planned to the free market economy in central and eastern Europe. CCEE, Countries of Central and Eastern Europe; EU, European Union; FSU, former Soviet Union. (Source: WHO *Health for all* data.)

plausible biological pathways actually operate; that is, not could they cause disease, but do they? The evidence on this is incomplete and is an important topic for current and future research, but it is sufficiently suggestive to point to hypotheses for testing.

The issue of biological plausibility is, of course, important as a contribution to discussion of whether the variety of associations observed in this book represent causation. To take one example: does low socio-economic status lead to poor health, or does poor health lead to low socio-economic status? This is variously described as health selection, reverse causation, or, for economists, endogeneity. There are various ways of designing studies or analysing data to address this question. One contribution is to set out a plausible model of how socio-economic status could influence health and then test the various stages of the model. We set out an example of such a model in this chapter. Part of the model describes how factors in the environment, acting through the central nervous system, could influence biology to cause ill health.

2.2 The personal and the social

In the past, the debate about stress and health has seen stress as a property of individuals. This has led to the view that what is stress for one person is stimulation for another. The approach we take is different. We relate the biological response of the individual to the social environment acting upon him or her. The response will clearly be influenced by previous experience and perhaps genetic make-up, but there is sufficient regularity of the response to suggest that the right approach is to understand how the social environment impacts on biology to cause disease.

Selye's approach calls the response of the organism 'stress' (Selye 1956). Others have used an engineering analogy, in which external demands are considered to be the stressor, and the biological response may or may not (depending on the resilience of the subject) have undesirable consequences. What is clearly known is the physiology of the fight-or-flight response. What has been more difficult to tie down is how the fight-or-flight response relates to chronic stress, and later on, to disease. The model elaborated by Sapolsky is that the fight-or-flight response is adaptive to acute stress, but may be maladaptive to chronic stress in today's urban environment (Sapolsky 1993). Thus, for example, the average life span of African-American men in Harlem is shorter than that of men in Bangladesh.

Psychosocial factors and their influences on health are active areas of research. There is now enough evidence to suggest that this is an important field for those concerned with improving public health in both economically developed and developing countries. Plausible mechanisms linking psychosocial factors to health are described in the first half of this chapter. We then look to the evidence from both human and animal literature to illustrate the ways in which social organization can influence our biology, and therefore the health of individuals and populations.

2.3 Biological pathways in a social context

Biological processes must be involved in the connection between social structure and health. But, perhaps even more than health, biology is thought of as an individual rather than a social attribute. Individuals develop some disturbance of their biology. They become sick so they go to see the doctor. The doctor treats individuals, except perhaps when there is an outbreak of infectious disease, or when a vaccination programme is undertaken. The individual, clinical view of health determinants is vitally important. It underlies medical training and biomedical science, and provides the framework for the treatment, cure, and amelioration of disease.

We can extend the conceptual framework to provide a public-health view in which the emphasis is on prevention rather than cure. Figure 2.2 is an example of such a framework, in which factors operating beyond the level of the individual, as well as individual characteristics, are recognized. Thus, social structure, top left of the diagram, influences well-being and health, bottom right. The influences of social structure operate via three main pathways. Material circumstances are related to health directly, and via the social and work environment. These in turn shape psychological factors and health-related

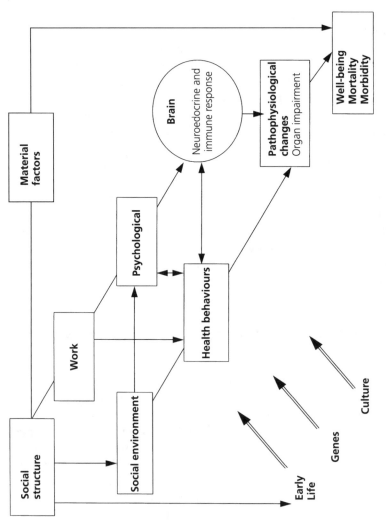

Fig. 2.2 Social determinants of health. The model links social structure to health and disease via material, psychosocial and behavioural pathways. Genetic, early life, and cultural factors are further important influences on population health.

behaviours. Early life experiences, cultural, and genetic factors also exert influences on health. Figure 2.2 is a generalization. A specific diagram for each disease category could be constructed, given the evidence. Further, the balance of influences on health depends on geographical location and historical circumstances of the population in question. For example, coronary heart disease is considerably more common in northern Europe than in the south of the continent, and within the UK and France similar north-south gradients exist. It should be noted however, that there is no evidence to suggest that lack of sunshine or northern latitude *per se* are risk factors for heart disease.

The left-hand side of Fig. 2.2 adds social causes to our picture of the determinants of health. The social and cultural environment, and organization of work, are among the upstream factors now re-emerging in thinking about public-health policy (Blane et al. 1996), partly as a response to the weaknesses of the education behaviour change model which dominated the field between the 1960s and the 1980s. Moving towards the right of Fig. 2.2, we encounter the psychological and biological dimensions. These downstream factors are, to use anatomical terminology, the proximal causes of disease which tend to be the main focus of medical attention. These factors are the intermediates on the pathway from the social level to well-being or disease in individuals. Put another way, there can be no doubt that the effects of social organization on population health are mediated by psychological and biological processes. The two big questions, outlined in the introduction, are, first, what are the processes involved and, secondly, given the plausibility of stress pathways, what is the importance of 'stress biology' in comparison with behavioural explanations which place factors such as smoking, exercise, and diet at centre stage?

The plausibility question is answered illustratively below. Even if the reader is initially sceptical about the pubic health importance of direct stress pathways operating independently of health-related behaviours, the social patterning of health-damaging habits, such as smoking, suggests that psychological and biological processes are at least indirectly important in understanding health differences within and between populations.

2.3.1 The fight-or-flight response

Humans evolved to rise rapidly to the challenge of external, potentially lethal, but short-term threats. Such threats may be physical, psychological, or biological, and often are a combination of all three. From a physiological point of view, the fight-or-flight response is very similar in all mammals, whether man, woman, mouse, or lion. Sensory information is the trigger – unless the threat comes from an invading virus or bacterium, when the alarm is sounded by other means – for a set of nerve and hormone signals which prepare the brain and body to respond to the emergency. The resulting physiological changes can be the key to survival in the face of a predator's attack or physical injury. For the mouse and particularly the lion, such stressors are brief and fairly unusual, and the accompanying disturbances to the body's internal status quo are likewise uncommon events. For humans, the contemporary environment is radically different. Physical and biological emergencies are comparatively rare, but instead life is filled with psychological demands and challenges which may activate the fight-or-flight response too hard and too often.

The mechanism of the fight-or-flight response involves two main pathways, which together co-ordinate an array of metabolic and physiological changes. Because these rely on parts of the nervous system and several hormonal or endocrine transmitters, they are known collectively as neuroendocrine pathways. Both are signal pathways that originate in the brain, where the threat is perceived and evaluated, and the resulting signal is initiated. The first pathway comes into action very rapidly, utilizing the sympathetic (as opposed to the parasympathetic) branch of the autonomic nervous system. The hormonal products of the pathway are noradrenaline, released at nerve endings, and adrenaline, secreted into the bloodstream by the medulla, or middle part, of the adrenal glands. This system is the sympatho-adrenal pathway. One effect of this involuntary reaction is known to us all: the unpleasant tightening of the gut we feel in response to a sudden shock. The second pathway comes into operation over minutes and hours instead of milliseconds. Its key components are three hormone-secreting glands, the hypothalamus and pituitary, respectively in and just below the brain, and the adrenal glands, located on the kidneys; hence the name of the second pathway, the hypothalamic–pituitary–adrenal axis. The adrenal glands secrete the important hormone cortisol, among other steroid hormones.

The sympatho-adrenal pathway

The almost instantaneous release of noradrenaline from sympathetic nerve endings and adrenaline from the adrenal medulla evoke responses throughout the body (Table 2.1). The effects are due, in varying degrees, to the presence of sympathetic nerves in the target organs, and to increased secretion of adrenaline into the circulation. One important target organ is the heart (Fig. 2.3) which is controlled directly by nerves of the autonomic nervous system, and indirectly by the level of adrenaline in the blood. The combined effects of sympatho-adrenal activation on the mind and body are psychological arousal and energy mobilization, and inhibition of functions which are irrelevant to immediate survival, such as digestion and growth. The precise nature of the activation varies according to the stressor and its duration, but its function is essentially to prepare for, or to maintain, physical exertion. The sympatho-adrenal pathway can be switched off rapidly. Even the circulating adrenaline has short-lived effects because its half-life is just a few minutes.

Table 2.1
Effects of circulating adrenaline and sympathetic nerve activity in the fight-or-flight response

Accelerate heart rate
Increase metabolic rate
Increase blood pressure
Increase sensory vigilance
Dilate pupils
Dilate airways
Constrict blood vessels in skin and gut
Dilate blood vessels in skeletal muscles
Inhibit salivation
Increase sweat secretion

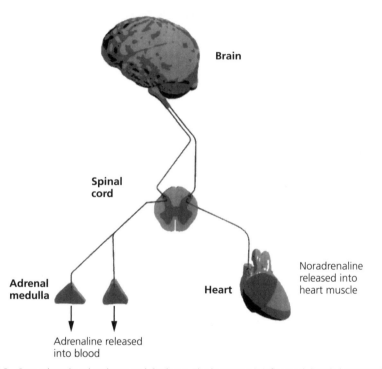

Fig. 2.3 Sympatho-adrenal pathway and the heart. The heart rate is influenced directly by sympathetic nerve impulses and indirectly by the circulating adrenaline level.

There is much evidence of wide variations between individuals in the size and duration of responses. These variations appear to be partly constitutional and partly due to social and individual differences in psychological coping resources. The impact of these variations on the development of chronic disease is uncertain.

The hypothalamic–pituitary–adrenal axis

The second, slow component of the stress response is the hypothalamic–pituitary–adrenal (HPA) axis. This pathway results in cortisol release into the bloodstream (Fig. 2.4) from the adrenal glands. The hormonal cascade starts in the brain with the release of corticotrophin releasing factor (CRF) into small vessels that carry it the few millimetres from the hypothalamus to the pituitary gland. Here, specialized cells respond to the presence of CRF by secreting the second hormone, adrenocorticotrophic hormone (ACTH) into the circulation.

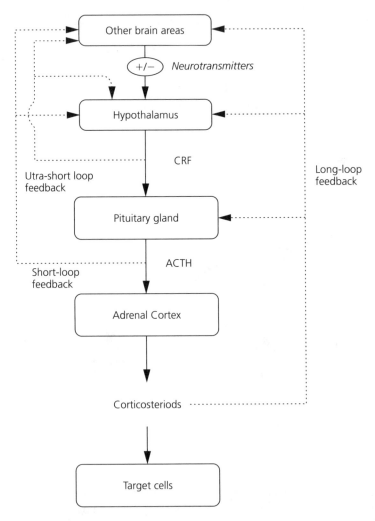

Fig. 2.4 The hypothalamic–pituitary–adrenal axis. The diagram shows how stimuli in the brain influence metabolic and immune functions in other parts of the body. The dotted lines show feedback controls which regulate release of cortisol and other corticosteroids from the adrenal cortex. CRF, corticotrophin releasing factor; ACTH, adrenocorticotrophic hormone. (Redrawn from Brown 1994.)

Within a few minutes, the level of ACTH in the adrenal cortex is sufficiently raised to stimulate cortisol release. As Fig. 2.4 shows, there are several feedback loops which regulate the activity of the HPA axis. The control system, involving each of the three hormones, provides sensitive mechanisms for adjustment of the circulating cortisol level during everyday life and in stress situations.

Cortisol and other related glucocorticoid hormones have both metabolic and psychological effects. They play a key role in the maintenance and control of resting and stress-related metabolic functions. As antagonists of the hormone insulin, they mobilize energy reserves by raising blood glucose and promoting fatty acid release from fat tissues. During an emergency this is a desirable effect, but in the physically inactive situation the superfluous availability of energy tends to increase output into the blood of cholesterol-carrying particles from the liver. The brain is also a target for glucocorticoids, which promote vigilance in the short term. However, a prolonged high level of cortisol, such as occurs in Cushing's syndrome, can provoke paranoia or depression. Some depressed patients respond to the drug metyrapone, which inhibits the production of cortisol within the adrenal gland (Checkley 1996), while in others, alterations of HPA axis functioning appear to override the effect of the drug, and cortisol output from the adrenal continues at a high level.

2.3.2 Acute and chronic stress

The neuroendocrine pathways outlined above, which generate the fight-or-flight response, are valuable properties of human biology because they provide the means by which to survive in the face of environmental challenge. From an evolutionary perspective it is easy to see that systems which gave survival advantage during the past million years, and have therefore been inherited by modern *homo sapiens*, may not be without a downside for the health of the present-day city dweller. The material and social environment has changed beyond recognition over the past 10 000 years since agriculture began, and in the past 200 years successive waves of industrial development have altered living conditions at a great pace. Yet our underlying biology is essentially the same as it was in ancient Babylon.

What, then, is the effect of living in social isolation on a shabby housing estate? Of growing up with parents who have no work and little self-respect? Of being a low-paid office worker surrounded by high-income executives? In advanced industrialized countries such groups of individuals will usually have adequate material circumstances, food, and clean water. Financial strain, lack of social support, and monotonous work may, however, produce a low level of psychosocial stress as a feature of daily life. Modern populations are largely free of the risks of fatal infectious disease, but not of the more subtle exposures which may repeatedly and frequently activate the fight-or-flight response over a period of decades. The increased risks of diabetes and cardiovascular disease among those lower down the social hierarchy fit this interpretation very well.

This is not to argue for stress counselling rather than poverty alleviation and social reform. The point is to dispel a common misconception that 'stress' is predominantly a health risk for senior managers, stockbrokers, and others in positions of corporate and public responsibility. Acute stress in such contexts provides challenges which often will be exciting, stimulating and, after the event, emotionally and intellectually satisfying. As Siegrist and his group have shown, high effort linked to high reward is generally health promoting (Siegrist 1996). In contrast, ill health is associated with prolonged exposure to psychological demands when possibilities to control the situation are perceived to be limited and chances of reward are small (Bosma et al. 1997). How might such repeated activation of the fight-or-flight response relate to the development of chronic disease?

2.3.3 The limits of stress reactivity

A principle of animal physiology is that an organism requires a stable internal environment in order to live successfully. Claude Bernard saw this to be true almost 150 years ago when he wrote '*La fixité du milieu interieur est la condition de la vie libre*'. Constant temperature, carbon dioxide concentration, and osmotic pressure are essential for the well-being of cells, tissues, and organs, and therefore for the integrity of the whole organism. At the same time, blood sugar, other circulating nutrients and waste products, blood pressure, and heart rate are also controlled, but the controls have wider margins. Variability in these factors is a fact of life, and the maintenance of a constant internal environment, termed homeostasis, is about balancing necessary variation against the need for physiological stability. Neuro-endocrine regulation, based on complex and interlocking positive and negative feedback mechanisms, is central to this function.

The nature and size of the biological response to psychological demands can influence health in several ways (Steptoe 1998). First, a particular type of response may be directly responsible for disease. Secondly, it might be that reactivity increases vulnerability to certain illnesses, such as colds or flu, but does not cause them. Thirdly, the pattern of reactivity may disrupt existing disease processes, and finally, it might act as trigger for acute events such as heart attack.

There is good evidence for the disruptive effect of stressors, such as life events, on existing medical conditions, including diabetes and rheumatoid arthritis, and for the precipitation of myocardial infarction by emotional trauma. But although a habitual pattern of high blood pressure reactivity has been seen to be a likely cause of hypertension, it has proved difficult to demonstrate that heightened blood pressure reactions are more common in those who go on to develop disease than in those who do not (Steptoe 1998).

An explanation for these findings may be found by considering the ways in which blood pressure may depart from and return to its baseline level. Figure 2.5 depicts three types of reactivity pattern which might apply to adrenaline and cortisol and other stress hormones, as well as to blood pressure. Time is on the horizontal axis, measured in minutes for adrenaline and blood pressure,' and hours in the case of cortisol. Blood pressure level (or hormone concentration) is on the vertical axis. In Fig. 2.5a, the stimulus produces a sharp reaction with a fast return to baseline; in Fig. 2.5b, the initial reaction is similar but the return to baseline is delayed, and there is a prolonged departure from the resting level. In Fig. 2.5c there is a blunted response and an elevated baseline. Other combinations of baseline and stimulated levels are also feasible, such as blunted response with a low basal level. The optimal reactivity pattern for each physiological system may be different.

For the blood pressure response to a psychological challenge, it appears that a large reaction may not be harmful, provided there is a fast return to baseline, as in Fig. 2.5a. If, however, such a response is provoked too frequently, the reactivity pattern may become like that shown in Figs 2.5b or c, and elevated blood pressure might follow. This example illustrates how feedback controls within the neuroendocrine system may be reset to a new level by environmental factors.

The allostatic load hypothesis (McEwen 1998) links the psychosocial environment to physical disease via neuroendocrine pathways. Allostatic load, or stress-induced damage, is considered relevant in cardiovascular disease, cancer, infection, and cognitive decline, and has been described as a sign of accelerated ageing. The concept of allostasis – the ability to achieve stability through change – extends the idea of homeostasis to include processes leading to disease. The price of adaptation to external and internal stress may be wear and tear on the organism, the result of chronic over- or

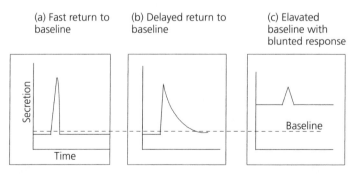

Fig. 2.5 Stress reactivity patterns. Idealized representations of neuroendocrine and metabolic reactivity. (a) Fast return to baseline: reactivity is responsive and flexible. (b) Delayed return to baseline: reactivity is responsive with slow recovery. (c) Elevated baseline with blunted response: weak reactivity and abnormal resting level.

underactivity of allostatic systems to produce allostatic load. For instance, the physiological system controlling blood glucose may be pushed towards diabetes. Allostatic load was investigated in a longitudinal study of older Americans (Seeman et al. 1997), where it was defined by measures of five established cardiovascular risk factors, plus urinary adrenaline and cortisol, and serum dehydroepiandrosterone sulphate (an adrenal androgen). Subjects with lower baseline allostatic load scores had better physical and mental functioning. Over the follow-up period the same group showed less decline in functioning and were less likely to develop cardiovascular disease.

The general description of stress reactivity in this section leads to many questions about individual and social differences in response to the same stimulus, which may or may not threaten homeostasis. This topic will be taken up later in the chapter.

2.3.4   The blood clotting system

Blood flow is vital for the transport of gases, nutrients, and waste materials to and from body tissues. It is also important that physical injury does not result in massive blood loss, and the clotting, or haemostatic, system provides the mechanism to prevent such a disaster. The sensitivity of this system to a variety of triggers suggests that it may be an important stress pathway in heart disease.

The change of blood from the liquid to the solid state involves a series of chemical reactions in which more than a dozen blood proteins take part. When the first protein is activated, it in turn activates the second protein, and so on. At the end of this cascade, the thrombin molecule catalyses the splitting of fibrinogen into fibrin. The fibrin molecules so produced condense to form threads which intermesh, trapping red blood cells and platelets, and very quickly a blood clot is formed. Major abnormalities of the haemostatic system are life-threatening; in haemophilia, for example, loss of blood after injury results from a defective clotting mechanism. An increased tendency for the blood to clot even in the absence of injury is very dangerous, and may be provoked in susceptible individuals by hormones such as those found in oral contraceptives.

The clotting system is, like other physiological systems, influenced by environmental stressors. The fight-or-flight response produces, via the increase in circulating adrenaline, increased 'stickiness' in platelets. The blood tends to become more concentrated and viscous at the same time, and stress-related hormones can increase the output of fibrinogen from the liver. It is plausible that, over decades, such small changes may add to the formation of arterial plaques, and therefore increase risks of heart disease and stroke.

2.3.5   Infection, inflammation, and immunity

Infectious disease continues to contribute to ill health, particularly among poorer groups, in developed as well as in developing countries. Standards of housing and sanitation, vaccination, and other infectious disease control programmes are crucial to reducing this public-health burden. Recent research suggests that infection and immunity may also be important in two poorly recognized ways. First, as a contributory cause of diseases not previously considered to be due to infection (Vallance et al. 1997), and secondly, because chronic stress may alter susceptibility to infection and its severity. Though the evidence is incomplete, immunity has been implicated in a variety of conditions, such as peptic ulcer, gastric, cervical and other cancers, and coronary heart disease. The brain is able to influence immune function. Nerves of the autonomic nervous system are found in all relevant tissues – bone marrow, thymus, spleen, and lymph nodes – and hormones, including cortisol, have large effects on the immune system.

It is now evident that long-term, but low-level, inflammatory processes resulting from undetected infection alter circulating levels of hormones and proteins in ways which increase the risk of heart disease by damaging the walls of blood vessels and promoting the development of atherosclerosis. Modification of these processes by stress is possible. For example, in the absence of infection the stress of space flight was shown to produce a rise in urinary output of interleukin-6 (Stein and Schluter 1994), a hormone considered to be important in immune and inflammatory responses.

2.3.6   Integration

The endocrine, immune, haemostatic, and nervous systems are often studied as distinct and separate entities. This simplification has been useful and probably essential because it allows laboratory scientists to focus on the details of their chosen mechanism. In this way, each discipline has come to understand the complexity of the relevant pathways, each with its set of feedforward and feedback controls. The reality, of course, is that there are not clear boundaries between these systems.

Figure 2.6 shows some of the interconnections between the neural, endocrine, and immune systems. The diagram shows how the brain and then the HPA axis are able to respond to non-cognitive stimuli, and conversely how the immune system has the capacity to respond to perception and emotion. The brain (central nervous system) cannot itself detect the presence of infection. One of the functions of the immune system is therefore to act as a sensory system, making the brain aware of infection by means of messengers of the immune system, the cytokines, which enter the brain via the bloodstream. Immune function responds to cognitive stimuli via the autonomic nervous system and the release of hormones from the hypothalamus

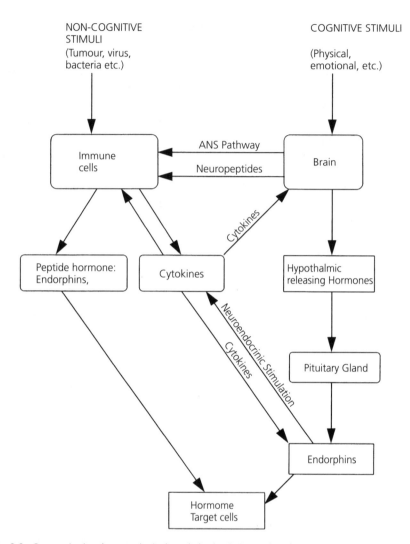

Fig. 2.6 Communications between brain, hypothalamic–pituitary–adrenal axis, and immune system. The brain perceives cognitive stimuli which can influence immune function via neuropeptides, the autonomic nervous system (ANS), and the HPA axis. The immune system responds to non-cognitive stimuli (infection and tumour growth) by secreting cytokines (immune messengers) and peptide hormones which act on the brain and neuroendocrine system. The immune system thus has a sensory function. (Redrawn from Brown 1994.)

and pituitary gland. In animals, isolation rearing, crowding, low dominance status, and social stress influence the effectiveness of defences against infection (Brown 1994).

This brief account has emphasized the roles of the autonomic nervous system and the HPA axis in the stress response. However, it is important to recognize that there are at least 15 neurotransmitter substances which convey sensory and cognitive information in the human nervous system. Among these, serotonin appears to be important in depression and hostility, and both psychological states have been linked with increased heart disease risk in a variety of studies. In animal studies, learned helplessness, the tendency to passivity in the face of repeated experimental stress, is associated with a reduced level of serotonin receptors in the hippocampus, an area of the brain which also responds to cortisol (Checkley 1996).

2.4 Human studies

The sections above have illustrated some of the major biological pathways that plausibly change risk of developing major disease according to social and psychological circumstances. Central to these processes is the concept of disturbance of homeostatic equilibrium and thus increased risk of ill health. We now turn to the second question posed at the beginning of the chapter: what is the evidence that these pathways do actually operate to produce or accelerate disease? Throughout this book there are numerous examples of the ways in which aspects of social organization are correlated with measures of health and disease. Here the aim is to examine some of the evidence for the biological pathways which intervene. The research findings are divided into two groups: those based on human subjects (discussed here), and those based on observational and experimental studies of animals (discussed later).

2.4.1 Psychological effect on growth

Psychogenic dwarfism is a rare syndrome associated with severe childhood deprivation. Psychosocial growth retardation of a less dramatic nature appears to have been documented in Widdowson's study of orphaned children in post-war Germany (Widdowson 1951). Under identical food rationing regimes, those who lived in the '*Bienenhaus*' orphanage, initially under the control of the stern and forbidding Fraülein Schwarz, gained less weight and grew more slowly than children cared for by the affectionate Fraulein Grün at the '*Vogelnest*' orphanage. By chance, Schwarz replaced Grün during the study and the growth rates reversed, despite the provision of extra food at '*Vogelnest*'. This controlled cross-over study provides evidence that adverse psychosocial circumstances in childhood can influence growth (although it is not clear whether this was the result of upset appetite and eating, or a direct psychosocial effect). Separately, there is evidence that attained height is a marker of health capital, or constitution, which is a protective factor for adult disease. Recent studies suggest that long-term effects on health may be produced by early deprivation, even among children born in the British welfare system of the 1950s (Montgomery et al. 1997; Power et al. 1998).

2.4.2 Social patterning of coronary risk factors in adults

Measures of social and economic status, including occupation, are extremely powerful predictors of premature heart disease. Employment grade proved, on its own, to be more powerful than the combination of classic risk factors including smoking, serum cholesterol, and blood pressure, in a follow-up study of 17 000 British civil servants (Marmot et al. 1984). This important observation prompted a new long-term study to investigate the possible psychosocial causes of heart disease and other important health problems. Biology is being given special attention in the Whitehall II study, in order to clarify the mechanisms involved.

At the baseline of the Whitehall II study in 1985–88 (Marmot et al. 1991) there was a stepwise relationship between civil service employment grade (1992 salary range £7400–£87 600) and the prevalence of several of health-related psychosocial factors: low control and lack of variety at work, lack of social contact with friends, distressing life events, difficulty paying bills, hostility, and health locus of control. These relationships were seen before employment security in the British civil service was reduced in the late 1980s (Ferrie et al. 1995) and it is likely that their prevalence is now higher, particularly within the lower grades of staff.

Biochemical and physiological risk factors were studied in detail at the second medical examination of Whitehall II subjects in 1991–93 (Brunner et al. 1997). Because total serum cholesterol levels were similar by employment grade, and resting blood pressure showed only a small differential in the expected direction at the baseline examination, we speculated that a particular pattern of risk factors might be associated with occupational status. This 'metabolic syndrome' pattern has previously been shown to predict diabetes and coronary disease in other populations, including South Asian migrants to the UK (McKeigue et al. 1991). Figure 2.7 shows that the metabolic syndrome is indeed linked with lower status in the sample of 4691 men and 1903 women.

As the grade hierarchy is descended, a progressively larger proportion of subjects exhibits adverse levels of each component of the metabolic syndrome (Fig. 2.8; moving from left to right in each block of histograms). The top four panels of Fig. 2.8 are components reflecting adverse homeostatic alterations in carbohydrate and lipid metabolism, and Fig. 2.8e shows that abdominal obesity, a fat pattern particularly associated with coronary risk, is also strongly associated with low status. Figure 2.8f shows that the blood clotting protein, fibrinogen, also shows a strong inverse social gradient (Brunner et al. 1996).

The findings for blood glucose are particularly interesting because they are based on a metabolic challenge rather than a measurement of fasting, or baseline, level. Subjects in the fasting state were given 75 g of glucose as a drink, and 2 hours later the level of blood glucose was measured. The results (Fig. 2.8a) show that the lower the position in the civil service, the greater was

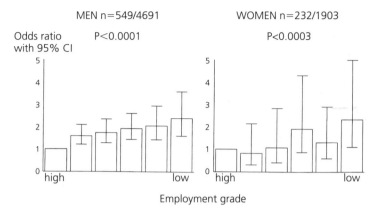

Fig. 2.7 Prevalence of the metabolic syndrome by employment grade in the Whitehall II study. Odds ratios and 95 per cent confidence interval (CI) adjusted for age and, in women, menopausal status. *P* values are for trend test across grades. (From Brunner et al. 1997).

the probability that a subject had difficulty in clearing the glucose into body tissues for storage or energy functions and returning to the optimal baseline state. This finding corresponds to the condition shown in Fig. 2.5b, or perhaps in Fig. 2.5c. It illustrates that the ability to mount a hormonal response to the glucose challenge, and thus to maintain homeostasis, appears in some way to depend on occupational status.

The social gradient in prevalence of the metabolic syndrome is consistent with a psychosocial explanation for the social pattern of coronary risk. The alternative life-style explanation was only weakly supported by statistical analysis. When grade differences in rates of smoking, physical inactivity, and alcohol consumption were taken into account, 90 per cent of the grade differential in metabolic syndrome prevalence remained. Further adjustment for overall obesity (body mass index) but not central obesity (waist–hip ratio), which is itself a component of the syndrome, as well as the behavioural factors, reduced the grade differential by only an additional 22 per cent in men and 1 per cent in women. How then does the metabolic syndrome develop? One possibility, which is the subject of current research (Fig. 2.9), is that this cluster of risk factors may be the product of altered activity of the HPA axis (section 2.3.1) in response to long-term exposure to adverse psychosocial circumstances (Bjorntorp 1991; McEwen 1998).

2.4.3   Socio-economic status and cortisol secretion in two cities

Middle-aged men in Lithuania and Sweden had similar coronary heart disease mortality rates in 1978. Subsequently, rates rose in Lithuania and fell in Sweden, so that by 1994 coronary mortality was fourfold higher in Lithuania. The divergence in life expectancy, in addition to coronary disease rates,

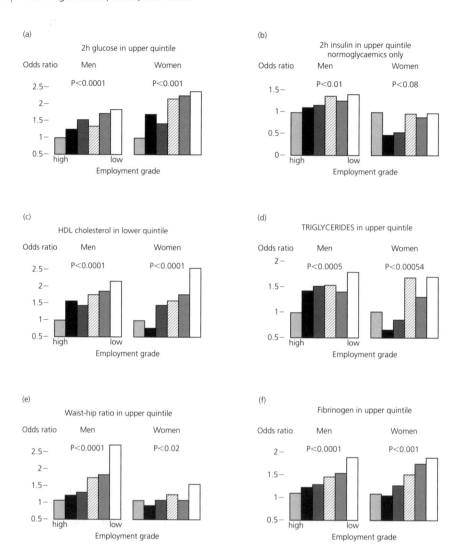

Fig. 2.8 Prevalence of adverse levels of metabolic syndrome variables and fibrinogen by employment grade in the Whitehall II study. Odds ratios and 95 per cent confidence interval for occupying top quintile (except HDL cholesterol: bottom quintile). Adjusted for age and, in women, menopausal status. *P* values are for trend test across grades. (From Brunner et al. 1997.)

between the countries of eastern and western Europe around the time of the collapse of the Soviet system illustrates the importance of socio-economic factors in health (Bobak and Marmot 1996). The widening East–West health gap prompts the thought of a possible analogy with the widening socio-economic inequalities in health within countries. Could it be that the psycho-social environment is part of this analogy?

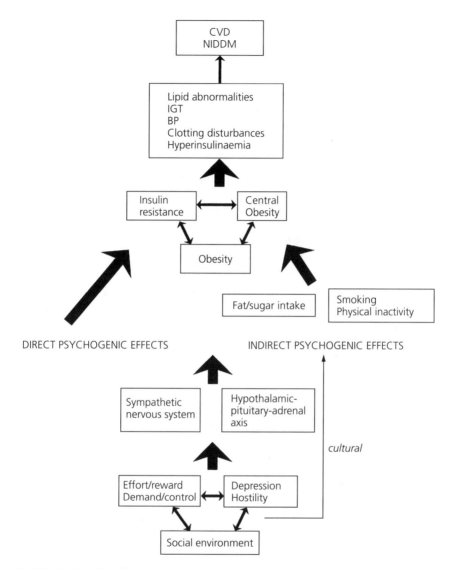

Fig. 2.9 Psychosocial and biological pathways in cardiovascular disease (CVD) and non-insulin-dependent diabetes (NIDDM). Hypothesized research model. IGT, impaired glucose tolerance; BP, blood pressure.

Kristenson et al. and co-workers examined the possible causes for the differences in coronary heart disease incidence between Lithuania and Sweden, and between men of high and low socio-economic status in each country (Kristenson et al. 1997, 1998). Random samples of 150 50 year-old men participated in each of two cities: Linköping in southern Sweden and Vilnius, the capital of Lithuania. Response rates were 82 and 76 per cent, respectively. The conventional risk factors (smoking, serum cholesterol, and blood pressure) did not provide a good explanation for national differences in risk, as was the case in the Whitehall study (Marmot et al. 1984). There were substantial differences in blood levels of antioxidant vitamins, suggesting that dietary differences are important both between and within countries. Psycho-social factors were found to follow precisely the predicted pattern. Vilnius men reported more social isolation, more job strain, and more depression than those in Linköping. The low-income groups in both cities likewise reported higher levels of isolation and vital exhaustion, and greater difficulties coping than those on higher incomes.

Here then is evidence from a cross-cultural study, conducted in 1993–95, that certain dietary and psychosocial factors are important in explaining the differences in coronary risk both between Swedes and Lithuanians, and between those with financial insecurity and their relatively well-off neighbours. Other measures also revealed marked differences between the two popula-tions. Quality of life and perceived health showed a large differential (one standard deviation) in favour of Linköping. Although depression was more common in Vilnius, the mean hostility score in Linköping was substantially higher than that in Vilnius. It may be that many men in Vilnius had a sense of defeat and a lack of confidence in their post-Soviet society.

The contrasting psychosocial environments in Linköping (population 130 000) and Vilnius (600 000) translate into different patterns of the HPA axis stress response. Subjects took a standardized laboratory stress test involving anger recall, mental arithmetic, and immersion of one hand in iced water. Subjects attended the test the morning after an overnight fast in order to standardize the biological measurements. Attending the clinic, and fasting, can be considered to be additional stressors, but since all men did the same it does not detract from the findings. Figure 2.10 shows that both the high- and low-income groups of Swedish men had what is considered to be an adaptive response to the experimental challenge: low baseline followed by a rise and fall in blood cortisol. The difference in findings with the Vilnius subjects is striking. The high-income group exhibited a low baseline level like the Swedes, but a relatively blunted response. However, the low-income group, showed a very different response from the other groups. There was a much higher baseline level of blood cortisol and a failure to respond to the challenge, corresponding to the condition shown in Fig. 2.5c.

The implications of these results, if confirmed in other studies, are dramatic. They highlight the significance of quality of life, in terms of the social and working environment, as key determinants of population health. The demon-stration of a biological mechanism, involving altered functioning of the main neuroendocrine stress pathway, is evidence that the psychosocial hypothesis is not only plausible, but that it is a significant social policy consideration. A study of 63 German army recruits given a mental stress test (Hellhammer et al. 1997) further supports the view that social rank is related to HPA axis

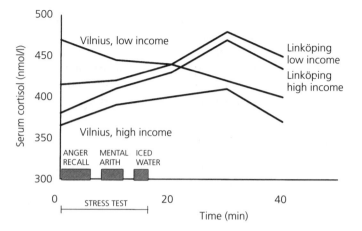

Fig. 2.10 Serum cortisol responses to a standardized stress test in Vilnius, Lithuania, and Linköping, Sweden, by income group. Low income: group with lowest 25 per cent of income. High income: group with highest 25 per cent of income. (Redrawn from Kristenson et al. 1998.)

functioning. Salivary cortisol levels showed a considerably larger response among psychologically dominant soldiers than subordinates.

An outstanding question is whether the apparently adverse cortisol responses are indeed responsible for future ill health, or are merely markers of psychological state. Related to this is the issue of reversibility, since a stress response pattern which becomes fixed early in life would have specific policy implications. Barker's group has demonstrated, for example, that lower birthweight is associated with higher morning plasma cortisol level among 59–70-year-old men (Phillips et al. 1998). Their findings give evidence that plasma cortisol levels within the normal range are among the determinants of blood pressure and glucose tolerance. However, in this group of men, fetal programming of the HPA axis was more important than the effect of current socio-economic position, suggesting that interventions after infancy may be ineffective. Nevertheless, it seems likely that both fetal growth and experiences during the life course will turn out to be of importance in shaping neuroendocrine function in later life.

2.5 Animal studies

Animal studies provide some added dimensions to our understanding of the connections between social organization, stress, and health. Referring to our general model in Fig. 2.2, it is clear that direct analogies are to be avoided. The human social environment is immensely and uniquely complex. From a psychological perspective, the faculties of abstract thought, emotion, and memory appear largely to be limited to our own species. However, many animals live within hierarchical social structures and mammalian biology is potentially comparable across species. An added value of such studies is that, unless required to by man, animals do not smoke, drink coffee or alcohol, take drugs, or sit in front of a computer all day. This truism means that we do not have the problem of separating these behavioural effects from purely psychosocial processes which may influence disease risks.

2.5.1 Genes, constitution, and destiny

With due attention to relevance, animal studies can tell us about the plausible links between psychosocial factors, biology, and health. Their value is not confined to the social gradient in health (see section 2.5.2), and is also a way to understand effects such as the interaction between genetic predisposition to disease and environmental factors. Our first example may provide a caution to those who view genetic susceptibility, in the absence of medical intervention, as an irreversible destiny.

The spontaneously hypertensive rat (SHR) is an animal model often used in the study of hypertension. An experiment in cross-fostering (Cierpial and McCarthy, 1987) shows the importance of early environment in expressing this characteristic. When pups of SHR rats were cross-fostered with Kyoto–Wistar mothers they did not develop hypertension as they matured. This 'pure' genetic characteristic did not manifest itself as the phenotype of hypertension in the absence of the appropriate environmental stimulus.

Another example of the impact of nurture on nature comes from Suomi's elegant long-term studies of rhesus monkeys (*Macaca mulatta*) (Suomi 1997). Some 20 per cent of any troop are 'high reactors' who are more likely than others to exhibit depressive responses to maternal separation, along with greater and prolonged activation of the HPA axis, more dramatic sympatho-adrenal arousal, and immunosuppression. These responses remain quite stable throughout development. The pattern of arousal appears to be determined genetically, but it can be reproduced in other non-susceptible animals by raising them without their mothers (suggesting that non-genetic inter-generational transmission may be an alternative explanation). Interestingly, the high reactors tend to end up at the bottom of the social hierarchy.

The genetic, or at least constitutional, high-reactor destiny can be interrupted by changing the environment. When reared with especially nurturing mothers, such animals showed no signs of the usual behavioural disorder. Instead, they showed signs of precocious behavioural development and rose to the top of the hierarchy as adults. Females adopted the maternal style typical of their especially nurturing mothers. Further evidence from the same research group (Suomi 1997) suggests that the consequences of experimental social isolation can be modified with timely intervention, and that long-term effects are most likely to be seen under stress conditions in adult life.

2.5.2 Social dominance among wild baboons

Determinants of circulating levels of the protective high-density lipoproteins (HDL), which promote 'reverse transport' of cholesterol away from the arterial wall, appear be important in explaining the social differential in coronary risk. We have seen above that the HDL cholesterol level in civil servants is strongly related to employment grade, and is a component of the cluster of factors making up the metabolic syndrome (Fig. 2.8). To our surprise, the same pattern of blood fat levels was found in the social hierarchy of wild male baboons (Sapolsky and Mott 1987).

The neuroscientist Sapolsky has been studying the behaviour and physiology of wild baboon troops in the Serengeti for many years. He argues the animals are ideal subjects for investigating psychosocial factors. Food is plentiful, predators are scarce, and infant mortality is low. Only some 4 hours/day are required for foraging, leaving the animals, who live in groups of 50–100, plenty of time to engage in social activity. Attainment and maintenance of social rank is a preoccupation which determines access to a variety of resources. On the basis of these behaviours, Sapolsky classified males of the troop into dominants and subordinates. Blood samples obtained following anaesthesia under controlled conditions showed, just as in Whitehall II men, that total and low-density lipoprotein cholesterol were similar by rank position, and that HDL levels were higher in the dominant compared to the subordinate males, again mirroring findings in civil servants. Subordinate baboons were found to have higher resting cortisol levels, and levels of the hormone were inversely correlated with HDL.

Do these parallels reflect the common psychosocial effects of position within the two primate hierarchies? That the baboons are non-smokers and non-drinkers is consistent with a psychosocial explanation, since smoking is known to lower, and alcohol consumption to raise, HDL levels. Production of the more favourable physiological profile in dominant baboons might be the direct consequence of their assertions of supremacy and consequent feelings of well-being, or alternatively the result of easier access to the best available food. Equally, these observational data are compatible with the view that the fittest attain the highest rank, but studies utilizing captive macaque monkeys suggest that this is not the case (Shively and Clarkson 1994). Initial rank in small groups of females fed an atherogenic diet was altered experimentally by switching animals between groups. The effects of manipulating social status were dramatic. Dominants who became subordinate had a five fold excess of coronary plaques compared with animals who remained dominant, while subordinates who became dominant had a two fold excess of atherosclerotic changes compared to those remaining subordinate.

2.6 Conclusions

Disturbance of usual homeostatic equilibrium by the repeated activation of the fight-or-flight response may be responsible for social differences in neuro-endocrine, physiological, and metabolic variables which are the precursors of ill health and disease. Social and individual differences in the response to social and environmental stressors appear to be determined by many factors, including birthweight and conditioned hypo- or hyper-responsiveness. It seems likely that the optimal stress response in relation to health in the long term is associated with living and working environments typical of the materially advantaged. This optimal response can be characterized as one with a rapid return to a resting level, and thus a high resistance to stress-related disorder (Fig. 2.11). The level of demands does not in itself pose a risk to health, provided that the individual has adequate coping resources and the opportunity to control his or her environment.

The causal role of psychosocial factors in coronary heart disease has been reviewed recently (Hemingway and Marmot 1999). The evidence from longitudinal studies involving more than 500 healthy subjects was strongest for social isolation, depression and anxiety, and low control at work.

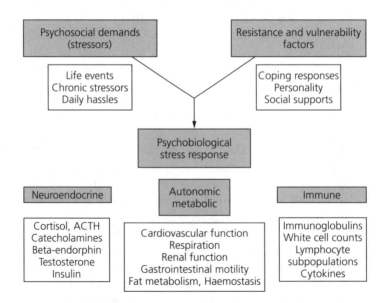

Fig. 2.11 The psychobiological stress response. Resistance and vulnerability factors influence the response to psychosocial stressors. The major hormonal, metabolic, and immune elements of the response are shown. (From Steptoe 1998.)

2.7 Summary

Stress has short-term effects on the human body and mind. The effects are positive if the situation is right, but everyone has his or her limits. We are now beginning to recognize that people's social and psychological circumstances can seriously damage their health in the long term. Chronic anxiety, insecurity, low self-esteem, social isolation, and lack of control over work appear to undermine mental and physical health.

The power of psychosocial factors to affect health makes biological sense. The human body has evolved to respond automatically to emergencies. This stress response activates a cascade of stress hormones which affect the cardiovascular and immune systems. The rapid reaction of our hormones and nervous system prepares the individual to deal with a brief physical threat. The heart rate rises; blood is diverted to muscles; anxiety and alertness increase. This response is highly adaptive: it may save life in the short term. But if the biological stress response is activated too often and for too long, there may be multiple health costs. These include depression, increased susceptibility to infection, diabetes, high blood pressure, and accumulation of cholesterol in blood vessel walls, with the attendant risks of heart attack and stroke.

These health problems increase progressively down the social strata in industrialized countries. Psychosocial and stress mechanisms have been studied in a variety of non-human primates, both in the wild and in captivity. In monkeys there is also a social hierarchy in cardiovascular damage. Submissive animals have a higher prevalence of atherosclerosis and a pattern of metabolic changes similar to that linked with increased cardiovascular risk in humans. In baboons, those of lower status in the troop have a higher level of the stress hormone cortisol, and this is associated with lower levels of protective high-density lipoprotein cholesterol in the blood.

Clustering and accumulation of psychosocial disadvantage, perhaps beginning with a poor emotional environment in early childhood, is a neglected area of public-health prevention and social policy. This is an area of active research.

References

Bjorntorp, P. (1991). Visceral fat accumulation: the missing link between psychosocial factors and cardiovascular disease? *J. Int. Med.* **230**, 195–201.

Blane, D., Brunner, E.J. and Wilkinson, R. (1996). The evolution of public health policy: an anglocentric view of the last fifty years. In: *Health and social organization: towards a health policy for the the 21st century* (ed. D. Blane, E. Brunner, and R.G. Wilkinson), pp. 120. Routledge, London.

Bobak, M. and Marmot, M.G. (1996). East–West mortality divide and its potential explanations: proposed research agenda. *BMJ* **312**, 421–5.

Bosma, H., Marmot, M.G., Hemingway, H., Nicholson, A., Brunner, E.J. and Stansfeld, S. (1997). Low job control and risk of coronary heart disease in the Whitehall II (prospective cohort) study. *BMJ* **314**, 558–65.

Brown, R.E. (1994). *An introduction to neuroendocrinology.* Cambridge University Press, Cambridge.

Brunner, E.J. (1997). Stress and the biology of inequality. *BMJ* **314**, 1472–6.

Brunner, E.J., Davey Smith, G., Marmot, M.G., Canner, R., Beksinska, M. and O'Brien, J. (1996). Childhood social circumstances and psychosocial and behavioural factors as determinants of plasma fibrinogen. *Lancet* **347**, 1008–3.

Brunner, E.J., Marmot, M.G., Nanchahal, K., et al. (1997). Social inequality in coronary risk: central obesity and the metabolic syndrome. Evidence from the Whitehall II study. *Diabetologia* **40**, 1341–9.

Checkley, S. (1996). The neuroendocrinology of depression and chronic stress. *Br. Med. Bull.* **52**, 597–617.

Cierpial, M.A. and McCarthy, R. (1987). Hypertension in SHR rats: contribution of maternal environment. *Am. J. Physiol.* **253**, H980–H984.

Ferrie, J.E., Shipley, M.J., Marmot, M.G., Stansfeld, S. and Davey Smith, G. (1995). Health effects of anticipation of job change and non-employment: longitudinal data from the Whitehall II study. *BMJ* **311**, 1264–9.

Hellhammer, D.H., Buchtal, J., Gutberlet, I. and Kirschbaum, C. (1997). Social hierarchy and adrenocortical stress reactivity in men. *Psychoneuroendocrinology* **22**, 643–50.

Hemingway, H. and Marmot, M. (1999). Psychosocial factors in the aetiology and prognosis of coronary heart disease: a systematic review of prospective cohort studies. *BMJ* **318**, **in press**.

Kristenson, M., Zieden, B., Kucinskiene, Z., et al. (1997). Antioxidant state and mortality from coronary heart disease in Lithuanian and Swedish men: concomitant cross sectional study of men aged 50. *BMJ* **314**, 629–33.

Kristenson, M., Kucinskiene, Z., Bergdahl, B. and Orth-Gomer, K. (1998). Risk factors for ischaemic heart disease in different socioeconomic groups of Lithuania and Sweden: the Livicordia study. In: Kristenson M. PhD thesis *The Livivcordia study* (medical dissertation no. 547), Linkoping University 1998, Sweden.

McEwen, B.S. (1998). Protective and damaging effects of stress mediators. *N. Engl. J. Med.* **338**, 171–9.

McKeigue, P.M., Shah, B. and Marmot, M.G. (1991). Relation of central obesity and insulin resistance with high diabetes prevalence and cardiovascular risk in South Asians. *Lancet* **337**, 382–6.

Marmot, M.G., Shipley, M.J. and Rose, G. (1984). Inequalities in death – specific explanations of a general pattern. *Lancet* **i**, 1003–6.

Marmot, M.G., Davey Smith, G., Stansfeld, S.A., et al. (1991). Health inequalities among British Civil Servants: the Whitehall II study. *Lancet* **337**, 1387–93.

Montgomery, S., Bartley, M. and Wilkinson, R.G. (1997). Family conflict and slow growth. *Arch. Dis. Child.* **77**, 326–30.

Phillips, D.I.W., Barker, J.P., Fall, C.H.D., et al. (1998). Elevated plasma cortisol concentrations: A link between low birth weight and insulin resistance syndrome? *J. Clin. Endocrinol. Metab.* **83**, 757–60.

Power, C., Matthews, S. and Manor, O. (1998). Inequalities in self-rated health: explanations from different stages of life. *Lancet* **351**, 1009–14.

Sapolsky, R.M. (1993). Endocrinology alfresco: psychoendocrine studies of wild baboons. *Recent Prog. Horm. Res.* **48**, 437–68.

Sapolsky, R.M. and Mott, G.E. (1987). Social subordinance in wild baboons is associated with suppressed high density lipoprotein–cholesterol concentrations: the possible role of chronic social stress. *Endocrinology* **121**, 1605–10.

Seeman, T.E., Singer, B.H., Rowe, J.W., Horwitz, R.I. and McEwen, B.S. (1997). Price of adaptation – allostatic load and its health consequences. *Arch. Intern. Med.* **157**, 2259–68.

Selye, H. (1956). *Stress of life.* McGraw-Hill, New York.

Shively, C.A. and Clarkson, T.B. (1994). Social status and coronary artery atherosclerosis in female monkeys. *Art. Thromb.* **14**, 721–6.

Siegrist, J. (1996). Adverse health effects of high-effort/low-reward conditions. *J. Occup. Health Psychol.* **1**, 27–41.

Stein, T.P. and Schluter, M.D. (1994). Excretion of IL-6 by astronauts during spaceflight. *Am. J. Physiol.* **266**, E448–E552.

Steptoe, A. (1998). Psychophysiological bases of disease. In: *Comprehensive clinical psychology. Volume 8: Health psychology*, (ed. D.W. Johnston and M. Johnston), pp. 3978. Pergamon, New York.

Suomi, S.J. (1997). Early determinants of behaviour: evidence from primate studies. *Br. Med. Bull.* **53**, 170–84.

Vallance, P., Collier, J. and Bhagat, K. (1997). Infection, inflammation, and infarction: does acute endothelial dysfunction provide a link? *Lancet* **349**, 1391–2.

Widdowson, E.M. (1951). Mental contentment and physical growth. *Lancet* **i**, 1316–18.

Acknowledgements

Dr Brunner's and Professor Marmot's research is supported by the British Heart Foundation.

3 Early life

Michael Wadsworth

3.1 Introduction

Associations of poverty and social inequality and social exclusion with child health are found in all countries, regardless of methods and delivery of medical care and of culture (Williams et al. 1994; Helman 1994; Williams et al. 1994). Child health is of the greatest importance for the future of health of a nation, not only because today's children grow up to become the next generation of parents and workers, but also because recent research in child health shows that early life health is, for each child, the basis of health in adult life. Therefore investment in health in early life has beneficial effects, specifically on the future health of a nation as well as on the future functioning of its citizens.

The purpose of this chapter is to describe the biological processes that affect child health and that determine adult health, and then to outline the nature of the social factors that affect these biological processes, both at the family level and in terms of the cultural social context. Conclusions are drawn about the policies needed to improve health in early life.

3.2 Biological processes affecting child health

3.2.1 Biological processes occurring before birth

Disruption and curtailment of growth *in utero* may be caused by poor nutrient supply to the fetus. This is not only a matter of the mother's diet, but also includes oxygen.

> The nutrients that get into the fetus . . . are clearly related to the many aspects of the mother's physiology, her preconceptual stores, her competence to sustain fetal growth and maybe to a minor extent what she eats in pregnancy, and whether the mother exercises in pregnancy. Delivery of nutrients to the fetus is a very complicated agenda.
> *(Barker 1994a, p. 238).*

Although the effects of serious malnutrition in the mother, and the stage in pregnancy at which it occurs, are well documented (Perry 1997), it seems likely that in reasonably well-nourished populations the interaction of diet 'with the mother's prepregnancy nutritional status, metabolism, and physiology' (Perry 1997, p. 159), is likely to affect fetal development. Fetal development is also disrupted by maternal smoking (Eskenzai and Bergmann 1995), alcohol consumption (Spohr et al. 1993), and experience of infection. These are complex processes, as Hall and Peckham (1997, p. 18) exemplify in the case of maternal infection.

> Damage may . . . occur as a result of interference with fetal growth producing disturbances in developmental pattern or structure, as in the case of congenital rubella. There may be a diminution of the normal number of fetal cells which interferes with the structure or function of selected organs or whole systems. Changes may be very subtle, for example in the brain they could affect later perception or learning ability. The changes produced may not manifest themselves unless the affected individual meets a specific challenge later in life, many years after the initial infection.
> *(p. 18)*

Retardation of fetal development is associated with suboptimal development of vital systems because:

> Many tissues and organs are largely or completely formed with regard to cell numbers at or shortly after birth. Most of postnatal growth is a consequence of the enlargement of pre-existing cells rather than the accretion of additional cells.
> *(Hales 1997, p. 115).*

Barker (1997, p. 100) argues that when undernutrition occurs in late gestation:

> the fetus uses an adaptive response present in mammals and diverts oxygenated blood away from the trunk to sustain the brain (Dicke 1987). This affects the growth of the liver, two of whose functions, regulation of cholesterol and of blood clotting, seem to be permanently perturbed (Barker et al. 1995; Barker et al. 1992). Disturbance of cholesterol metabolism and blood clotting are both important features of coronary heart disease.
> *(p. 100)*

It is also argued also that airway and alveolar growth is similarly affected by poor fetal nutrition at critical developmental stages (Shaheen 1997), and so too is insulin resistance (Barker 1997; Hales 1997).

3.2.2 Biological processes occurring during infancy

The major risk factors in early life are malnutrition and infection. Each is associated with poor social circumstances, and each can threaten the child's survival as well as development. Malnutrition adversely affects not only bodily growth, but also cognitive development and educational attainment (Horwood et al. 1998; Stinson 1998), and breast feeding of 3 months or more seems to be associated with improved cognitive performance (Rodgers 1978; Lucas et al. 1992). Infection can also carry long-term developmental risks (Hall and Peckham 1997). For example, damage may occur to postnatal development processes and, in the case of lung and airway development, may restrict growth and, increase 'airway responsiveness to allergens, viruses and air pollutants in later childhood or adult life (Martinez 1994); . . . the age related decline in respiratory function which commences in mid adult life may be more rapid or reach a critical threshold at an earlier age in those in whom maximal fetal and early childhood growth potential has not been achieved (Brown and Weiss 1991).' (Dezateux and Stocks 1997, p. 42).

Postnatal damage may also occur in systems already fully developed. For example, Martyn (1997) suggests that early life damage from infection that affects the neurological system, for example from poliovirus, may result in neurone loss, with consequent increased central nervous system vulnerability. He showed how cohorts exposed in infancy and childhood to poliovirus epidemics in the 1930s in England and Wales were at raised risk of motor-neuron disease when they were aged 55–74 years. It was hypothesized that the experience of subclinical forms of poliomyelitis would result in substantial loss of motorneurons, so that motorneuron disease 'might be a delayed sequel either because of further neuronal loss through ageing or as a result of a second insult' (Martyn 1997, p. 31).

3.2.3 Biological programming

From such evidence, as outlined above, it has been concluded that there is a process of biological programming, through which malnutrition at critical phases of development before birth 'may permanently reduce the number of cells in particular organs (Widdowson and McCance 1975; McCance and Widdowson 1974)' (Barker 1997, p. 96) (Fig. 3.1). Thus organs and systems adapted in this way to function maximally only at a reduced level, carry a programmed raised risk, that may be triggered by a risk encountered in later life. For example, a high risk of non-insulin-dependent diabetes and impaired glucose tolerance was found in people who showed signs of fetal malnutrition, being small in size at birth, who then added the further risk of obesity as adults (Hales et al. 1992; Lithell et al. 1996). Similarly, Barker argues that impaired kidney development before birth may not become a problem unless 'the system is stressed, for example by high salt intake and thereby becomes unable to maintain the volume and composition of body fluids' (Barker 1994*b*, p. 123). Martyn's (1997) hypothesis about the relationship of childhood neurological damage to raised risk of neurological illness in adulthood also requires a later event to trigger the onset of illness.

3.3 Biological processes and social factors

The biological processes outlined above all take place in a social context. The health of mothers during pregnancy depends on their health throughout all of

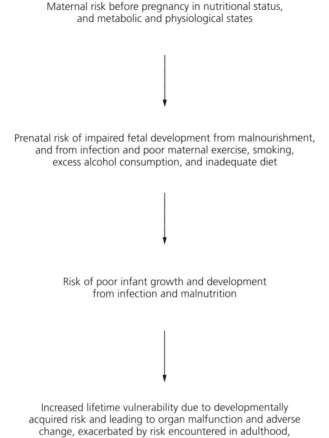

Maternal risk before pregnancy in nutritional status,
and metabolic and physiological states

Prenatal risk of impaired fetal development from malnourishment,
and from infection and poor maternal exercise, smoking,
excess alcohol consumption, and inadequate diet

Risk of poor infant growth and development
from infection and malnutrition

Increased lifetime vulnerability due to developmentally
acquired risk and leading to organ malfunction and adverse
change, exacerbated by risk encountered in adulthood,
such as obesity or smoking

Fig. 3.1 Summarized health risk arising from biological programming.

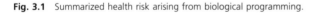

life before their first pregnancy, and that will vary according to their social and family circumstances, which in turn will affect not only their diet, smoking, exercise, and alcohol consumption, but also their mental well-being and coping skills. Similarly, the infant's health will depend on the mother's social and economic circumstances, as well as her health-related knowledge and confidence. The hypothesized biological programming processes require a later-life additional risk to push individuals beyond their biologically programmed safe working envelope, and these additional risks are also socially determined. Smoking and obesity, for example, are each strongly socially determined.

The processes of social determination in the health of mothers and children comprise family factors that are economic, educational, and psychological, and which form a dynamic process that affects lifetime opportunities, coping strategies, and outlook. These are described in the following sections and are summarized in Fig. 3.2.

Each of the factors that make up these family circumstances, and all aspects of the biological processes already described, are located in and affected by a broader social context. For instance, educational opportunity, parental divorce, the risk of poverty, and the likelihood of smoking or becoming obese are each dependent on cultural and historical circumstances, which vary over time. Therefore the third of the following sections is concerned with these aspects of the social context.

3.3.1 Family determinants of health in early life

The family context of early life sets the trajectory into adulthood. The socio-economic circumstances of the family relate strongly to the child's educational opportunities (Douglas 1964; Douglas et al. 1968; Wadsworth 1991), which in turn are associated with subsequent occupation and income (Kuh and Wadsworth 1991; Montgomery et al. 1996). Parental concern for and interest in the child's education are also powerful factors in determining educational attainment (Douglas 1964; Douglas et al. 1968; Wadsworth 1991), and educational attainment is important because of its association with such health-related habits as smoking, exercise, and dietary choice; occupation is similarly associated with health-related habits (Wadsworth 1996).

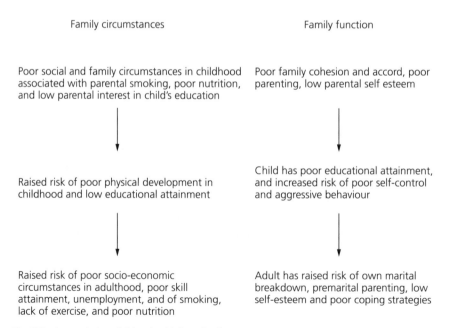

Family circumstances   Family function

Poor social and family circumstances in childhood associated with parental smoking, poor nutrition, and low parental interest in child's education

Poor family cohesion and accord, poor parenting, low parental self esteem

Raised risk of poor physical development in childhood and low educational attainment

Child has poor educational attainment, and increased risk of poor self-control and aggressive behaviour

Raised risk of poor socio-economic circumstances in adulthood, poor skill attainment, unemployment, and of smoking, lack of exercise, and poor nutrition

Adult has raised risk of own marital breakdown, premarital parenting, low self-esteem and poor coping strategies

Fig. 3.2 Accumulation of risk to health from family sources.

Family socio-economic circumstances are also associated with child growth, probably because of nutrition and exercise. Rising socio-economic status of the father was shown in one longitudinal study to be associated with increased height growth in the study child, compared with other study children whose fathers did not rise from the same socio-economic level (Douglas 1964; Kuh and Wadsworth 1989).

Emotional disruption in family life can reduce the child's likelihood of good educational attainment, but whereas parental divorce and separation have been shown to be associated with reduced educational attainment (Ely et al. 1999), a continuing high level of parental interest in the child's education, which is itself associated with parental education, may reduce that effect (Wadsworth and MacLean 1986). Childhood or adolescent experience of parental divorce or separation can also be associated with raised risk of subsequent premarital parenting, frequent job-changing, and own marital breakdown (Rodgers 1994), as well as with raised risk of premature death (Schwartz et al. 1995). Family conflict, with or without parental separation, is related to reduced growth in childhood (Montgomery et al. 1997; Eiben 1998), to reduced health in adolescence, and to lower self-esteem and psychological well-being (Sweeting and West 1995). In considering the association between family life in childhood and labour market position, Sweeting and West (1995, p. 174) concluded that:

> The mechanism may therefore simply be that more family-centred families and/or those with the closest relationships are also those where more time is spent on homework or academic interests. Thus, the link between family functioning and subsequent labour market position, which in turn sets up a chain of circumstances involving greater or lesser risks to future health, is forged.

At a further extreme in family life, neglected and abused children are at raised risk of antisocial or criminal behaviour and substance abuse in adolescence and adulthood (Widom and White 1997), and child abuse is itself associated with parental low self-esteem (Court 1970; Stratton and Swaffer 1988). It is also possible that in childhood interactional and response styles may be acquired which will affect later-life chances. Low self-control, which is associated with raised risk in adulthood of accidental injury as well as criminal behaviour (Tremblay et al. 1995), may also be associated with adverse child experiences at home (Pulkkinen and Hamalainen 1995). Caspi et al. (1991, p. 28) observed that 'childhood ill-temperedness predicts an early exit from formal schooling. Likewise, childhood shyness predicts delayed entry into family and work roles'. McCord and Ensminger (1997) observe that it is an illusion that poor or stressful home conditions predict all kinds of problems. They found specific outcomes associated with specific risks: early experience of aggression predicted violence and also, in women, depression; frequent beating predicted alcoholism, but not depression or violence. In general, parental behaviour is more important than family structure (McCord

1991), and positive experience of family interaction and stimulation in child-hood is associated with better attainment (Sylva 1997).

3.3.2 Social programming

It is necessary, therefore, to ask whether there are critical periods in social and psychological development, as there are in biological development. It seems more likely that there are sensitive rather than critical periods in development. Sylva (1997, p. 187) gives as examples the child's particular sensitivity to caretaking at ages 6–8 months, when children 'must develop their core attach-ment to their parents', and ages 12–13 months as a sensitive period of intellectual and linguistic development.

It is likely also that, as in the biological programming model, a behavioural or social risk established in childhood may need a trigger in adulthood to reactivate the risk. Thus, as adult-onset obesity seems to be at least part of the trigger mechanism for turning prenatally established developmental risk into raised blood pressure (Barker 1994*b*), so there may be a social and behavioural parallel. For example, Rodgers (1994) has shown that adult depression was associated with childhood experience of parental divorce when own divorce had also occurred.

Therefore it may be that a principal process in the association of childhood social factors with adult illness is the accumulation of vulnerability during childhood and adult life. In that case, the childhood social factors may either be an immediate risk, or the beginning of a long-term process of accumulation of vulnerability, or both. For example, parental smoking is a risk to the development of the child's respiratory capacity (Dezateux and Stocks 1997), and so is the infant experience of such lung diseases as bronchitis or pneumonia (Mann et al. 1992). Both are greater risks to children who live in poor socio-economic circumstances. But children in such circumstances are also at raised risk of smoking later in life, and in this instance this is the additional trigger to respiratory vulnerability in adult life (Mann et al. 1992).

These processes of social determination of health can be described in part as acquisition of personal social capital (Wadsworth 1996; Kuh et al. 1997), and in part as pathways of development of risk and protective factors (Robins and Rutter 1990). The element of personal social capital, like that of biological capital, comprises parental socio-economic status and education, parental self-esteem and the degree of family accord, as well as area of residence. The nature of the subsequent pathways to adulthood depends both on the element of personal social capital, and on subsequent individual character-istics (some associated with the development of personal capital) exemplified by Kuh et al. (1997, p. 176) as 'self-esteem, coping strategies and cognitive and social skills', and by Lundberg (1993, p. 1051) as 'a chain of unhealthy living conditions'. Peer-group pressures are also of considerable importance (Michell and West 1996).

A fundamental factor in each of these processes is the current social context, which determines opportunity both for personal capital and for pathways.

3.3.3 The social context

Family processes associated with health and the processes of biological programming are strongly mediated by their social context; examples of such effects are shown in Table 3.1. The most powerful aspect of social context associated with health is poverty because, as discussed elsewhere in this volume, it is often associated with poor diet and consequent poor likelihood of growth and development (Barker 1998), with raised risk of infection, with raised risk of smoking in mothers, and reduced parental self-esteem. In countries without a medical care scheme, that is in most countries, poverty is also associated with low availability of medical care, but even in countries with a national health service, where medical care is available to all, as in Britain, there is still an increasingly raised risk of poor health as poverty deepens. In Britain and the USA, family poverty, particularly in families with children, is increasing (Fuchs and Reklis 1992; Joseph Rowntree Foundation 1995; Hills 1996). Historical studies show that in Britain those born in areas of most dire poverty at times of great differentiation of poverty and wealth, carry into adult life a high risk of premature illness and death compared with those born in less poor areas (Barker 1998).

Unemployment is associated with raised risk to physical and mental health in adults (Montgomery et al. 1996). Because unemployment is more likely among those with low educational attainment and least skill, and because in many countries employment defines status, then experience of unemployment tends to bring not only low income but also social isolation and reduced self-esteem. It may be that the social gradient associated with health among those in employment owes something to these attributes of self-esteem and status. It seems likely that these effects of unemployment on adults will impact on

Table 3.1 The social context of raised risk to health in early life

- Poverty, maldistribution of income, particularly for families
- High rates of unemployment of both parents
- High rates of family discord
- Gender biassed and generally restricted opportunities for education, and low levels of literacy, especially in women
- Low levels of contraception and of breast feeding
- Isolation of women from the mainstream of social participation, and from legal and social security

children. Studies of the psychological effects of periods of mass unemployment, such as the American Great Depression, on adults and those who were
children at that time, show the adverse effects on temperament and
subsequent child rearing among those who had this experience (Elder et al.
1984). Graham (1984, p. 18) observed that:

> Family poverty is inextricably linked to employment policy and the policies
> for income maintenance for those not in paid employment. Since families
> outside the labour market are particularly vulnerable to poverty, employment
> remains the most effective guarantee against both poverty and the ill health
> with which it is associated.

The apparent effects of parental separation and divorce have already been
described, and the rising rates of these salient events in the lives of children
and parents are likely to bring increased health and behavioural problems. At
present Britain has the highest rate of divorce in Europe, at 3.1 per thousand
population, compared with the average for countries in the European
Community of 1.7 per thousand (Church and Summerfield 1996).

Similarly, another form of fundamental disruption of life, namely migration, can bring associated health risks. This has been shown among migrants
from the Tokelau Islands (Beaglehole et al. 1979), from Japan (Marmot et al.
1975), and from southern Asia (McKeigue et al. 1989). Explanations have
been given in terms of genetic differences, social differences, dietary and
psychological change, and the effect of 'cultural bereavement' (Eisenbruch
1988; Helman 1994). In terms of biological programming, poor nutrition in
the pre- and postnatal life of these individuals develops the body's system and
organs to deal with that level of nutrition. Subsequent migration to a richer
society then greatly increases the risks to health associated with obesity and
with glucose intolerance.

Low levels of education are associated with poor health-related behaviour,
for example in terms of diet and exercise, and in raised risk of overweight and
obesity, as already described, and arguably also in terms of self-esteem. In
many countries the education of women has lagged seriously behind that of
men. Watkins (1995) notes that the estimated proportion of children aged
6–11 years who will not be receiving education in the year 2000 will be 51 per
cent in sub-Saharan Africa, 12 per cent in East Asia, and 20 per cent in
southern Asia; and that of the 960 million illiterates in the world two-thirds
are women. In Britain, it was not until the 1970s that women entered
universities in a proportion equal to that of men. Thus the consequent
health-related value to children of higher education in mothers would not
have been seen until after that time, and the health value in terms of pre-
motherhood (i.e. adolescent) health would not have been seen until the
generation born to those mothers.

Two further important elements of social context are custom and fashion.
Deeply ingrained customs in family life and in the division of labour can
impact strongly on the health of mothers and children. Some of the most

striking examples are found in programmes that endeavour to introduce new methods of contraception. Barroso and Correa (1995, p. 302) note that whereas contraceptive programme planners make assumptions about choice and rationality, in practice 'conception is linked to sex – a meeting place for reason, passion, desire, ecstasy, cultural norm, religion, God and the devil, as well as the pleasure of taking risks so typical of games of chance'. Williams et al. (1994, p. 29) observe that 'in Lesotho, sexual intercourse is taboo while the woman is breast feeding, so migrant male workers bring home formula cans to their wives, who can then bottle feed their babies and have sex'. Customs that commonly prohibit female inheritance or even ownership of land and resources, as well as the opportunity of more than the most elementary education, also keep levels of women's health low through the effects of poverty, lack of civil rights, and low self-esteem. Women in some developing countries work a particularly arduous form of 'double day', because of their customary agricultural or industrial labour as well as the care of the family (Pearce 1995). Although in many countries women now form an increasing part of the labour force, 'labour laws seldom give them adequate protection against discrimination, or protect their rights to employment and social security during illness and pregnancy' (Watkins 1995, p. 27).

Fashion in health-related habits can also affect health in early life. It was, for example, neither fashionable nor customary for women to smoke until the late 1920s in Britain, when women in the upper social classes established the habit as fashionable. The habit spread to other social classes, accelerated by the acceptance of smoking as a relaxant during the Second World War, and has subsequently become a habit more frequent in women in socially dis-advantaged circumstances and those with young children (Graham 1984), and is high in men and women living in poverty (Flint and Novotny 1997). There are similarly relevant fashion changes in physical exercise, which is currently becoming increasingly fashionable in Britain, and in the consumption of alcohol, which is growing rapidly. Why the view of what is fashionable changes, and what drives the individual acceptance or rejection of what is fashionable, are important questions which are only now beginning to be studied (Lindbladh et al. 1997).

3.4 Policy implications

There have been experimental intervention studies or long-term reviews of outcomes in each of the areas discussed, which begin to show how health and social policies might systematically help improve health in early life.

In terms of biological programming, Barker (1998) recommends that the most effective long-term methods of preventing coronary heart disease in western urbanized countries would be to improve body composition and diet of girls and young women, and to prevent childhood obesity. Shaheen

(1997) argues that better infant nutrition would improve lung development, and thus help to prevent respiratory ill health in adulthood. Reduction in parental smoking would have a similar effect. In developing countries Barker (1998) recommends that the emphasis in nutritional programmes should be on health in young children:

> In rural India and other developing countries girls are thin and under-nourished, while in towns they are becoming overweight but remain short in stature. Children in many developing countries remain stunted but are now becoming obese. It is not known to what extent this reflects low lean body mass, low intakes of high energy food or hormonal changes associated with stunting. The likely benefits of improving the body composition and nutrition of girls and young women in developing countries include both a reduction in the rising epidemics of coronary heart disease and non-insulin-dependent diabetes and, it seems, an improvement in immune status and consequent lessening of infectious disease (Moore et al. 1997).
> *(Barker 1998, pp. 208–9)*

Williams et al. (1994, p. 13) emphasize the need for concern also with 'maternal depletion syndrome' in developing countries:

> The nutritional strain of reproduction on the mother requires emphasis. Females may be in a constant state of nutritional drain from girlhood through early teenage marriage, until their premature death from exhaustion in their early thirties.

Shaheen (1997, p. 68) notes that tobacco consumption is 'rising dramatically in the developing world . . . and if the lung function of young adults in these countries is compromised by poor pulmonary growth then the additional damage from cigarette smoking may lead to an epidemic of chronic airflow obstruction in the next few decades'.

At the family level, elements of an effective baseline for prevention of health problems have been demonstrated in a number of projects. In Britain a study of resilience to childhood stressful situations, and to physical and sexual abuse, showed the long-term value and effectiveness of having a close relationship with a stable adult as a protection against depression in adult life, reducing depression in women who had experienced abusive childhoods from 42 per cent among those who had no support of this kind to 19 per cent in those who had received support (Bifulco and Moran 1998). Werner (1995, p. 161) shows that protective factors for children living in poverty or in psychologically stressful family circumstances in the Kauai longitudinal study, and in others, may be characterized in three ways. First are the protective factors that are characteristics of the individual. Werner describes these individuals as engaging to others, 'they have good communication and problem-solving skills, including the ability to recruit substitute care givers . . . they have faith that their own actions can make a positive difference in their lives'. Secondly, these resilient children also had family relations or friends who provided affectional ties that 'encouraged trust, autonomy, and initiative'. Thirdly, such children also had relationships with others in the community who provided positive role models and reinforced and rewarded 'competencies of resilient children'.

Intervention designs have been developed from these kinds of observational studies. For example, an intervention study in Britain took the form of a programme administered by health visitors (community nurses), designed to offer support to new parents during the first year of their child's life, by giving them a sense of control over their lives. In this programme 'Considerable emphasis is also laid on the health and well-being of the mother, in her role as a woman with her own interests and future and not merely as a mother of her children. The role of the father or other male partner is brought into this context, with strategies for increasing the child-rearing and domestic contributions of that partner' (Barker et al. 1992, p. 5). Although the emphasis of this programme is not specifically to target child abuse, its effect was shown to reduce abuse substantially, by up to 50 per cent. Other pre-school intervention studies of infants living in low socio-economic circumstances and with mothers with low IQ were strikingly effective in raising children's IQ in comparison with those among controls (Garber and Heber 1981). Cognitive development of children of low birthweight has been raised by intervention (Achenbach et al. 1990), and among children of low birthweight and poor social circumstances (McCormick et al. 1993). One of the most striking intervention studies, the High/Scope Perry Pre-school Programme, was undertaken in the pre-school years with poor urban American children. This programme:

> ... enables children to better carry out the first school tasks that they encounter. This better performance is visible to everyone involved – the child, the teacher, the parents and other children. Realising they have the ability to achieve classroom success, children believe and act accordingly, thereby developing a stronger commitment to schooling. Teachers recognise better school performance and react to it with higher expectations.
> *(Schweinhart et al. 1993, p. 18)*

Children who experienced the programme were compared at age 27 years with others who had not had this experience but who came from similar social circumstances, and the results were striking. Programme children had significantly higher earnings, a higher percentage of home ownership, and higher levels of completed years of schooling, and a lower percentage received help from social services, and there were significantly fewer arrests. Like the High/ Scope Perry Project, most intervention studies show benefits across a range of outcomes including health, behaviour, and cognition. Reviews of such programmes are given by Schweinhart et al. (1993) and by Hertzman and Wiens (1996).

Intervention experiences have helped to improve the lot of individuals and families who are in poor circumstances, reduction of the causes of the poor circumstances themselves requires intervention on a political scale. When that has been attempted it has produced notable results. For instance Watkins

(1995) found that the Indian state of Kerala has a birth rate half that of the national average, and infant mortality rates a quarter below those of the national average. This he attributes to investment in health, education, and more equitable social relations; 'while in India as a whole, one in two girl children drops out of primary school, in Kerala completion is almost universal' (Watkins 1995, p. 30). From two other Asian countries there are comparable reports of successful intervention.

> By promoting the productive use of labour . . . countries have furnished opportunities for the poor, and by investing in health and education they have enabled the poor to take full advantage of the new possibilities. In Indonesia and Malaysia this approach has brought about a substantial reduction in poverty along with improvements in nutrition, under five mortality, and primary enrolment.
> *(Wallace et al. 1995, p. 42)*

3.5 Conclusions

Evidence for the long reach of childhood has been demonstrated over many years in psychology (Sugarman 1993), in mental health (Robins and Rutter 1990), and in studies of social circumstances (Douglas et al. 1968; Wadsworth 1991). It is now becoming evident also in physical health in terms of biological programming, and the long-term effects of childhood social circumstances. In view of the educational intervention studies, it seems logical to conclude that a useful next step in early child health would be experimental intervention. Barker (1998) has argued for improvement of girls' health in preparation for future motherhood.

However, health intervention studies have at best an inconsistent track record, for example those targeted at nutrition in pregnancy (Rush et al. 1980; Barker 1994b) and more broadly at smoking (Rose et al. 1983; Jarvis et al. 1984). By contrast the educational intervention studies and intervention studies on the larger social scale have had much greater success, as outlined above. This may be because they target young children, who are arguably at their most susceptible, and because they are at a sensitive period for learning, But it is certainly also because most educational and social intervention programmes have taught, in childhood, a range of basic ways of coping, cognitive skills, and the reinforcement of self-esteem. In comparison, the health programmes have targeted adults, and endeavoured to teach that something was good for them, which in many cases may well have gone against the grain, and the socially supported habit.

It may be concluded that three kinds of intervention would be valuable in the care of health in early life. The first would be designed to improve the wider social context, namely the improvement in opportunities, particularly educational, for girls. This could only be achieved through pressure for political change. The proverb quoted by Bali (1995, p. 216) aptly summarizes the importance of such intervention for the health and development of children: ' If you plan for one year grow rice, if you plan for ten years grow trees, if you plan for 100 years educate women.'

The second kind of intervention, intended as Barker (1998) recommends to improve diet and growth in girls, is necessary but needs to be delivered in the least didactic way possible. Whereas in some countries this might take the form of teaching about diet from an early age, it might also be necessary elsewhere to supplement diet. The educational intervention studies show that effective teaching is usually greatly enhanced by parental involvement. Growth monitoring would also be necessary. This kind of intervention is difficult to achieve successfully, and certainly needs the support of the third kind of intervention.

The third intervention is concerned with the development of cognitive and coping skills, which can be taught successfully, as the educational intervention studies show. This intervention would, in effect, build a basis of future confidence and self-esteem, which would help individuals to take control of their health and to make positive choices in health.

The effectiveness for health of this last proposed intervention can be tested, and by doing so it would throw light on recent epidemiological work on coronary heart disease. Adult epidemiological studies of coronary heart disease in relation to work circumstances consistently show raised risk of such illness in relation to the individual's experience of work stress, with particular risk associated with low control over the work process (Johnson et al. 1996; Bosma et al. 1998). On the other hand, the child intervention studies show success in teaching control over environment in terms of behaviour and economic and social attainment, even among children who begin life in very poor circumstances (Schweinhart et al. 1993). It would clearly be of value now to revisit populations who experienced childhood intervention of the kind described earlier, and the controls, in order to study health as an outcome. To do so would benefit the coronary heart disease work, and demonstrate the effectiveness of this broad-based intervention for health outcomes.

These proposals for intervention studies and for greater involvement in political pressure for educational improvements are some way from the conventional medical agenda about long-term preventive health care. But, as an influential clinical epidemiologist observed, 'the primary determinants of disease are mainly economic and social, and therefore its remedies must also be economic and social. Medicine and politics cannot and should not be kept apart' (Rose 1992).

References

Achenbach, T., Phares, V., Howell, C.T., Rauh, V. and Nurcombe, B. (1990). Seven year outcome of the Vermont intervention program for low birth-weight infants. *Child Devel.* **61**, 1672–81.

Bali, P. (1995). Health problems and needs of women in developing countries. In: *Health care of women and children in developing countries*, (ed. H.M. Wallace, K. Giri and C.V. Serrano) (2nd edn), pp. 209–17. Third Party Publishing, Oakland.

Barker, D.J.P. (1994a). Fetal growth and adult disease. In: *Early fetal growth and development* (ed. R.H.T. Ward, S.K. Smith and D. Donnai), pp. 197–209 and 238. RCOG Press, London.

Barker, D.J.P. (1994b). *Mothers, babies, and disease in later life.* British Medical Journal Publishing Group, London.

Barker, D.J.P. (1997). Fetal nutrition and cardiovascular disease in later life. In: *Fetal and early childhood environment* (ed. M.G. Marmot, and M.E.J. Wadsworth). *Br. Med. Bull.* **53**, 96–108.

Barker, D.J.P. (1998). *Mothers and babies and health in later life* (2nd edn). Churchill Livingstone, Edinburgh.

Barker, D.J.P., Meade, T.W., Fall, C.H.D., et al. (1992). Relation of fetal and infant growth to plasma fibrinogen and factor VII concentrations in adult life. *BMJ* **304**, 148–52.

Barker, D.J.P., Martyn, C.N., Osmond, C. and Wield, G.A. (1995). Abnormal liver growth *in utero* and death from coronary heart disease. *BMJ* **310**, 703–4.

Barker, W., Anderson, R. and Chalmers, C. (1992). *Child protection; the impact of the child development programme.* Early Childhood Development Unit, Bristol.

Barroso, C. and Correa, S. (1995). Public servants, professionals and feminists: the politics of contraceptive research in Brazil. In: *Conceiving the New World order* (ed. R. Ginsburg and R. Rapp), pp. 292–306. University of California Press, Berkeley.

Beaglehole, R., Eyles, E. and Prior, I. (1979). Blood pressure and migration in children. *Int. J. Epidemiol.* **8**, 5–10.

Bifulco, A. and Moran, P. (1998). *Wednesday's child.* Routledge, London.

Bosma, H., Peter, R., Siegrist, J. and Marmot, M. (1998). Two alternative job stress models and the risk of coronary heart disease. *Am. J. Publ. Hlth* **88**, 68–74.

Brown, R.D. and Weiss, S.T. (1991). The influence of lower respiratory illness on childhood asthma. *Semin. Resp. Infect.* **6**, 225–34.

Caspi, A., Elder, G.H. and Herbener, E.S. (1991). Childhood personality and the prediction of life-course patterns. In: *Straight and devious pathways from childhood to adulthood*, (ed. L. Robins and M. Rutter). Cambridge University Press, Cambridge.

Church, J. and Summerfield, C. (ed.) (1996). *Social trends*, p. 57. HMSO, London.

Court, J. (1970). Psychosocial factors in child battering. *J. Med. Women. Fed.* **52**, 99–104.

Dezateux, C. and Stocks, J. (1997). Lung development and early origins of childhood respiratory illness. In: Fetal and early childhood environment, (ed. M.G. Marmot and M.E.J. Wadsworth). *Br. Med. Bull.* **53**, 40–57.

Dicke, J.M. (1987). Poor obstetrical outcome. In: *Clinical obstetrics* (ed. C.J. Pauerstein), pp. 421–39. Churchill Livingstone, Edinburgh.

Douglas, J.W.B. (1964). *The home and the school*. MacGibbon and Kee, London.

Douglas, J.W.B., Ross, J.M. and Simpson, H.R. (1968). *All our future*. Peter Davies, London.

Eiben, O.G. (1998). Growth and maturation in Eastern Europe. In *Human biology and social inequality* (ed. S.S. Strickland and P.S. Shetty), pp. 132–50. Cambridge University Press, Cambridge.

Eisenbruch, M. (1988). The mental health of refugee children and their cultural development. *Int. Migration Rev.* **22**, 282–300.

Elder, G.H., Liker, J.R. and Cross, C.E. (1984). Parent–child behaviour in the Great Depression; life course and intergenerational influences. In: *Life-span development and behaviour* (ed. P.B. Baltes and O.G. Brim), pp. 109–57. Academic Press, New York.

Ely, M., Richards, M.P.M., Wadsworth, M.E.J. and Elliott, B.J. (1999). Secular change in the association of parental divorce and children's educational attainment: evidence from three British birth cohorts. *J. Soc. Policy*, in press.

Eskenzai, B. and Bergmann, J.J. (1995). Passive and active maternal smoking during pregnancy, as measured by serum cotinine and postnatal smoke exposure. *Am. J. Epidemiol.* **142** (Suppl.), S8–10.

Flint, A.J. and Novotny, T.E. (1997). Poverty status and cigarette smoking prevalence and cessation in the United States 1983–1993: the independent risk of being poor. *Tobacco Control* **6**, 14–18.

Fuchs, V.R. and Reklis, D.M. (1992). America's children: economic perspectives and policy options. *Science* **255**, 41–6.

Garber, H.L. and Heber, R. (1981). The efficacy of early intervention with family rehabilitation. In: *Psychosocial influences in retarded performance*, Vol. 2 (ed. M.J. Begab, R.C. Haywood and H.L. Garber), pp. 71–88. University Park Press, Baltimore.

Graham, H. (1984). *Women, health and the family*. Harvester Press, Brighton.

Hales, C.N. (1997). Non-insulin-dependent diabetes mellitus. In: Fetal and early childhood environment, (ed. M.G. Marmot and M.E.J. Wadsworth). *Br. Med. Bull.* **53**, 109–22.

Hales, C.N., Barker, D.J.P. and Clark, P.M.S. (1992). Fetal and infant growth and impaired glucose tolerance at age 64. *BMJ* **303**, 109–22.

Hall, A.J. and Peckham, C.S. (1997). Infections in childhood and pregnancy as a cause of adult disease – methods and examples. In: *Fetal and early childhood environment* (ed. M.G. Marmot and M.E.J. Wadsworth). *Br. Med. Bull.* **53**, 10–23.

Helman, C. (1994). *Culture, health and illness* (3rd edn). Butterworth Heinemann, London.

Hertzman, C. and Wiens, M. (1996). Child development and long-term outcomes: a population health perspective and summary of successful interventions. *Soc. Sci. Med.* **43**, 1083–95.

Hills, J. (ed.) (1996). *New inequalities: the changing distribution of income and wealth in the United Kingdom.* Cambridge University Press, Cambridge.

Horwood, L.J., Mogridge, N. and Darlow, B.A. (1998). Cognitive education and behavioural outcomes at 7 to 8 years in a national very low birthweight cohort. *Arch. Dis. Child.; Fetal Neonatal Edn* **79**, F12–20.

Jarvis, M., West, R., Tunstall Pedoe, H. and Vesey, C. (1984). An evaluation of the intervention against smoking in the multiple risk factor intervention trial. *Prevent. Med.* **13**, 501–9.

Johnson, J.V., Stewart, W., Hall, E.M., Fredlund, P. and Theorell, T. (1996). Long-term psychosocial work environment and cardiovascular mortality among Swedish men. *Am. J. Publ. Hlth* **86**, 324–31.

Joseph Rowntree Foundation (1995). *Inquiry into income and wealth.* Joseph Rowntree Foundation, York.

Kuh, D. and Wadsworth, M.E.J. (1989). Parental height, childhood environment and subsequent adult height in a national birth cohort. *Int. J. Epidemiol.* **18**, 663–8.

Kuh, D., Power, C., Blane, D. and Bartley, M. (1997). Social pathways between childhood and adult health. In: *A life course approach to chronic disease epidemiology* (ed. D. Kuh and Y. Ben Shlomo), pp. 169–98. Oxford University Press, Oxford.

Lindbladh, E., Lyttkens, H., Hanson, B.S. and Ostergren, P.-O. (1997). The diffusion model and the social-hierarchical process of change. *Hlth Promot. Int.* **12**, 323–30.

Lithell, H.O., McKeigue, P.M., Berglund, L., Mohnsen, R., Lithell, U.-B. and Leon, D. (1996). Relation of size at birth to non-insulin dependent diabetes and insulin concentrations in men aged 50–60 years. *BMJ* **312**, 406–10.

Lucas, A., Morley, R., Cole, T.J., Lister, G. and Leeson-Payne, C. (1992). Breast milk and subsequent intelligence quotient in children born preterm. *Lancet* **339**, 261–4.

Lundberg, O. (1993). The impact of childhood living conditions on illness and mortality in adulthood. *Soc. Sci. Med.* **36**, 1047–52.

McCance, R.A. and Widdowson, E.M. (1974). The determinants of growth and form. *Proc. R. Soc. London (Biol.)* **185**, 1–17.

McCord, J. (1991). Long-term perspectives on parental absence. In: *Straight and devious pathways from childhood to adulthood*, (ed. L.N. Robins and M. Rutter), pp. 116–34. Cambridge University Press, Cambridge.

McCord, J. and Ensminger, M.E. (1997). Mulitple risks and comorbidity in an AfricanAmercian population. *Crim. Behav. Mental Hlth* **7**, 339–52.

McCormick, M.C., McCarton, C, Tonascia, J. and Brooks-Gunn, J. (1993). Early educational intervention for very low birth weight infants: results from the infant health and development program. *J. Pediatr.* **123**, 527–33.

McKeigue, P.M., Miller, G.J. and Marmot, M.G. (1989). Coronary heart disease in South Asians overseas: a review. *J. Clin. Epidemiol.* **42**, 597–609.

Mann, S.L., Wadsworth, M.E.J. and Colley, J.R.T. (1992). Accumulation of factors influencing respiratory illness in members of a national birth cohort and their offspring. *J. Epidemiol. Commun. Hlth.* **46**, 286–92.

Marmot, M.G., Syme, S.L. and Kagan, A. (1975). Epidemiologic studies of CHD and stroke in Japanese men living in Japan, Hawaii and California; prevalence of coronary and hypertensive heart disease and associated risk factors. *Am. J. Epidemiol.* **102**, 514–25.

Martinez, F.D. (1994). Role of viral infections in the inception of asthma and allergies during childhood: could they be protective? *Thorax* **49**, 1189–91.

Martyn, C.N. (1997). Infection in childhood and neurological diseases in adult life. In: Fetal and early childhood environment (ed. M.G. Marmot and M.E.J. Wadsworth). *Br. Med. Bull.* **53**, 24–39.

Michell, L. and West, P. (1996). Peer pressure to smoke: the meaning depends on the method. *Hlth Educ Res: Theory and Practice* **11**, 39–49.

Montgomery, S.M., Bartley, M.J., Cook, D.G. and Wadsworth, M.E.J. (1996). Health and social precursors of unemployment in young men in Great Britain. *J. Epidemiol. Commun. Hlth* **50**, 415–22.

Montgomery, S.M., Bartley, M.J. and Wilkinson, R.G. (1997). Family conflict and slow growth. *Arch. Dis. Child.* **77**, 326–30.

Moore, S.E., Cole, T.J., Poskitt, E.M.E., et al. (1997). Season of birth predicts mortality in rural Gambia. *Nature* **388**, 434.

Pearce, T.O. (1995). The health of working women in developing countries. In: *Health care of women and children in developing countries*, (ed. H.M. Wallace, K. Giri and C.V. Serrano) (2nd edn), pp. 218–24. Third Party Publishing, Oakland.

Perry, I.J. (1997). Fetal growth and development: the role of nutrition and other factors. In: *A life course approach to chronic disease epidemiology* (ed. D. Kuh and Y. Ben Shlomo), pp. 145–68. Oxford University Press, Oxford.

Pulkkinen, L. and Hamalainen, M. (1995). Low self-control as a precursor to crime and accidents in a Finnish longitudinal study. *Crim. Behav. Mental Hlth* **5**, 424–38.

Robins, L.N. and Rutter, M. (ed.) (1990). *Straight and devious pathways from childhood to adulthood.* Cambridge University Press, Cambridge.

Rodgers, B. (1978). Feeding in infancy and later ability and attainment. *Develop. Med. Child Neurol.* **20**, 421–6.

Rodgers B. (1994). Pathways between parental divorce and adult depression. *J. Child Psychol. Psychiat.* **35**, 1289–308.

Rose, G. (1992). *The strategy of preventive medicine.* Oxford University Press, Oxford.

Rose, G., Tunstall Pedoe, H.D. and Heller, R.F. (1983). UK heart disease prevention project: incidence and mortality results. *Lancet* **1**, (8333) 1062–6.

Rush, D., Stein, Z. and Susser, M. (1980). A randomized controlled trial of prenatal nutritional supplementation in New York City. *Pediatrics* **65**, 683–97.

Schwartz, J.E., Friedman, H.S., Tucker, J.S., et al. (1995). Sociodemographic and psychosocial factors in childhood as predictors of adult mortality. *Am. J. Publ. Hlth* **85**, 1237–45.

Schweinhart, L.J., Barnes, H.V. and Weikart, D.P. (1993). *Significant benefits: the High/Scope Perry Preschool Study through age 27 years.* High/Scope Press, Ypsilanti.

Shaheen, S. (1997). The beginnings of chronic airflow obstruction. In: Fetal and early childhood environment (ed. M.G. Marmot and M.E.J. Wadsworth). *Br. Med. Bull.* **53**, 58–70.

Spohr, H.L., Willms, J. and Steinhausen, H.C. (1993). Parental alcohol exposure and long-term developmental consequences. *Lancet* **341**, 907–10.

Stinson, S. (1998). Educational potential and attainment: long-term implications of childhood undernutrition. In: *Human biology and social inequality*, (ed. S.S. Strickland and P.S. Shetty), pp. 132–50. Cambridge University Press, Cambridge.

Stratton, P. and Swaffer, R. (1988). Maternal causal beliefs for abused and handicapped children. *J. Reprod. Infant Psychol.* **6**, 201–16.

Sugarman, L. (1993). *Life-span development: concepts, theories and interventions.* Routledge, London.

Sweeting, H. and West, P. (1995). Family life and health in adolescence: a role for culture in the health inequalities debate? *Soc. Sci. Med.* **40**, 163–75.

Sylva, K. (1997). Critical periods in childhood learning. In: Fetal and early childhood environment (ed. M.G. Marmot and M.E.J. Wadsworth). *Br. Med. Bull.* **53**, 185–97.

Tremblay, R.E., Boulerice, B., Jungner, M. and Arsenault, L. (1995). Does low self-control during childhood explain the association between delinquency and accidents in early adolescence? *Crim. Behav. Mental Hlth* **5**, 439–51.

Wadsworth, M.E.J. (1991). *The imprint of time: childhood, history and adult life.* Oxford University Press, Oxford.

Wadsworth, M.E.J. (1996). Family and education as determinants of health. In: *Health and social organisation* (ed. D. Blane, E. Brunner and R. Wilkinson), pp. 152–70. Routledge, London.

Wadsworth, M.E.J. and Maclean, M. (1986). Parents' divorce and children's life chances. *Child. Youth Services Rev.* **8**, 145–59.

Wallace, H.M., Giri, K. and Serrano, C.V. (1995). *Health care of women and children in developing countries* (2nd edn). Third Party Publishing, Oakland.

Watkins, K. (1995). *The OXFAM Poverty Report*. OXFAM, Oxford.

Werner, E. (1995). Resilience in development. *Curr. Direct. Psychol. Sci.* **32**, 159–62.

Widdowson, E.M. and McCance, R.A. (1975) A review: new thought on growth. *Pediatr. Res.* **9**, 154–6.

Widom, K.S. and White, H.R. (1997). Problem behaviours in abused and neglected children grown up: prevalence and co-occurence of substance use, crime and violence. *Crim. Behav. Mental Hlth* **7**, 287–310.

Williams, C.D., Baumslag, N. and Jelliffe, D.B. (1994). *Maternal and child health* (3rd edn). Oxford University Press, Oxford.

Acknowledgement

Professor Wadsworth's research is funded by the Medical Research Council.

4 The life course, the social gradient, and health

David Blane

4.1 Introduction

The life-course perspective on health and its social determinants sees a person's biological status as a marker of their past social position and, through the structured nature of social processes, as liable to selective accumulation of future advantage or disadvantage. A person's past social experiences become written into the physiology and pathology of their body. The social is, literally, embodied; and the body records the past, whether as an ex-officer's duelling scars or an ex-miner's emphysema. The duelling scar as a mark of social distinction, in turn, predisposes to future advancement and social advantage, while the emphysema robs the employee of their labour power and predisposes to future deprivation and social disadvantage. From a life-course perspective, the social distribution of health and disease results from these processes of accumulating advantage or disadvantage.

A number of scientific developments have contributed to an understanding of the usefulness of a life-course approach (Wadsworth 1997). The chronic natural history of most of the prevalent causes of death in affluent societies has generated an interest in cumulative developmental stresses throughout life (Wilkinson 1996; Kuh and Ben Shlomo 1997; van de Mheen et al. 1998). The maturing of the British birth cohort studies has demonstrated how health in adulthood is influenced by circumstances in the earlier phases of life (Kuh and Wadsworth 1993 Power et al. 1998). A series of studies has demonstrated the long-term influence of childhood socio-economic circumstances on adult, particularly cardiovascular, health (Notkola et al. 1985; Lynch et al. 1994; Gliksman et al. 1995; Brunner et al. 1996). Research into the idea of bio-logical programming has shown an association between intra-uterine and infant circumstances and the prevalent diseases of late middle age and older (Barker 1994; Marmot and Wadsworth 1997). And these developments, in turn, have stimulated an interest in the range of methodologies that can be used to study life-course influences on health (Caselli et al. 1991; Salhi et al. 1995; Berney and Blane 1997; Giele and Elder 1998).

4.2   Social structure and the life course

The life course may be regarded as combining biological and social elements which interact with each other. Individual biological development takes place within a social context which structures life chances so that advantages and disadvantages tend to cluster cross-sectionally and accumulate longitudinally. Exposure to one environmental hazard is likely to be combined with exposure to other hazards and these exposures are likely to accumulate over the course of life (Blane et al. 1997).

Cross-sectionally, advantage or disadvantage in one sphere of life is likely to be accompanied by similar advantage or disadvantage in other spheres. A person whose working environment is free of hazards is likely to reside in good-quality housing, to live in an area of little air pollution, and to have an income that permits a varied diet. In contrast, someone who is exposed to physicochemical and psychosocial hazards during work is at greater risk of occupying damp and inadequately heated accommodation, of being exposed to industrial and traffic exhaust atmospheric pollution in their area of residence, and of earning an income that restricts dietary choice.

Social organization also structures advantage and disadvantage longitudinally. Advantage or disadvantage in one phase of the life course is likely to have been preceded by and to be succeeded by similar advantage or disadvantage in the other phases of life. A child raised in an affluent home is likely to succeed educationally, which will favour entry to the more privileged sectors of the labour market, where an occupational pension scheme will provide financial security in old age. At the other extreme, a child from a disadvantaged home is likely to achieve few educational qualifications and, leaving school at the minimum age, to enter the unskilled labour market where low pay and hazardous work combine with no occupational pension, which ensures reliance on welfare payments in old age.

4.3   Health and the life course

These social processes interact with health in a number of ways. The relationship may be direct and disease-specific. For example, periconceptual intake of folic acid influences strongly the risk of fetal neural tube defects (MRC Vitamin Study Research Group 1991) and the sharp social gradient in these defects most plausibly arises from low incomes and the consequent restriction of dietary choice (Smithells et al. 1976). More general relationships are also possible. For instance, parental social class is a predictor of birthweight (Drever and Whitehead 1997) and, as noted, birthweight is associated with a range of health outcomes in later life. Part of this association may be due to 'biological programming' (Barker 1994): marginally incomplete fetal development, of which low birthweight is a non-specific marker, which later in life is manifest as specific types of organ failure, such as respiratory disease, diabetes, or hypertension. Any effect of this biological programming will be interwoven with ongoing social processes.

4.3.1 Social accumulation

The underlying dynamic of this ongoing social process is the continuity of social circumstances from parental social class to social conditions during childhood and adolescence and, eventually, to adult socio-economic position. What appears to be important is not any one factor which has a major long-term influence on health, but a number of comparatively small differences which become linked into a chain of disadvantage. To pursue the present example, parents' social class influences birthweight (Drever and Whitehead 1997); and adult health is influenced, independently of any long-term effect of birthweight, by social conditions during childhood and adolescence as well as during adulthood (Kuh and Ben Shlomo 1997). Birthweight, in consequence, acts as a marker of social conditions in later life.

Data on the male members of the 1958 British birth cohort have been used to demonstrate this relationship (Bartley et al. 1994). Birthweight, divided into those weighing above and below 6 pounds (2721 g) at birth, was examined in relation to a range of social data collected later at ages – 7, 11, 16, and 23 years. These analyses found that low birthweight babies, subsequently, are more likely to spend their childhood in less affluent families and poor-quality residential accommodation. For example, at age 7 years, 43 per cent of low birthweight babies, compared with 35 per cent of those weighing 2721 g or more, had fathers in clerical or manual social classes and lived in overcrowded homes; in contrast, 17 per cent of low birthweight babies, but 22 per cent of those born weighing 2721 g or above, had fathers in professional social classes I and II. This association was observed throughout childhood; $P = 0.01$, 0.01, and 0.13 at ages 7, 11, and 16 years, respectively. When not having access to, or sole use of, a set of household amenities (inside toilet, hot-water supply, bathroom) was substituted in the analysis for overcrowding, virtually identical results were obtained.

The relationship between birthweight and later socio-economic circumstances is graded in a stepwise fashion across the whole birthweight distribution; and does not simply reflect the existence of an exceptionally disadvantaged low birthweight group. In these same analyses, dividing the birthweight distribution into fifths produced a graded relationship with the number of occasions (from zero to three, at ages 7, 11, and 16 years) on which the cohort members had lived in inadequate housing (overall test of association: $P = 0.0009$) (Table 4.1). The number of times cohort members had experienced financial hardship either in their parents' home, between birth and 16 years, or as young adults at age 23 years, also showed a graded relationship across the birthweight distribution (test for trend: $P = <0.001$).

Table 4.1
Birthweight and subsequent social circumstances in male members of the 1958 British birth cohort study; percentage of each fifth of the birthweight distribution who later experienced housing inadequacy[a] and financial difficulties[b]; (n = 4321) (source: Bartley et al. (1994); adapted from tables III and IV)

Birthweight (fifths)	Housing inadequacy[a]	Financial difficulties[b]
Highest (>136 oz)	18.1	31.6
Fourth (125–135 oz)	20.4	33.7
Third (116–124 oz)	20.4	35.0
Second (106–115 oz)	22.0	36.3
Lowest (<105 oz)	26.6	39.2

[a] Housing inadequacy: overcrowding and/or either no use or shared use of basic household amenities (inside toilet, hot-water supply, bathroom) at each of ages 7, 11, and 16 years.
[b] Financial difficulties: one or more of the following: father in social class V at birth; parents reported family financial problems at subject's age 7 years; in receipt of free school meals at subject's age 11 or 16 years; in receipt of supplementary or unemployment benefit at age 23 years.

Broadly similar relationships were also found among the female members of the 1958 cohort (Power et al. 1996).

As well as short-term effects on health, these types of disadvantage have less obvious longer-term effects. The 1958 British birth cohort study allows the same example to be pursued further. A series of analyses investigated the predictors of unemployment among young men, operationalized as those who had experienced more than 1 year of unemployment between the ages of 22 and 32 years (Montgomery et al. 1996). Height at age 7 years proved a powerful predictor of the subsequent risk of unemployment (Table 4.2). When the distribution of height at age 7 years was divided into fifths, the relationship of later unemployment across the distribution of childhood height was graded in a stepwise manner, with the chances of later unemployment in the shortest fifth of children being nearly three times (relative odds 2.90; 95 per cent confidence interval (CI) 1.84-4.57) that in the tallest fifth. Adjustment for a series of possible confounders such as social class at birth, educational qualifications, and parental height, had little effect; the relative odds reduced from 2.90 to 2.41 (95 per cent CI 1.43-4.04) and the graded relationship across the whole distribution remained. Adult height was a weaker predictor of unemployment risk than height at age 7 years; and adjustment for possible confounders removed the association between adult height and unemployment risk.

Height at age 7 years in these results was interpreted as a measure of delayed growth during childhood, caused by the socio-economic and psycho-social adversity entailed in factors such as poor nutrition and disrupted sleep patterns (Montgomery et al. 1997). Poor nutrition and disrupted sleep relate directly to the financial hardship and crowded residential accommodation

Table 4.2
Childhood height and subsequent social experience in male members of the 1958 British birth cohort; relative odds of each fifth of the childhood height distribution experiencing later unemployment during early adulthood[a]; (n = 2256) (source: Montgomery et al. (1996); adapted from table 2)

Height at age 7 years	Relative odds of unemployment[a]	
	Unadjusted	**Adjusted[b]**
Shortest	2.9	2.41
Second	2.02	1.81
Third	1.3	1.23
Fourth	1.19	1.2
Tallest	1	1

[a] Unemployment: more than 1 year of unemployment between ages 22 and 32 years.
[b] Adjusted for parental height; social class at birth; residential crowding and region at age 7 years; social adjustment at age 11 years; and educational qualifications and height at age 23 years.

which have been discussed earlier. When put together, these analyses of the 1958 British birth cohort suggest a plausible chain: parental disadvantage and low birthweight; some or all of, financial hardship and poor nutrition, crowded residential accommodation and disrupted sleep patterns, and delayed growth during childhood; and the social circumstances which delay childhood growth predispose to labour market disadvantage, as indexed by prolonged or frequent spells of unemployment. Slow childhood growth may identify a particularly disadvantaged subgroup within each social class, who obtain lower educational qualifications and grades than their social class peers. These educational disadvantages subsequently weaken their labour market position which, in turn, exposes them to the health hazards of un-employment and casual employment in the poorly regulated secondary labour market. It is probably unusual for any of these factors on their own to have a major impact on health, but an effect on health becomes plausible when these factors are assembled into an accumulating chain of disadvantage.

4.3.2 Social mobility

Social mobility provides a further mechanism by which health and social factors can accumulate across the life course. Parental socio-economic position influences many aspects of childhood which, in turn, influence the chances and direction of social mobility into a different social class where further advantage or disadvantage accumulates. This process has been explored in the male members of the West of Scotland Collaborative Study (Blane et al. 1999a) (Table 4.3). Adult height, the chances of having left full-time education at the statutory minimum age, and the number of siblings in

Table 4.3
Physical and social characteristics and social mobility in male members of the West of Scotland Collaborative Study; regression coefficients in mutually adjusted regression analysis; (n = 5645) (source: Blane et al. (1999a); adapted from tables 3 and 4)

	Height (cm)	Education[a]	Number of siblings
Father's social class	−0.82	1.91	0.39
Upward mobility	1.02	1.28	0.97
Downward mobility	0.98	0.80	1.05
Own social class	−1.44	2.48	0.59

[a] Education: (a) class: left education at age 14 years or younger; (b) mobility: years of education completed.

the family of origin are all independently associated ($P < 0.0001$) with father's social class, based on the father's main occupation during the study subject's childhood. Those from working-class homes in this data set are more likely than those from middle-class homes to have been brought up in a large family, to have left school early, and to have stopped growing at a short final height. Each of these factors is subject to a range of influences; for example, height is influenced by parental height, education by the quality of local schools, and number of siblings by parental religion. Collectively, however, these factors represent the clustering of various dimensions of advantage and disadvantage during childhood: adult height indexes childhood health and growth; education indexes the cultural environment; and number of siblings, the material conditions of the family of origin. Each of these factors is also associated independently ($P < 0.001$) with the chances and direction of social mobility. They are also associated independently ($P < 0.0001$) with the subject's own social class during adulthood; and in each case the increase in the size of the regression coefficients shows that the association with adult class is stronger than with father's class. Height, years of education, and number of siblings are measures of, and result from, childhood advantage or disadvantage. They also indicate the chances and direction of social mobility, so that their association with other types of social advantage or disadvantage strengthens as the life course unfolds.

The effect of these life-course selective processes, somewhat counter-intuitively, is to constrain rather than widen adult inequalities. The contribution of social mobility to the size of social inequalities can be observed in a social mobility table by comparing the size of inequalities among the socially stable with the size of inequalities in the whole population, which consists of both socially stable and socially mobile. If the former is larger than the latter, the effect of social mobility has been to constrain the size of the inequalities. Such constraint is observed intergenerationally in the West of Scotland Collaborative Study, in relation to height, years of education, and number of siblings (Blane et al. 1999*a*), and has been described intragenerationally in the ONS Longitudinal Study in relation to both limiting long-term illness (Bartley and Plewis 1997) and premature death (Blane et al. 1999*b*). The constraining effect occurs because although the upwardly mobile are more advantaged than those they leave behind (socially stable in their class of origin), they are less advantaged in terms of accumulated lifetime privilege than those they join (socially stable in class of destination). Similarly, the downwardly mobile are disadvantaged in comparison with those they leave, but in terms of accumulated lifetime privilege are more advantaged than those they join. This constraining effect couterbalances the accumulation of advantage and disadvantage and prevents inequalities from widening over the life course.

Data which demonstrate this phenomenon are far from new. Nearly 40 years ago, for example, Morris' famous study of coronary heart disease in London busmen demonstrated that the measured physique of the upwardly mobile bus conductors who became bus drivers was midway between the measured physique of the direct-entry bus drivers, who can be regarded as socially stable members of class IIIM, and the measured physique of those who remained bus conductors and hence can be regarded as socially stable members of class IV (Heady et al. 1961). In the past those interpreting such data have tended to concentrate on the half of the picture which shows that the upwardly mobile are more advantaged than those they leave behind and, on this basis, to conclude that social mobility widens social inequalities. The innovation has been to see the whole picture, including the half which shows that the upwardly mobile are less advantaged than those they join, and to realize that the overall effect of these processes will not be to widen inequalities but to constrain their growth.

4.3.3 Social protection

Social protection provides a third mechanism by which health and social advantage or disadvantage interact over the life course. Previous socio-economic circumstances condition the impact of new disadvantage, minimizing its impact among the advantaged and amplifying its effect among the disadvantaged; and the importance of this conditioning effect increases as the wider external environment becomes more hazardous. Analyses of General Household Survey data have illustrated this mechanism (Bartley and Owen 1996).

In the General Household Survey, men of working age who report a limiting long-standing illness are more likely than those who report good health to be unemployed or economically inactive. The likelihood that chronic ill health will be associated with exclusion from employment varies with socio-economic position (Fig. 4.1). Employment rates among the chronically ill in the advantaged socio-economic groups are higher than among those with

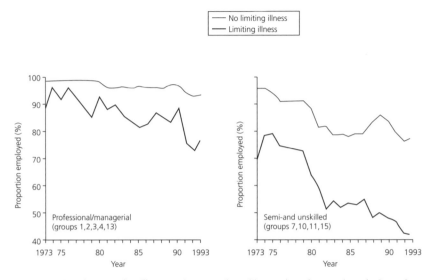

— No limiting illness
— Limiting illness

Fig. 4.1 Limiting long-standing illness, socio-economic position, and employment in male General Household Survey subjects, 1973–93. (From Bartley and Owen 1996; adapted from Figure 2.)

similarly poor health in the less advantaged socio-economic groups. When chronic disease develops, the previous level of general social advantage, as indexed by socio-economic group, can be interpreted as either, in the case of professionals and managers, protecting against the further disadvantage of labour market exclusion; or, in the case of semi- and unskilled manual workers, as adding the further disadvantage of unemployment to the pre-existing disadvantages of chronic disease and the standard of living obtainable with an unskilled manual wage.

This protective or amplifying effect was present in General Household Survey data during the relatively full employment of the mid-1970s. The effect became stronger, in the sense that social class differences in the labour market effects of chronic disease became wider, with the economic recession of the 1980s when unemployment levels and rates of economic inactivity rose. In other words, the 'social protection' type of interaction between health and social circumstances becomes more important when the general external environment becomes more hostile.

4.4　Life-course influences on health and mortality at older ages

Much of the best-quality information about life-course influences on health comes from the British birth cohort studies. These studies started in 1946, 1958, and 1970 so the members of even the oldest of the cohorts have yet to reach the high morbidity and mortality age groups. Consequently, they are as yet silent about life-course influences on premature mortality and contain comparatively sparse data on serious morbidity. For the present one must look elsewhere in order to investigate life-course influences on the health outcomes relevant to the older age groups.

4.4.1   US National Longitudinal Survey

One source is the National Longitudinal Survey of Labour Market Experience of Mature Men (NLS) in the United States; a panel survey of some 5000 men aged 45–59 years in 1966. The data set contains retrospective occupational, educational, and family histories, and a range of prospective information, including deaths, during the follow-up period from 1966 to 1983. These deaths, at ages 45–76 years, have been analysed in relation to preceding life-course events (Mare 1990).

The chance of premature death in this data set is graded in the expected direction, with length of schooling, father's occupation, first occupation on entering the labour market, occupation in middle age, and family assets in middle age. Controlling for education largely eliminates the association between father's occupation and later mortality risk, which suggests that the influence of childhood socio-economic circumstances is transmitted mainly through later experiences and, particularly, educational attainment. Multivariate analysis further suggests that about half of the mortality differential associated with education results from the occupational and financial advantage enjoyed subsequently by men with more schooling. First occupation retains an independent effect on mortality risk at least 25 years later, especially if the first occupation was professional or managerial. Most of the effect of occupation in middle age on subsequent mortality risk appears to result from the differences in wealth and family assets associated with occupation. In summary, the risk of premature death during late middle age or early old age in the NLS is influenced independently by factors across the life course, most importantly length of schooling, type of first occupation and, in middle age, family wealth and assets and type of occupation.

4.4.2   Norwegian linked data

A second source is provided by analyses of a Norwegian longitudinal data set composed of linked information from the national censuses of 1960, 1970, and 1980, and vital registration statistics up to 1985. The approximately 180 000 deaths during this period have been examined in relation to lifetime socio-economic variables, expressed as both the type of social circumstances and the temporal sequencing of these circumstances (Wunsch et al. 1996).

Mortality risk among men is highest for life courses which combine an education which ended at primary level, manual occupations followed by early retirement from work, and housing conditions which were poor in earlier life and often remain poor through to later life. Unfavourable life courses for women similarly involve low education, starting in poor housing conditions, and economic inactivity. Favourable life courses for women, in contrast, are characterized by initially good housing conditions and rarely working in manual occupations; neither high educational level nor high-level employment appear to be important. The life courses associated with low mortality risk among men combine education to secondary level or higher, initial white-collar employment followed by promotion to high-level employment, or a move to self-employment and good housing conditions in later life. These results, despite using different methods to analyse different data from a different continent, are broadly similar to those from the US National Longitudinal Survey.

4.4.3 West of Scotland Collaborative Study

A third source is the West of Scotland Collaborative Study which, in the early 1970s, screened some 5500 male employees, mostly aged 35–64 years, in a representative range of workplaces. Information on cardiovascular health and cardiovascular disease risk factor status was collected, as well as a limited amount of data concerning the earlier stages of life. Twenty-one years of follow-up mortality data are available.

In this data set the conventional risk factors vary in their relationship to the life course (Blane et al. 1996). The behavioural risk factors (recreational exercise and cigarette smoking) are related to the subjects' own social class during adulthood, but are not related to their father's social class when they were children. In contrast, most of the physiological risk factors (diastolic blood pressure, serum cholesterol concentration, and forced expiratory volume in one second) are associated with both father's and own social class, but in such a way that the associations are stronger with adulthood than with childhood. One physiological risk factor, body mass index, was related to the father's social class during the subject's childhood, but not to adult class. These results can be interpreted as showing that behaviour is determined primarily by current social context, probably the norms of the person's significant others, while physiological status reflects the accumulated influences of both past and present.

The life-course dimension to these analyses was taken a step further by including social class based on first occupation (Davey Smith et al. 1997). Each individual now could be assigned to three social class positions: social class during childhood, based on father's occupation; social class at labour market entry, based on own first occupation; and social class during adulthood, based on own occupation at the time of screening. The number of times, between zero and three, that subjects were assigned to manual as opposed to non-manual social classes was related to many aspects of physiological status, with the best health being found among those who had been in non-manual social classes at all three stages of life (Table 4.4). Systolic blood pressure, diastolic blood pressure, serum cholesterol concentration, height, body mass index, forced expiratory volume in one second (FEV_1), and the symptoms of angina and chronic bronchitis were all related in a graded, stepwise fashion to this measure of cumulative lifetime social class. Each move away from thrice non-manual produced worsening health. All-cause mortality during the 21 years of follow-up showed the same relationship with lifetime cumulative class, being more than 50 per cent higher in the group assigned to the manual social classes on all three occasions than in those assigned thrice to non-manual classes. Most importantly, adjustment for a range of behavioural and physiological risk factors produces only rather modest attenuation in the increased risk of death in relation to cumulative social class (see also: Stronks et al. 1996).

Further analyses of these mortality data show that specific diseases and causes of death relate to the life course in different ways (Davey Smith et al. 1998). Some causes of death (cancers, apart from stomach and lung, and accidents and violence) are related to adult, but not to childhood, social class. Most of the other prevalent causes of death (coronary heart disease, stroke, lung cancer, stomach cancer, and respiratory disease) are related independently to both childhood and adult social class. Adjustment for adult socio-economic circumstances and risk factors eliminates the association between lung cancer and childhood class and attenuates the relationship of childhood class with death due to coronary heart disease and respiratory disease, but it does not alter the relationship between childhood class and stroke and stomach cancer. Stroke and stomach cancer mortality in adulthood appear to be associated to an unusual extent, and independently of any continuity of social disadvantage throughout life, with adverse socio-economic circumstances during childhood.

Table 4.4
Cumulative social class at three stages of life and all-cause mortality among men in the West of Scotland Collaborative Study; relative death rates; ($n = 5766$) (source: Davey Smith et al. (1997); adapted from Table 6)

Cumulative social class	Age adjusted	Age and risk factor adjusted[a]
All three non-manual	1.00	1.00
Two non-manual, one manual	1.29	1.30
Two manual, one non-manual	1.45	1.33
All three manual	1.71	1.57

[a] Risk factors: cigarette smoking, diastolic blood pressure, serum cholesterol concentration, body mass index, adjusted FEV_1, angina, bronchitis, and electrocardiogram ischaemia.

The fall during the twentieth century in deaths due to stomach cancer and stroke is unexplained, although refrigeration, with the consequent diminution in consumption of salted, smoked, and pickled foods, has long been suspected (Charlton and Murphy 1997). A different explanation, however, is suggested by the finding that these causes of death during adulthood are related strongly to childhood deprivation. A concern with childhood poverty has been a constant theme of twentieth-century social policy and social science, stretching from:

(1) at the turn of the century, Rowntree's surveys of poverty, the 1904 Inter-Departmental Committee and the introduction of school meals; to

(2) in the 1930s, Eleanor Rathbone's Family Endowment Society and its campaign for family allowances, and the study of child nutrition by the British Medical Association and Boyd Orr at the Rowett Institute; to

(3) during the Second World War, food rationing policy and the Beveridge Report; and

(4) post-war, to the welfare state (Hall et al. 1978).

If adult mortality due to stomach cancer and stroke is unusually sensitive to previous deprivation in childhood, the long fall in mortality from these causes could be an unintended consequence of the series of scientific studies and policy initiatives which have progressively reduced childhood deprivation.

4.4.4 In summary

The US National Longitudinal Survey, the Norwegian record linkage data set, and the West of Scotland Collaborative Study lack the rich information which has been collected by successive sweeps of the birth cohort studies. Analyses are consequently limited by, and to, the range of variables available. Nevertheless, these studies provide the first information about the types of life course which are associated with physiological damage and premature death in late middle age and early old age. Most of the characteristics of these life courses are familiar from cross-sectional studies: childhood circumstances, educational attainment, first occupation, and occupation and level of affluence in adulthood.

New insights have emerged, however. There does not appear to be a stage or phase of life which has special priority for later health or the risk of premature death in the high morbidity–mortality age groups. Each phase of life appears capable of adding its own protection or disadvantage. Behaviour may be the most malleable of these, in the sense that it can respond to the norms of the person's current social context, while physiological status accumulates the results of past events, habits, and hazardous exposures. The elements of the life course appear to be interdependent; educational attainment is a major transmission belt for the long-term effects of childhood circumstance; and family assets are a major component of the effects of adult occupation. Finally, the general advantage or deprivation associated with a social class position would appear to have a sizeable long-term influence, over and above the effect of the generally recognized risk factors, and the various phases of the life course may have different weights for different diseases and causes of death.

4.5 Policy implications

The life-course perspective has important implications for social policy. Bartley and colleagues have drawn on the concept of 'critical periods' during biological development when, if anything goes wrong, permanent damage can result, to coin the analogous concept of critical social transitions, by which is meant life-course changes in social status whose outcome can have long-term effects on future life chances (Bartley et al. 1997). Such transitions include the move from primary to secondary school, labour market entry, establishing own residence, occupational change, onset of chronic illness, and retirement from paid employment. The life course relates in two ways to these critical social transitions.

First, previous levels of accumulated advantage or disadvantage influence whether or not some types of transition, such as those associated with tertiary education, redundancy, and early chronic disease, will occur. The relationship between parental social class and the chances of admission to a university education (Halsey 1988) and the considerably higher risk of redundancy associated with manual as opposed to non-manual employment (Gershuny and Marsh 1994) are well documented. The 1946 British birth cohort study provides a more detailed understanding of the life-course antecedents of the transition to physical disability during early middle age (Kuh et al. 1994). Father's social class during the subject's childhood is the strongest early life predictor of the chances of being physically disabled by age 43 years and this early disadvantage is transmitted into later life primarily through educational attainment and occupational social class location in early adulthood. The effects, in terms of loss of income and employment, of becoming physically disabled in early middle age are, in turn, considerably greater for those with less advantaged pasts.

Previous levels of accumulated advantage or disadvantage also influence whether a critical transition results in a favourable or an unfavourable out-come. As mentioned, previous disadvantage makes labour market exclusion more likely after the early onset of chronic disease (Bartley and Owen 1996). Similarly, the more favourable routes out of redundancy, such as retraining, new skills, and re-employment in a perhaps better-paid occupation, are more likely among those with educational qualifications and a family and social network which can offer encouragement and temporary financial support.

Conversely, redundancy following previous disadvantage is more likely to result in either long-term unemployment or casual re-employment in the insecure and hazardous secondary labour market (Walker et al. 1985).

In the past, social policy has implicitly assumed that these critical social transitions are distributed randomly and, over the long term, approximately equally among the population; and consequently, that protection against them can be financed by social insurance, in which everyone saves a little during the good times to prevent destitution if and when misfortune strikes. A life-course perspective identifies the traditional flaw in this 'safety net' approach to social welfare. Those at greatest risk of misfortune, say redundancy and unemployment, are least likely to have previously enjoyed stable employment and hence are least likely to have accumulated sufficient insurance contributions to finance the welfare benefits that they require (Sinfield 1981). As a result, those most in need of a safety net are least able to provide one.

The life-course perspective goes further than simply explaining the limitations of social insurance, because it also shows that the 'safety net' approach is inadequate. Adversity is not randomly distributed; instead it tends to cluster and to accumulate present on top of previous disadvantage. Consequently, any single misfortune tends to identify the most vulnerable individuals who have accumulated the greatest number of previous handicaps. What is required is not so much a safety net which allows the individual to re-establish their habitual life, but a 'springboard' which repairs the damage caused by past disadvantage and equips the individual to enter, perhaps for the first time, a socially normal life.

A modernized social policy which took account of life-course influences would recognize that:

(1) critical social transitions identify at-risk individuals who, in the absence of effective interventions, are likely to require frequent and, cumulatively over a lifetime, considerable welfare, health, and social support;

(2) effective policy interventions require not only safety nets, to prevent the accumulation of further disadvantage, but also springboards to repair past damage and set people on a more advantaged life trajectory.

The second main policy implication of a life-course perspective is that each of the phases of the life course is equally important and that none can be prioritized. Disadvantage is cumulative, so the move to a more advantaged trajectory can be made at any age. Late middle age and early old age are key age groups for social policy because of their impact on health and welfare expenditure. What is important in terms of the least physiological damage and the lowest risk of premature death at these ages, the evidence suggests, is the proportion of the life course spent in advantaged social positions. Best is life-long advantage; worst is life-long disadvantage; and intermediate is anything which for some proportion of life has shifted the life course from the latter to the former trajectory. In this sense, it is never too late, and always good sense, for social policy to offer a 'helping hand'.

References

Barker, D.J.P. (1994). *Mothers, babies and disease in later life.* British Medical Journal Publishing, London.

Bartley, M. and Owen, C. (1996). Relation between socioeconomic status, employment and health during economic change, 1973–93. *BMJ* **313**, 445–9.

Bartley, M. and Plewis, I. (1997). Does health-selective mobility account for socioeconomic differences in health? Evidence from England and Wales, 1971 to 1991. *J. Hlth Soc. Behav.* **38**, 376–86.

Bartley, M., Power, C., Blane, D., Davey Smith, G. and Shipley, M. (1994). Birth weight and later socioeconomic disadvantage: evidence from the 1958 British cohort study. *BMJ* **309**, 1475–8.

Bartley, M., Blane, D. and Montgomery, S. (1997). Health and the life course: why safety nets matter. *BMJ* **314**, 1194–6.

Berney, L.R. and Blane, D. (1997). Collecting retrospective data: accuracy of recall after 50 years judged against historical records. *Soc. Sci. Med.* **45**, 1519–25.

Blane, D., Hart, C.L., Davey Smith, G., Gillis, C., Hole, D.J. and Hawthorne, V.M. (1996). Association of cardiovascular disease risk factors with socio-economic position during childhood and during adulthood. *BMJ* **313**, 1434–8.

Blane, D, Bartley, M. and Davey Smith, G. (1997). Disease aetiology and materialist explanations of socioeconomic mortality differentials. *Eur. J. Publ. Hlth* **7**, 385–91.

Blane, D., Davey Smith, G. and Hart, C. (1999*a*). Some social and physical correlates of intergenerational social mobility: evidence from the West of Scotland Collaborative Study. *Sociology* **33**, 169–183.

Blane, D., Harding, S. and Rosato, M. (1999*b*). Does social mobility affect the size of the socioeconomic mortality differential? Evidence from the Office for National Statistics Longitudinal Study. *J. R. Stat. Soc.* **162**, 59–70.

Brunner, E., Davey Smith, G., Marmot, M., Canner, R., Beksinska, M. and O'Brien, J. (1996). Childhood social circumstances and psychosocial and behavioural factors as determinants of plasma fibrinogen. *Lancet* **347**, 1008–13.

Caselli, G., Duchene, J., Egidi, V., Santini, A. and Wunch, G. (1991). A matter of life and death: methodologies for studying the life history analysis of adult mortality. In: *Socioeconomic differential mortality in industrialised countries*, Vol. 7, pp. 242–77. Comité International de Cooperation dans les Recherches Nationales en Demographie (CICRED), Paris.

Charlton, J. and Murphy, M. (ed.) (1997). *The health of adult Britain*. HMSO, London.

Davey Smith, G., Hart, C.L., Blane, D., Gillis, C. and Hawthorne, V.M. (1997). Lifetime socioeconomic position and mortality: prospective observational study. *BMJ* **314**, 547–52.

Davey Smith, G., Hart, C., Blane, D. and Hole, D. (1998). Adverse socioeconomic conditions in childhood and cause specific adult mortality: prospective observational study. *BMJ* **316**, 1631–5.

Drever, F. and Whitehead, M. (1997). *Health inequalities*. The Stationery Office, London.

Gershuny, J. and Marsh, C. (1994). Unemployment in work histories. In: Social change and the experience of unemployment, (ed. D. Gallie, C. Marsh, and C. Vogler), pp. 66–114. Oxford University Press, Oxford.

Giele, J.Z. and Elder, G.H. (ed.) (1998). *Methods of life course research: qualitative and quantitative approaches*. Sage, London.

Gliksman, M.D., Kawachi, I., Hunter, D., Colditz, G.A., Manson J.A.E. and Stampfer, M.J. (1995). Childhood socioeconomic status and risk of cardiovascular disease in middle aged US women: a prospective study. *J. Epidemiol. Commun. Hlth* **49**, 10–15.

Hall, P., Land, H., Parker, R. and Webb, A. (1978). The introduction of family allowances. In: *Change choice and conflict in social policy* (ed. P. Hall, H. Land, R. Parker, and A. Webb), pp. 157–230. Heinemann, London.

Halsey, A.H. (1988). *British social trends since 1900*. Macmillan, Basingstoke.

Heady, J.A., Morris, J.N., Kegan, A. and Raffle, P.A.B. (1961). Coronary heart disease in London busmen. *Br. J. Prevent. Soc. Med.* **15**, 143–53.

Kuh, D.L.J. and Ben Shlomo, Y. (ed.) (1997). *A life course approach to chronic disease epidemiology*. Oxford University Press, Oxford.

Kuh, D.J.L. and Wadsworth, M.E.J. (1993). Physical health status at 36 years in a British national birth cohort. *Soc. Sci. Med.* **37**, 905–16.

Kuh, D.L.J., Wadsworth, M.E.J. and Yusuf, E.J. (1994). Burden of disability in a post war birth cohort in the UK. *J. Epidemiol. Commun. Hlth* **48**, 262–9.

Lynch, J.W., Kaplan, G.A., Cohen, R.D., Kauhanen, J., Wilson, T.W. and Smith, N.L. (1994). Childhood and adult socioeconomic status as predictors of mortality in Finland. *Lancet* 343, 524–7.

Mare, R.D. (1990). Socioeconomic careers and differential mortality among older men in the United States. In: *Measurement and analysis of mortality: new approaches* (ed. J. Vallin, S. D'Souza and A. Palloni), pp. 362–87. Clarendon Press: Oxford.

Marmot, M.G. and Wadsworth, M.E.J. (ed.) (1997). Fetal and early childhood environment: long-term health implications. *Br. Med. Bull.* **53**, (Issue 1).

Montgomery, S.M., Bartley, M.J., Cook, D.G. and Wadsworth, M.E.J. (1996).

Health and social precursors of unemployment in young men in Great Britain. *J. Epidemiol. Commun. Hlth* **50**, 415–22.

Montgomery, S., Bartley, M. and Wilkinson, R. (1997). Family conflict and slow growth. *Arch. Dis. Child.* **77**, 326–30.

MRC Vitamin Study Research Group (1991). Prevention of neural tube defects: results of the Medical Research Council Vitamin Study. *Lancet* **338**, 131–7.

Notkola, V., Punsar, S., Karvonen, M.J. and Haapakoski, J. (1985). Socio-economic conditions in childhood and mortality and morbidity caused by coronary heart disease in adulthood in rural Finland. *Soc. Sci. Med.* **21**, 517–23.

Power, C., Bartley, M., Davey Smith, G. and Blane, D. (1996). Transmission of social and biological risk across the life course. In: *Health and social organisation*, (ed. D. Blane, E. Brunner and R. Wilkinson), pp. 188–203. Routledge, London.

Power, C., Matthews, S. and Manor, O. (1998). Inequalities in self rated health: explanations from different stages of life. *Lancet* **351**, 1009–14.

Salhi, M., Caselli, G., Duchene, J., et al. (1995). Assessing mortality differentials using life histories: a method and applications. In: *Adult mortality in developed countries: from description to explanation*, (ed. A.D. Lopez, G. Caselli, and T. Valkonen), pp. 57–79. Clarendon Press, Oxford.

Sinfield, R.A. (1981). *What unemployment means*. Martin Robertson, Oxford.

Smithells, R.W., Sheppard, S. and Schorah, C.J. (1976). Vitamin deficiencies and neural tube defects. *Arch. Dis. Child.* **51**, 944–50.

Stronks, K., van de Mheen, H. and Looman, C.W.N. (1996). Behavioural and structural factors in the explanation of socioeconomic inequalities in health: an empirical analysis. *Sociol. Hth Illness* **18**, 653–74.

van de Mheen, H., Stronks, K. and Mackenbach, J. (1998). A life course perspective on socioeconomic inequalities in health. In: *The sociology of health inequalities* (ed. M. Bartley, D. Blane and G. Davey Smith), pp. 193–216. Blackwell, Oxford.

Wadsworth, M.E.J. (1997). Health inequalities in the life course perspective. *Soc. Sci. Med.* **44**, 859–70.

Walker, A., Noble, I. and Westergaard, J. (1985). From secure employment to labour market insecurity. In: *New approaches to economic life*, (ed. B. Roberts, R. Finnegan, and D. Gallie), pp. 1947. Manchester University Press, Manchester.

Wilkinson, R.G. (1996). *Unhealthy societies: the afflictions of inequality*. Routledge, London.

Wunch, G., Duchene, J., Thiltges, E. and Salhi, M. (1996). Socioeconomic differences in mortality: a life course approach. *Eur. J. Popn* **12**, 167–85.

Acknowledgements

Dr Blane's research is supported by the Economic and Social Research Council's Health Variations Programme, Grant Number L128251033.

5   Living in a high-unemployment economy: understanding the health consequences

Mel Bartley, Jane Ferrie, and Scott M. Montgomery

5.1   Introduction

This chapter assembles evidence on the impact of high unemployment on population health. It takes an approach informed by the most recent research done on the basis of longitudinal data and, where possible, from studies that include objective measures of both physical and psychological health at more than one point in time. The availability of such data helps to overcome some of the major problems in deciding whether there is a health impact of unemployment and job insecurity sufficient to justify policy debate and response.

Research has shown repeatedly a higher prevalence of ill health (Daniel and Stilgoe 1979; Moylan and Davies 1980; Cook et al. 1982; Moylan et al. 1984) and excess mortality (Moser et al. 1984 1987; Morris et al. 1994) in men and women who are unemployed. Figures 5.1 and 5.2 show rates of poor self-rated health by employment status in men and women in England in 1998. Men who are unemployed, and women who are either unemployed or keeping house full time, are more likely to describe their health as generally fair or poor.

Damage to psychological health is also found by the vast majority of studies, an effect that appears to be independent of pre-existing health and to be reversed on re-employment in many cases (Banks and Jackson 1982; Warr 1984 1987; Isaakson 1989; Montgomery et al. 1999). However, it is not a simple step from this observation to a causal relationship between unemployment and health. Those who are ill may be more likely to lose their jobs and find it harder to regain employment. Or there may be indirect effects whereby men and women with other characteristics such as lower levels of education, which are known to be related to health risks, are also less likely to be employed. When considering the policy implications of the relationship of

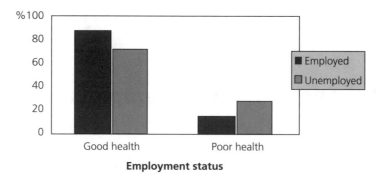

Fig. 5.1 Employment status and health: men.

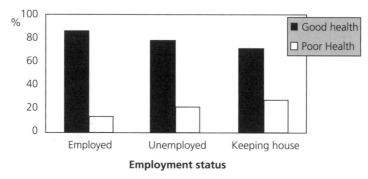

Fig. 5.2 Employment status and health: women.

unemployment to health, it is obviously essential to assess the possibility that this is a consequence of selection.

5.2 Selection

Although there is a cross-sectional association of unemployment with illness, physical health does not necessarily decline during a spell of unemployment; a number of studies failed to find an increase in morbidity amongst those who were continuously unemployed for up to 18 months (Bartley 1987). Indeed, it has been reported that physical health may actually improve during a period of unemployment (Ramsden and Smee 1981). Those who are ill may be more likely to lose their jobs and find it harder to regain employment, because of their illness: this is known as selection (Fig. 5.3).

The 'direct health selection' hypothesis asserts that poorer health itself increases the risk of unemployment (Stern 1983; Cook 1985; Wadsworth, 1986; Wagstaff 1986; Robinson et al. 1989). Ill health has been clearly shown to be a risk for both initial job loss and for subsequent chances of

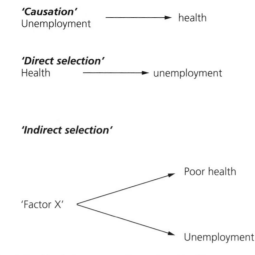

'Causation'
Unemployment ————————→ health

'Direct selection'
Health ————————→ unemployment

'Indirect selection'

'Factor X' → Poor health

→ Unemployment

Fig. 5.3 Possible relationships between unemployment and health.

re-employment (Clausen et al. 1993). A test of the 'direct selection' hypothesis can be made by using longitudinal data on unemployment and mortality (Moser et al. 1984). There are not very many longitudinal studies of un-employment and mortality, as such data sets require a great deal of effort and cost to collect and maintain. However, in those that do exist, people who are unemployed at the beginning of any follow-up period are always found to have higher mortality than those who are employed. The question is: could this be because the unemployed also have more life-threatening illnesses which precede their unemployment? One way of deciding whether this is the case is to examine the trend in mortality over a long period of time. If high mortality in the unemployed was found only because life-threatening diseases were more prevalent in the unemployed than the employed, longitudinal data would show high mortality in the unemployed in the early periods of follow-up, with a sharp decline in mortality rate with increasing length of time. This is because those amongst the unemployed who were ill would eventually all die: if they were the sole reason for the excess risk of death, then the excess should disappear at this point in time. Research using linked census-based data from England and Wales (the ONS Longitudinal Study: Goldblatt et al. 1990; Bethune 1997) and from the Nordic countries (Martikainen 1990; Iversen et al. 1987) have not identified this pattern of mortality. On the contrary, the unemployed display a higher risk of mortality no matter how long the cohorts are followed. This finding makes it rather unlikely that direct selection into unemployment of those with life-threatening disease can account for the relationship between unemployment and excess mortality.

There may still be some tendency for those who remain unemployed to be 'different' to those who do not, even if this difference does not take the form of a life-threatening disease. Perhaps people at high risk of unemployment may also have certain personality characteristics (this could be the 'factor X' in Fig. 5.3). However, this is a more complex hypothesis, and not necessarily the same as 'selection'. These ideas have to be considered alongside other evidence on the life-course accumulation of social and health disadvantage. Whether or not we consider that there may be differences in the previous life histories of those at higher and lower risk of unemployment, we need to consider the mechanisms through which a relationship to health may occur. The indirect selection hypothesis states that characteristics such a personality traits are 'confounders'. In this case, the mechanism would be a that both unemployment and health are related to a certain personality trait. This makes it appear that unemployment is related to health, whereas in fact the true causal relationship is that by which the personality trait affects both health and unemployment separately. If this is the mechanism, we would find that those with the personality trait were equally likely to develop poor health whether or not they became unemployed, and there should be no greater illness in people who do not possess the relevant trait whether they are employed or unemployed.

One study which has been able to test this hypothesis in relation to mental health is the 1958 British birth cohort study (Montgomery et al. 1999). The study contains extensive data on psychological development throughout the school years and young adult life, as well as complete employment histories from leaving school to age 33. It can therefore address the possibility that the high level of psychological morbidity found in unemployed men and women is due to a pre-existing vulnerability to poor mental health (Catalano et al. 1981 1985). The researchers were able to date the onset of symptoms of depression and anxiety which required medical care in cohort members, and relate this to both recent unemployment and a measure of the total amount of unemployment which an individual had accumulated since first entering the labour market.

Even after taking into account pre-existing mental health, recent unemployment was clearly related to the onset of symptoms, although in the cohort as a whole, the amount of accumulated past unemployment was not. However, when those with a prior tendency to depression were excluded from the analysis, this had the effect of strengthening the relationship between longer-term accumulation of unemployment and the onset of episodes of depression and anxiety. This showed that it is not only men with pre-existing poor mental health who are vulnerable to the psychologically damaging consequences of job loss. It provides strong evidence that longer-term unemployment causes deterioration in mental health in those who were previously healthy. It was recent unemployment, rather than the total amount of unemployment a person experienced, which put him at risk for deterioration in mental health. This indicates that interventions need initially to be targeted at those who have recently lost their jobs, when the decline in mental health may be steepest.

What might be the reasons for this effect of unemployment? Several have been put forward, and here we will consider three of these: poverty, the fact that unemployment is a stressful life event, and changes in health-related behaviours at the time of unemployment.

5.2.1 Poverty

Some research into the relationship between unemployment and ill health has argued for putting poverty back into the centre of the enquiry (Fryer 1992). Low living standards are not an inevitable consequence of unemployment; this is a result of the levels at which benefits are set. During the 1980s levels of income replacement for the unemployed were lowered. It was argued that under conditions of increasing automation of unskilled and semi-skilled work, levels of benefit available to the unemployed exceeded the market worth of their labour (Gaffikin and Morrisey 1992), that is, the wage rate which employers were willing to pay. If the level of pay at which an unemployed person will accept new work – the 'reservation wage' – is too high, employers will not take them on. If benefit levels are too high, the state is raising the reservation wage and therefore may be contributing to the problem of high unemployment (Benjamin and Kochin 1979; Minford 1990).

In the UK, benefits were cut in a number of ways from the early 1980s, and this was indeed followed by a decrease in the real value of the lowest wages, and a general redistribution of income away from the poorest sections of society, so that between 1979 and 1991, while the average household experienced an increase in real income of 36 per cent, that of the poorest tenth fell by 14 per cent after housing costs (Sinfield 1993). In 1981 the households in the lowest 10 per cent of the income distribution shared out 4.1 per cent of total income (including benefits and net of direct taxation) in the population between them; this had fallen to 2.9 per cent by 1993, while the richest 10 per cent shared out 21.3 per cent in 1981 and 26.2 per cent in 1993 (Goodman et al., 1997). Job insecurity, in addition, has the desired effect (according to this model) of aiding the imposition of the 'right to manage'. As well as exerting downward pressure on wages, a shortage of jobs may reduce the propensity of employees to question health and safety provisions, or otherwise assert employment rights.

Many studies link the health effects of unemployment directly to financial problems. Jackson and Warr reported that the proportional change in family income between employment and unemployment predicted subjects' scores on the General Health Questionnaire (GHQ), a widely used measure of psychological health (Jackson and Warr 1984). In studies by White and colleagues, long-term unemployed people who had to borrow money in the past year had a risk of depression, as measured by the GHQ score (4.5) which was more than double that of those who did not have to borrow (2.0). These researchers also found that those obliged to borrow were also more likely to report deterioration in physical health (White 1994). Others have documented the ways in which increasing financial pressures, as savings are used up and worn-out items need to be replaced, are responsible for the growing inactivity and social isolation of many unemployed people (Bradshaw et al. 1983; Clarke 1978). In the OPCS/DSS survey of living standards in unemployment, GHQ scores were related to debt (Heady and Smyth 1989). In the Medical Research Council's 1946 cohort study, after financial hardship was controlled for the relationships between unemployment and psychological symptoms in both men and women were weakened or disappeared (Rodgers 1991). Figures 5.4 and 5.5 show that among unemployed men, and among both unemployed women and those keeping house only, rates of car and home ownership are lower, and fewer households had central heating in the English health survey in 1993.

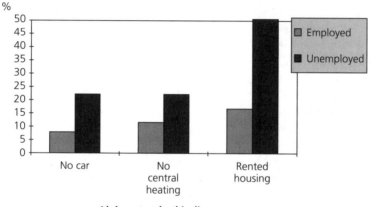

Fig. 5.4 Employment status and living standards: men.

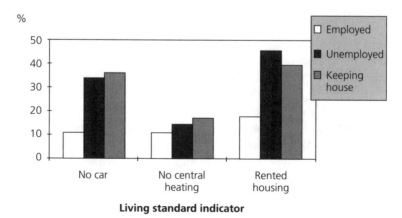

Fig. 5.5 Employment status and living standards: women.

These British findings are echoed in other countries. Kessler et al. found that financial strain was the strongest mediating factor between unemployment and reported ill health in their American study, being far more important than reduced social integration or an increased number of life events (Kessler et al. 1988). A Dutch study found similarly that present or anticipated financial problems, as well as loneliness, were the major mediating factors between unemployed status and reported health problems in both men and women (Leeflang et al. 1992a,b). Eventually, it seems, many of the unemployed adapt to straitened financial and social circumstances. Several studies agree that there appears to be no further deterioration in psychological well-being after a period of between 1 year and 18 months (Warr and Jackson 1985; Banks and Ullah 1987; Hamilton et al. 1993). This adds weight to the argument for providing early assistance to those who become unemployed. Other evidence suggests that adaptation to unemployment is accompanied by lowered expectations of oneself, and perhaps a degree of alienation and cynicism. In Warr and Jackson's study, GHQ scores did not deteriorate between 18 and 27 months of continuous unemployment, although they remained at a level far above those of comparable employed samples (Warr and Jackson 1987). The authors compare the adaptive process to that found in institutionalized inmates of prisons or hospitals.

5.2.2 Unemployment as a stressful life event

Research shows job loss to be a highly stressful life event, which has been characterized as a form of bereavement (Fagin and Little 1984). In modern welfare states, starvation and physical privation are no longer thought to accompany the loss of paid work (Stern 1982; Gravelle 1985). Many researchers have suggested that work has a number of non-financial benefits to the individual, termed by Jahoda 'latent consequences', and it is the loss of these which results in the threatening character of unemployment. Jahoda's latent consequences of employment included giving a time structure to the day, self-esteem, and the respect of others (Jahoda 1942 1979; Fryer 1987). Warr has developed a somewhat similar 'vitamin theory' of the benefits of work for mental health, which include physical and mental activity, use of skills, decision latitude, interpersonal contact, social status, and 'traction' – a reason to go on through the day and from one day to the next (Warr 1987).

Figure 5.6, based on the English National Health Survey for 1993, shows low levels of psychological well-being, as measured by the GHQ, in both men and women who were unemployed. In the Scandinavian countries, where benefits are relatively generous and financial effects might not be expected to be as great, the psychological effects are similar. A study in Stockholm of men with irregular work histories and a variety of problems which required frequent social service assistance found that those who were employed, even in low-paid casual jobs, were all more active and integrated (and psychologically

% depressed

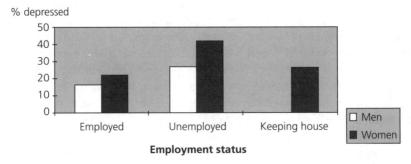

Fig. 5.6 Employment status by depression on GHQ: men and women.

healthier) than the unemployed (Isaakson 1989). Amongst unemployed industrial workers in Finland, those who regained work experienced a considerable improvement in psychological health regardless of their financial circumstances either before or after re-employment (Lahelma 1992*a,b*). Italian workers laid off from their jobs experienced raised amounts of both psychological and physical illness despite receiving the whole of their normal wage (Rudas et al. 1991). These studies provide evidence of the non-financial benefits of work for psychological health. 'Stress' may affect physical health as well as psychological health as a result perhaps of chronically increased levels of anxiety (Kaplan 1991).

5.2.3   Health-related behaviour

There is evidence that unemployment is associated with some forms of health-damaging behaviour, although previous research has yielded inconsistent findings on the relationship between unemployment and health-related behaviour (Wilson 1980; Cook et al. 1982; Lee et al. 1990 1991; Power and Estaugh 1990; Morris et al. 1992). While the evidence that people actually increase their hazardous health behaviours while they are unemployed is not overwhelming (Morris and Cook 1991), associations between unemployment and health behaviours need to be seen in the context of the longer-term development of health behaviours (Wadsworth 1991). Few studies have been able to examine unemployment over time, or to adjust for health behaviour prior to starting work, i.e. before any experience of unemployment. Because of its longitudinal nature, the 1958 birth cohort study was able to consider the relationship of unemployment between the ages of 23 and 33 not only to health behaviours at 33, but also to behaviours at 16 years of age, a period when behaviour patterns were being established (Montgomery et al. 1998). Men who experienced unemployment were more likely to smoke, to have a low weight for their height, and to consume less alcohol at age 16 years. However, even after taking account of these pre-existing differences, and of material and cultural circumstances in childhood, there were significant associations of health behaviour and body weight, both with recent un-employment at age 33 years and with the amount of unemployment since age 23 years. Men who experienced more unemployment tended to have lower body weight, were less likely to have given up cigarette smoking and slightly more likely to have taken it up, and were more likely to have a high CAGE score (indicating problem drinking).

At the age of 33 years, the NCDS cohort members were too young for a significant proportion to have become clinically obese, but in later years these findings indicate that unemployment may be associated with further weight gain. Just as being too fat can be a risk to health, the low body weight among some of the young unemployed may be a cause for concern, as low weight and weight loss have been associated with later adverse health outcome through stress-mediated mechanisms (Arnetz et al. 1991). Periods in and out of un-employment result in stress-related alternations of weight loss and weight gain, which has been reported to be a significant risk for cardiovascular disease (Bosello et al. 1993)

By its nature, the relationship of unemployment to illegal drug-taking is difficult to investigate. Young unemployed people in Lothian region had more experience of drugs such as cannabis, opiates, and LSD, reflecting national trends (Peck and Plant 1986). A study of young people in Norway produced similar findings but concluded that drugs were not being used to combat stress; rather drug use was part of the adoption of an alternative cultural identity (Hammer 1992).

More directly self-destructive behaviour amongst unemployed men has been widely investigated (Platt 1984). In the ONS Longitudinal Study, men unemployed at the 1971 census had an standardized mortality ratio (SMR) for suicide of 236: this excess risk was greatest in those aged 35–44 (Moser et al. 1984). More recently, the possible link between unemployment and national trends in suicide amongst younger men have given cause for concern (Pritchard 1992). However, male suicide continued to rise as unemployment fell in the late 1980s (Charlton et al. 1992). Parasuicide ('attempted suicide') has also been found to be higher in unemployed men (Platt and Kreitman 1984 1985; Hawton and Rose 1986). There seems to be agreement that it is not unemployment *per se* that precipitates suicidal behaviour (Platt 1986). Rather, as Kessler et al. have also found in their American studies, unemployment increases the likelihood of other adverse life events and lessens the psychological and social resources needed to cope with these (Kessler et al. 1988). Longitudinal research in England and Wales also shows that spells of unemployment have longer-term effects, such as loss of home and marriage breakdown (Fox 1986; Fox and Shewry 1988).

5.3 Job insecurity and job quality

One of the most consistently replicated findings in this area is that health begins to be affected at the time when people anticipate unemployment but are still at work (Cobb and Kasl 1977; Iversen and Clausen 1981; Beale and Nethercott 1985). Job insecurity and threat of job loss have been found to result in increased psychological disturbance (Arnetz et al. 1988) and physiological changes (Cobb et al. 1966), as well as increased consumption of medical care (Beale and Nethercott 1985, 1987). In a study in Malmo, Sweden, the relationship between threatened redundancy and psychological and physiological health measures appeared to vary according to the degree of future financial uncertainty. Male shipyard workers threatened with redundancy aged over 58, who knew that they would be offered relatively generous early retirement settlements, experienced no deterioration in psychological health and a rise of only 0.09 mmol/l in measured serum cholesterol. In younger men with no such reassuring prospects, cholesterol rose by 0.28 mmol/l. By contrast, in members of the control group not involved in the shipyard closure at all, the rise in men over 58 years of age was greater than that in younger men (Matthiasson et al. 1990).

Studies in both Britain and Australia have suggested that not all jobs, regardless of quality, can protect physical or mental health: in some cases unsatisfactory jobs can be as depressing as unemployment (Winefield et al. 1988 1991; Graetz 1993). In the British Social Change and Economic Life Initiative, those with insecure work who had been obliged to take lower-status jobs in the recent past had a score on the GHQ not significantly different from that of the unemployed (Burchell 1996). Insecure jobs also tend to be ones that involve high exposure to work hazards such as heavy lifting, falls, and dangerous chemicals (Robinson 1986).

In order fully to understand the links between unemployment, ill health, and mortality, it is necessary to look beyond the experience of unemployment itself. Even within the adult work history, spells of unemployment are not randomly distributed interludes (Stern 1979; Sinfield 1981) and have longer-term effects even after they are over (Ferman and Gardner 1979; Daniel 1983 1990). Once a person has become unemployed for the first time, their risk of further unemployment is greatly increased (Westergaard et al. 1989). Losing a job can precipitate the individual into a self-perpetuating series of negative events, such as occupational downgrading, loss of pay and status, less-secure employment, well into the future, even after work has been regained (White 1983; Fox 1986; Harris 1987; Fox and Shewry 1988).

Job insecurity may also constitute a psychosocial hazard in itself. A recent investigation of the effects of privatization in the British civil service took advantage of the availability of detailed physical and psychological screening over a 10-year period during which some departmental functions were sold to the private sector and others were converted into agencies in preparation for privatization. In the department which was entirely sold off to the private sector, a deterioration in health status was seen during the 'period of anticipation' before the finalization of the change (Ferrie et al. 1995). Immediately before the sale, significant increases were also seen in cardio-vascular risk factors (Ferrie et al. 1998*a*). After the sale of this department to the private sector, a follow-up survey found that 40 per cent of respondents were out of employment, and 50 per cent of those in employment were in insecure jobs (Ferrie 1997) (Fig. 5.7). Amongst the other departments in the study which were not completely privatized, the workers most threatened by job insecurity were found to have experienced increases in reported symptoms, long-term illness, and adverse sleep patterns. Those whose civil service departments had been transferred to agency status were also found to have relatively higher blood pressure than those untouched by the changes (Ferrie et al. 1998*b*).

5.4 Unemployment in the life course

Having considered selection, poverty, stress, health behaviours and insecurity as mechanisms through which unemployment may influence health, we may consider the evidence that unemployment and work insecurity are part of a process through which health disadvantage is accumulated over the life course. Research taking this perspective turns away from any simple opposition between 'selection and causation', and shows that unemployment occurs as part of a much longer-term sequence of events in the life of the individual, stretching back into childhood. This means that those most likely to experience unemployment may also be more vulnerable to excess mortality and morbidity both because of earlier experience of hardship and disadvantage, and of their experience of unemployment (Valkonen and Martikainen 1995).

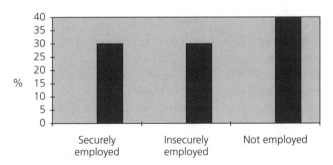

Fig. 5.7 Employment status after PSA privatization.

5.4.1 Early life

It is known that unemployment is more common in those young people who have previously experienced less favourable family circumstances and educational attainment (Power et al. 1991; Montgomery et al. 1996). We know that material, educational, psychological, and cultural circumstances during childhood are related to many aspects of adult life opportunity (Douglas et al. 1968; Pilling 1990; Wadsworth 1991), including occupational attainment (Elias and Blanchflower 1987; Payne et al. 1994). We are also beginning to understand the ways in which physical and psychological development in early life, and the acquisition of health-related habits in childhood and adolescence, may be associated with health in later life (Wadsworth 1991; Barker 1994). Poor growth during early childhood has been shown to be associated with increased risks to adult health (Tanner 1955; Douglas et al. 1968; Preece and Holder 1982; Preece 1985) and shorter stature in adolescence has been associated with future experience of unemployment. The importance of variations in the development of psychological health potential during childhood has been similarly demonstrated (Zoccolillo et al. 1992; Harrington et al. 1994), and it has been shown to be a source of risk and protection in terms of adult life adversity (Cherry 1976; Block and Gjerde 1989).

Because more longitudinal data from childhood to adulthood are now available, it is possible to describe some of the ways in which unemployment fits into patterns of disadvantage accumulated from early in life. Some of these data include detailed physiological measures which allow fuller account to be taken of pre-existing health when considering the impact of job loss and insecurity. Using data on the lifetime experience of people born in 1958, who passed through the recession of the 1980s in their young adult years, it has been shown that material hardship in the family of origin, such as overcrowding and low social class, were significant predictors of greater labour market difficulty during the crisis of the 1980s. Growth up to age 7 years and measures of psychological adjustment at age 11 years were also related to the amount of unemployment that young men later experienced during the recession, up to the age of 33. Men who were relatively short for their age at age 7 were found to be more likely to experience over 12 months of unemployment during the period 1981–91, independent of the effects of adult height, hardship in their family of origin (although they often went together), and of educational attainment or psychological adjustment during the school years. Men who were shorter as adults were also more likely to suffer longer and more frequent periods of unemployment. It has been suggested that this may be because employers are more impressed by taller men, which improves their chances of obtaining and keeping employment. However, longitudinal data have shown that this is not true. Adult short stature is only associated with more unemployment among men who grew relatively slowly during childhood. Although employers can clearly only discriminate on the basis of *adult* height, shorter men who grew at a normal rate have no significantly increased risk of unemployment (Montgomery et al. 1997). Short adult stature is not a true risk for unemployment, but slow growth in childhood is (Fig. 5.8). Slow childhood growth may be related to future unemployment for a number of reasons: growth may be a sensitive indicator of material hardship, operating through factors such as increased infectious load and poor diet. In a modern society such as Great Britain, the most important factor explaining the relationship between slow growth in childhood and later unemployment is likely to be psychosocial stress. Even after material and cultural factors have been taken into account, there is evidence that chronic psychosocial stress in families slows the growth of children The stress indicated by slow growth also influences neuroendocrine development, slowing and impairing cognitive development (Sapolsky 1997). It is this effect on cognitive and personality development which may influence the future risk of unemployment. This shows that those most at risk of unemployment are often those whose early life has resulted in an accumulation of hardship and lower levels of physical and psychological health resources.

This same study also showed that unemployment between labour market entry and 1985 contributed to greater social and economic disadvantage in 1958 cohort members, *whatever their level of human resources in 1981* (Wadsworth et al. 1999). In this way, unemployment actually appeared to change the course of people's lives, causing a 'depreciation' of human resources. For the same levels of social and cultural (family of origin), intellectual (measured ability), and educational (qualifications) input, young

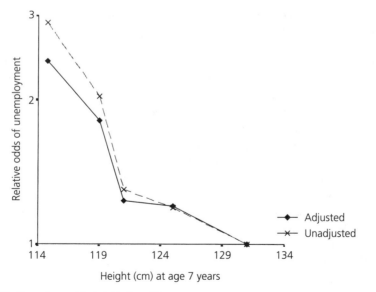

Fig. 5.8 Unemployment by height at age 7.

men with moderate or large amounts of unemployment were appreciably less likely than those with none to attain higher levels of social and economic advantage (as indicated by income, occupational level, and home ownership) by the age of 33 in 1991. This was true even of those who had been steadily employed for at least 6 years prior to the outcome measure. This depreciation effect was particularly marked in those who had suffered a total amount of 12 months or more of unemployment in the period 1981–86.

5.5   Effect of unemployment on population health

These findings suggest that unemployment may have effects well beyond the experiences of those undergoing a spell without work. Societies with higher levels of employment may actually produce different sorts of life histories in individual members than those with high levels of unemployment and job insecurity.

It has been all too easy to take for granted some of the effects of quasi-full employment on the wider society, one of the most important of which was that employers carried many of the social overhead costs of labour power. In order to recruit and retain skilful workers in a tight labour market where there are plenty of jobs, most large firms undertook extensive training, recruiting school leavers at an early age into apprenticeships. Schools therefore had far fewer restless and unmotivated teenagers to deal with than would otherwise have been the case: benefiting all children in the school. 'Internal labour markets' (the availability of promotion within a firm based on experience rather than on qualifications) offered people the chance to advance in their jobs even in the absence of school qualifications, from a later starting point. Increasing numbers of firms offered occupational pensions, thus raising the living standards of the retired population at little cost to the state (Sinfield 1981). As unemployment has risen, the costs of training and of supporting those who are no longer able to work are now increasingly being borne by the individual (the disappearance of apprenticeships and the appearance of student loans, critical illness policies, and private pensions are examples).

A reduction in the demand for labour results in more than unemployment. There is a parallel increase in the numbers of persons who become economically inactive, which in many countries far exceeds the increase in the numbers officially unemployed and seeking work. In the UK, between 1975 and 1993, the proportion of the population of working age who were classified as in full-time tenured work fell from 55.5 per cent to 35.9 per cent (Gregg and Wadsworth 1995). By 1996 the 1.5 million unemployed men were accompanied by 2.8 million economically inactive, i.e. neither in work nor classified as unemployed (Convery 1996).

When considering the social and economic costs of unemployment, the effects of labour market deregulation on levels of economic inactivity are seldom considered. It has been assumed that men of working age are inactive because they are ill, and women are keeping house, so that the state of the labour market is not responsible (as it is for unemployment). However, we know that in times of low unemployment, the great majority of men with long-term illness are in fact employed, and thus deriving most of their income from paid work. As unemployment rises, men with some degree of illness are increasingly forced into economic inactivity, and thus into dependency on benefits (Bartley and Owen 1996). The effect of home responsibilities on women's labour force participation is also known to vary widely according to the demand for labour and the supply of child care.

A full audit of the health impact of rising job insecurity needs to locate paid employment in the life trajectory of individual men and women. The idea of a 'healthy worker', or of a worker with no other demands on their physical and mental resources than employment, is a myth. There is no clear dividing line between good and bad health, even at a single time point. When jobs are scarce, trivial physical or psychological factors may become sources of discrimination (as was found in the 1930s for the wearing of spectacles, Bartley 1987). When looking more realistically at human beings passing through the life course, the distinction between 'healthy workers' and 'unhealthy non-workers' seems even more artificial. The approach adopted here is that individuals are located on a continuum of 'health resources' which are built up, used, and replaced over the life course. These include:

(1) basic biological endowment at birth;

(2) development of physical strength and vitality;

(3) development of cognitive function;

(4) development of psychological capacities such as self-esteem, coping, secure identity;

(5) human capital (education and work experience);

(6) social capital (socially supportive relationships and networks).

Biological endowment and material and emotional experiences during childhood confer varying amounts of 'health resources' or 'health potential' to the young person (Dahl and Kjaersgaard 1993). From the end of childhood, individuals are constantly engaged in processes that may act to develop and sustain the health and social resources they bring with them, or to jeopardize them.

Of these health resources, physical strength and vitality are unique in being inevitably 'used-up' or depreciated by work. Physical strength must be replaced on a regular basis, hence the importance of reasonable working hours, breaks, and holidays during which energies are renewed. However, leisure time is of less benefit in the renewal of physical health if it is experienced in poor conditions and at the expense of low resources and social stigmatization, as is the case during unemployment. In the real world, the occupations with more adverse working conditions and lower rates of pay also tend to have higher rates of job insecurity and unemployment (Robinson 1986; Bartley 1991). It is of no surprise therefore that the ageing process itself is known to take place at differential rates according to the employment history of the individual: more arduous work being associated with faster ageing (House et al. 1994).

Unlike physical resources, psychological and social resources are more likely to be increased than depreciated by the experiences involved in employment: deterioration in psychological health during unemployment is therefore more immediate, and improvement on re-employment happens quickly. Stable employment contributes to building up skills, work experience, and social networks, although some forms of work will also have a psychological cost. In youth, important considerations of establishing an independent identity arise, followed by the complex socio-emotional agendas involved in the formation of partnerships. When these processes break down, mental health is at risk, and the risks of accidental and self-inflicted harm are increased (Platt 1984).

Work is known to aid the development of secure identity and self-esteem in men, and to facilitate the formation of stable relationships (Wadsworth 1991). Men living outside of partnerships are at increased health risk, and unemployment is a major risk factor for relationship breakdown (Fox 1986). Little research has been done to relate directly the high risk of partnership breakdown in households affected by unemployment to health outcomes, although what there is points clearly to increases in risk for both men and women (Moser et al. 1984). Likewise, we know very little about the effects of unemployment in the household on the health of children and their chances of educational and occupational attainment, although, once again, what we do know is disquieting (Johnson and Reed 1996).

5.6 Policy implications

Recent studies have added a considerable amount to our understanding of why unemployment is associated with poor health. We are beginning to see that unemployment takes place as part of a process of accumulation of disadvantage which may begin in childhood, and that a spell of unemployment often occurs as part of a more general pattern of hazardous and insecure work. Rather than making an oversimplified distinction between 'having a job' and being unemployed, we are beginning to see that there are degrees of insecurity in the work conditions people experience, so that health effects are not limited to those with no employment at all. Rather than labelling effects as 'causal' or 'selective' we can begin to see how advantage and disadvantage accumulate over the life course.

In policy terms, the implications are rather wide-reaching. The old assumptions behind the notion of a social insurance or welfare state 'safety net' are seen to be too simple. To use a metaphor, the people most likely to fall into the net bear a heavier weight of disadvantage than those who are less likely to need its support. Becoming unemployed may be a stressful and disturbing event to anyone, and the factory closure studies, where job loss is indiscriminate, show that this is the case. Short-term health service implications of large-scale redundancy need to be addressed. In the UK it has been traditional to weight health needs indices using unemployment as one factor in planning services. However, if policies are designed using average needs indices which take no account of the impact of chronic job insecurity, this may be insufficient. Income support levels are determined, as discussed above, with the intention of meeting only the most basic material needs. This takes no account whatever of the fact that those who experience greater amounts of unemployment are likely to carry with them additional burdens produced by earlier disadvantage and hardship. There is a need for 'spring boards' rather than mere 'safety nets': positive help in the shape of social and emotional as well as improved financial support, as well as the opportunity for education and training.

The benefits of such policies would extend beyond individuals themselves during a single spell of unemployment. Policies designed as 'springboards' would automatically work counter to the tendency of unemployment to lower the value of the human resources an individual brings with them to the labour market. Attention to the psychosocial problems which often go along with unemployment would also have the effect of lowering the threat to family stability, with benefits which could stretch forward into the next generation, just as the costs do at the present time.

References

Arnetz, B.B., Brenner, S., Hjelm, R., Levi, L. and Petterson, I. (1988). *Stress reaction in relation to threat of job loss and actual unemployment: physiological, psychological and economic effects of job loss and unemployment.* Stress Research Reports No. 206, Karolinska Institute, Stockholm.

Arnetz, B.B., Brenner, S.O., Levi, L., et al. (1991). Neuroendocrine and immunological effects of unemployment and job insecurity. *Psychother. Psychosom.* **55**, 76–80.

Banks, M.H. and Jackson, P.R. (1982). Unemployment and the risk of minor psychiatric disorder in young people: cross-sectional and longitudinal evidence. *Psychol. Med.* **12**, 189–98.

Banks, M.H. and Ullah, P. (1987). *Youth unemployment: social and psychological perspectives.* Department of Employment Research Paper No. 61. HMSO, London.

Barker. D.J.P. (1994). *Mothers, babies and disease in later life.* British Medical Journal Publications, London.

Bartley, M.J. (1987). Unemployment and health: selection or causation? *Sociol. Hlth Illness* **10**, 41–67.

Bartley, M. and Owen, C. (1996). Relation between socioeconomic status, employment and health during economic change 1973–93. *BMJ* **313**, 445–9.

Beale, N. and Nethercott, S. (1985). Job loss and family morbidity: a study of a factory closure. *J. R. Coll. Gen. Pract.* **35**, 510–14.

Beale, N. and Nethercott, S. (1987). The health of industrial employees four years after compulsory redundancy. *J. R. Coll. Gen. Pract.* **37**, 390–4.

Benjamin, D.K. and Kochin, L.A. (1979) Searching for an explanation of unemployment in interwar Britain. *J. Polit. Econ.* **82**, 441–78.

Bethune, A. (1997). Unemployment and mortality. In: *Health inequalities* (ed. F. Drever and M. Whitehead). HMSO, London.

Block, J. and Gjerde, P.F. (1989). Depressive symptoms in late adolescence: a longitudinal perspective on personality antecedents. In: *Risk and protective factors in the development of psychopathology* (ed. J. Rolf, A.S. Masten, D. Cicchetti, K.H. Nuechterlein and S. Weintraub). Cambridge University Press, Cambridge.

Bosello, O., Zamboni, M., Armellini, F. and Todesco, T. (1993). Biological and clinical aspects of regional body fat. *Diabet. Nutrit. Metab.* **6**, 163–71.

Bradshaw, J., Cooke, K. and Godfrey, C. (1983). The impact of unemployment on the living standards of families. *J. Soc. Policy* **12**, 433–52.

Burchell, B. (1996). Who is affected by unemployment? Job insecurity and labour market influences on psychological health. In: *Unemployment and social change* (ed. D. Gallie, C. Marsh, C. Vogler). Oxford University Press, Oxford.

Catalano, R., Dooley, D. and Jackson, R. (1981). Economic predictors of admissions to mental health facilities in a nonmetropolitan community. *J. Hlth Soc. Behav.* **22**, 284–97.

Catalano, R., Dooley, D. and Jackson, R. (1985). Economic antecedents of help seeking: reformulation of time series tests. *J. Hlth Soc. Behav.* **26**, 141–52.

Charlton, J., Kelly, S., Dunnell, K., Evans, B. and Jenkins, R. (1993). Suicide deaths in England and Wales: trends in factors associated with suicide deaths. *Popn Trends* **71**, 34–42.

Cherry, N. (1976). Persistent job changing – is it a problem? *J. Occupat. Psychol.* **49**, 203–21.

Clarke, M. (1978). The unemployed on supplementary benefit: living standards and making ends meet on a low income. *J. Soc. Policy* **7**, 385–410.

Clausen, B., Bjorndal, A. and Hjort, P.F. (1993). Health and re-employment in a two year follow-up of long term unemployed. *J. Epidemiol. Commun. Hlth* **47**, 14–18.

Cobb, S. and Kasl, S.C. (1977). *Termination: the consequences of job loss.*

DHEW-NIOSH Publication no. 77–224, US National Institutes for Occupational Safety and Health, Cincinnati.

Cobb, S., Brooks, G.W., Kasl, S.V. and Connelly, W.E. (1966). The health of people changing jobs. *Am. J. Publ. Hlth* **56**, 1476–81.

Convery, P. (1996). How many people are unemployed? *Working Brief* **78**, 23–6.

Cook, D.G. (1985). A critical view of the unemployment and health debate. *The Statistician* **34**, 73–82.

Cook, D.G., Cummins, R.O., Bartley, M.J. and Shaper, A.G. (1982). Health of unemployed middle aged men in Great Britain. *Lancet* **i**, 1290–4.

Dahl, E. and Kjaersgaard, P. (1993). Social mobility and inequality in mortality. *Eur. J. Publ. Hlth* **3**, 124–32.

Daniel, W.W. (1983). How the unemployed fare after they find new jobs. *Policy Studies* **??**, 246–60.

Daniel, W.W. (1990). *The unemployed flow*, Chapters 2 and 3. Policy Studies Institute, London.

Daniel, W.W. and Stilgoe, E. (1979). Where are they now? A follow up study of the unemployed. *Political and Economic Planning*, London.

Douglas, J.W.B., Ross, J.M. and Simpson, H.R. (1968). *All our future*. Peter Davies, London.

Elias, P. and Blanchflower, D. (1987). *The occupations, earnings and work histories of young adults – who gets the good jobs?* Department of Employment Research Paper No. 68. HMSO, London.

Fagin, L. and Little, M. (1984). *The forsaken families*. Harmondsworth, Penguin Books.

Ferman, L. and Gardner, J. (1979). Economic deprivation, social mobility and mental health. In: *Mental health and the economy*, (ed. L. Ferman and I. Gordus (eds.). W.E. Upjohn Institute for Employment Research, Kalamazoo, Michigan.

Ferrie, J. (1997). Labour market status, insecurity and health. *J. Hlth Psychol.* **2**, 373–97.

Ferrie, J.E., Shipley, M.J., Marmot, M.G., Stansfeld, S. and Davey Smith, G. (1995). Health effects of anticipation of job change and non-employment: longitudinal data from the Whitehall II study. *BMJ* **311**, 1264–9.

Ferrie, J.E., Shipley, M.J., Marmot, M.G., Stansfeld, S.A. and Smith, G.D. (1998*a*). An uncertain future? The health effects of threats to employment security in white collar men and women. *Am. J. Publ. Hlth* **88**, 1030–6.

Ferrie, J.E., Shipley, M.J., Marmot, M.G., Stansfeld, S. and Davey Smith, G. (1998*b*). The health effects of major organizational change and job insecurity. *Soc. Sci. Med.* **46**, 243–54.

Fox, A.J. (1986). Socio-demographic consequences of unemployment: a study of changes in individuals' characteristics between 1971 and 1981. City University, Social Statistics Research Unit, mimeo.

Fox, A.J. and Shewry, M. (1988). New longitudinal insights into relationships between unemployment and mortality. *Stress Med.* **4**, 11–19.

Fryer, D. (1987). Monmouthshire and Marienthal: sociographies of two un-employed communities. In: *Unemployed people*, (ed. D. Fryer and P. Ullah). Open University Press, Milton Keynes.

Fryer, D. (1992). A plea for a greater emphasis on the role of poverty in psychological research on unemployment and mental health in the social context. In: *On the mysteries of unemployment*, (ed. C.H.A. Verhaar and J.G. Janussen). Kluwer Academic Publishers, Amsterdam.

Gaffikin, F. and Morrisey, M. (1992). *The new unemployed: joblessness and poverty in the market economy.* Zed Books, London.

Goldblatt, P., Fox, J. and Leon, D. (1990). Mortality of unemployed men and women. In: *Mortality and social organisation*, (ed. P. Goldblatt). HMSO, London.

Goodman, A., Johnson, P. and Webb, S. (1997). *Inequality in the UK.* Oxford University Press, Oxford.

Graetz, B. (1993). Health consequences of employment and unemployment: longitudinal evidence for young men and women. *Soc. Sci. Med.* **36**, 715–24.

Gravelle, H.S.E. (1985). *Does unemployment kill?* Portfolio No. 9, Nuffield, York.

Gregg, P. and Wadsworth, J. (1995). A short history of labour turnover, job tenure and job security 1975–1993. *Oxford Rev. Econ. Policy* **11**, 73–90.

Hamilton, V.L., Hoffman, W.S., Broman, C.L. and Rauma, D. (1993). Un-employment, distress and coping: a panel study of autoworkers. *J. Person. Soc. Psychol.* **65**, 234–47.

Hammer, T. (1992). Unemployment and use of drug and alcohol among young people: a longitudinal study in the general population. *Br. J. Addict.* **87**, 1571–81.

Harrington, R., Bredenkamp, D., Groothues, C., Rutter, M., Fudge, H. and Pickles, A. (1994). Adult outcomes of childhood and adolescent depression – links with suicidal behaviors. *J. Child Psychol. Psychiat. All. Discip.* **35**, 1309–19.

Harris, C.C. (1987). *Redundancy and recession.* Blackwell, Oxford.

Hawton, K. and Rose, N. (1986). Unemployment and attempted suicide among men in Oxford. *Hlth Trends* **18**, 29–32.

Heady, P. and Smyth, M. (1989). *Living standards during unemployment.* HMSO, London.

House, J.S., Lepowski, J.M., Kinney, A.M., Mero, R.P., Kessler, R.C. and Herzog, A.R. (1994). The social stratification of aging and health. *J. Hlth Soc. Behav.* **35**, 213–34.

Isaakson, K. (1989). Unemployment and mental health and the psychological function of work in male welfare clients in Stockholm. *Scand. J. Soc. Med.* **17**, 165–9.

Iversen, L. and Klausen, H. (1981). *The closure of the Nordhavn shipyard.*

Mel Bartley et al. 101

Institute of Social Medicine. Kobenhavns Universitet Publikation 13, FADL, Copenhagen.

Iversen, L., Andersen, O., Andersen, P.K., Christoffersen, K. and Keiding, N. (1987). Unemployment and mortality in Denmark. *BMJ* **295**, 879–84.

Jackson, P.R. and Warr, P.B. (1984). Unemployment and psychological ill-health: the moderating role of duration and age. *Psychol. Med.* **14**, 605–14.

Jahoda, M. (1942). Incentives to work – a study of unemployed adults in a special situation. *Occupat. Psychol.* **16**, 20–30.

Jahoda, M. (1979). The impact of unemployment in the 1930s and the 1970s. *Bull. Br. Psychol. Soc.* **32**, 309–14.

Johnson, P. and Reed, H. (1996). *Two nations? The inheritance of poverty and affluence.* Institute for Fiscal Studies Commentary No. 53. IFS, London.

Kaplan, H.B. (1991). Social psychology of the immune system: a conceptual framework and review of the literature. *Soc. Sci. Med.* **33**, 909–23.

Kessler, R.C., Turner, J.B. and House, J.S. (1988). Effects of unemployment on health in a community survey: main, modifying and mediating effects. *J. Soc. Issues* **44**, 69–85.

Lahelma, E. (1992a). Paid employment, unemployment and mental well-being. *Psychiatr. Fenn.* **23**, 131–44.

Lahelma, E. (1992b). Unemployment and mental well-being: elaboration of the relationship. *Int. J. Hlth Serv.* **22**, 261–74.

Lee, A.J., Crombie, I.K., Smith, W.C. and Tunstall-Pedoe, H.D. (1990). Alcohol consumption and unemployment among men: the Scottish Heart Health Study. *Br. J. Addict.* **85**, 1156–70.

Lee, A.J., Crombie, I.K., Smith, W.C. and Tunstall-Pedoe, H.D. (1991). Cigarette smoking and employment status. *Soc. Sci. Med.* **32**, 1309–12.

Leeflang, R.L.I., Klein-Hesselink, D.J. and Spruit IP. (1992a). Health effects of unemployment II: Men and Women. *Soc. Sci. Med.* **34**, 351–62.

Leeflang, R.L.I., Klein-Hesselink, D.J. and Spruit, I.P. (1992b). Health effects of unemployment I: Long term unemployed men in a rural and an urban setting. *Soc. Sci. Med.* **34**, 341–50.

Martikainen, P. (1990). Unemployment and mortality among Finnish men. *BMJ* **301**, 407–11.

Matthiasson, I., Lindgarde, F., Nilsson, J.A. and Theorell, T. (1990). Threats of unemployment and cardiovascular risk factors: longitudinal study of quality of sleep and serum cholesterol concentrations in men threatened with redundancy. *BMJ* **301**, 461–6.

Minford, P. (1990). Corporatism, the natural rate and productivity. In: *Trade Unions and the economy: into the 1990s,* (ed. J. Philpot). Employment Institute, London.

Montgomery, S.M., Bartley, M.J., Cook, D.G. and Wadsworth, M.E.J. (1996). Health and social precursors of unemployment in young men in Great Britain. *J. Epidemiol. Commun. Hlth* **50**, 415–22.

Montgomery, S.M., Bartley, M.J. and Wilkinson, R.G. (1997). Family conflict and slow growth. *Arch. Dis. Child.* **77**, 326–30.

Montgomery, S.M., Cook, D.G., Bartley, M.J. and Wadsworth, M.E.J. (1998). Unemployment, cigarette smoking, alcohol consumption and body weight in young British men. *Eur. J. Publ. Hlth* **8**, 21–7.

Montgomery, S.M., Cook, D.G., Bartley, M.J. and Wadsworth, M.E.J. (1999). Unemployment in young men pre-dates symptoms of depression and anxiety resulting in medical consultation. *Int. J. Epidemiol.* **28**, 95–100.

Morris, J.K. and Cook, D.G. (1991). A critical review of the effect of factory closures on health. *Br. J. Indust. Med.* **48**, 1–8.

Morris, J.K., Cook, D.G. and Shaper, A.G. (1992). Non-employment and changes in smoking, drinking and body weight. *BMJ* **304**, 536–41.

Morris, J.K., Cook, D.G. and Shaper, A.G. (1994). Loss of employment and mortality. *BMJ* **308**, 1135–9.

Moser, K.A., Fox, A.J. and Jones, D.R. (1984). Unemployment and mortality in the OPCS Longitudinal Study. *Lancet* **ii**, 1324–8.

Moser, K.A., Goldblatt, P.O., Fox, A.J. and Jones, D.R. (1987). Unemployment and mortality: comparison of the 1971 and 1981 Longitudinal Study Samples. *BMJ* **294**, 86–90.

Moylan, S. and Davies, R. (1980). The disadvantages of the unemployed. *Employ. Gaz.* **88**, 830–2.

Moylan, S., Millar, J. and Davies, R. (1984). *For richer, for poorer – DHSS Cohort Study of Unemployed Men.* HMSO, London.

Payne, J., Payne, C. and Connolly, S. (1994). Long-term unemployment: individual risk factors and outcomes (an analysis of data from the National Child Development Study). Report to the Employment Department from the Policy Studies Institute (unpublished).

Peck, D.F. and Plant, M.A. (1986). Unemployment and illegal drug use: concordant evidence from a prospective study and national trends. *BMJ* **293**, 929–32.

Pilling, D. (1990). *Escape from disadvantage.* The Falmer Press, London.

Platt, S. (1984). Unemployment and suicidal behavior: a review of the literature. *Soc. Sci. Med.* **19**, 93–115.

Platt, S. (1986). Parasuicide and unemployment. Editorial. *Br. J. Psychiat.* **149**, 401–5.

Platt, S. and Kreitman, N. (1984). Trends in parasuicide and unemployment among men in Edinburgh: 1968–82. *BMJ* **289**, 1029–32.

Platt, S. and Kreitman, N. (1985). Parasuicide and unemployment among men in Edinburgh 1968–1982. *Psychol. Med.* **15**, 113–23.

Power, C. and Estaugh, V. (1990). Employment and drinking in early adulthood: a longitudinal perspective. *Br. J. Addict.* **85**, 487–94.

Power, C., Manor, O. and Fox, A.J. (1991). *Health and class: the early years.* Chapman and Hall, London.

Preece, M.A. (1985). Prepubertal and pubertal endocrinology. In: *Human growth* (2nd edn), Vol. 2. (ed. J. Falkner and J.M. Tanner). Plenum Press, London.

Preece, M.A. and Holder, A.T. (1982). The somatomedins: a family of serum growth factors. In: *Recent advances in endocrinology and metabolism,* Vol. 2 (ed. J.L.H. O'Riordan). Churchill Livingstone, Edinburgh.

Pritchard, C. (1992). Is there a link between suicide in young men and unemployment? *Br. J. Psychiat.* **160**, 750–6.

Ramsden, S. and Smee, C. (1981). The health of unemployed men: DHSS Cohort Study. *Employ. Gaz.* **89**, 397–401.

Robinson, J.C. (1986). Job hazards and job security. *J. Hlth Politics, Policy Law* **11**, 117.

Robinson, N., Yateman, N.A., Protopapa, L.E. and Bush, L. (1989). Unemployment and diabetes. *Diabet. Med.* **6**, 797–803.

Rodgers, B. (1991). Socio-economic status, employment and neurosis. *Soc. Psychiatry Psychiat. Epidemiol.* **26**, 101–4.

Rudas, N., Tondo, L., Musio, A. and Mosia, M. (1991). Unemployment and depression. Results of a psychometric evaluation. *Min. Psichiatr* **32**, 205–9.

Sapolsky, R.M. (1997). The importance of a well-groomed child. *Science* **277**, 1620–1.

Sinfield, R.A. (1981). *What unemployment means.* Martin Robertson, Oxford.

Sinfield, A. (ed.) (1993). *Poverty, inequality and justice.* New Waverley Papers No. 6, quoting *Hansard* written answers 18 October 1993 cols 1667, Edinburgh.

Stern, J. (1979). Who bears the burden of unemployment? In: *Slow growth in Britain,* (ed. W. Beckermann). Clarendon, Oxford.

Stern, J. (1982). Does unemployment really kill? *New Society* 10 June, 421–2.

Stern, J. (1983). The relationship between unemployment, morbidity and mortality in Britain. *Popn Studies – J. Demog.* **37** (1), 61–74.

Tanner, J.M. (1955). *Growth at adolescence.* Blackwell, Oxford.

Valkonen, T. and Martikainen, P. (1995). The association between unemployment and mortality: causation or selection? In: *Adult mortality in developed countries: from description to explanation* (ed. A.D. Lopez, G. Caselli, and T. Valkonen). Clarendon, Oxford.

Wadsworth, M.E.J. (1986). In *Class and health* (ed. R.G. Wilkinson), pp. 5074. Tavistock, Cambridge.

Wadsworth, M.E.J. (1991). *The imprint of time: childhood history and adult life.* Clarendon Press, Oxford.

Wadsworth, M.E.J., Bartley, M.J. and Montgomery, S.M. (1999). Unemployment, health and human resources. *Soc. Sci. Med.,* forthcoming.

Wagstaff, A. (1986). Unemployment and health: some pitfalls for the unwary. *Hlth Trends* **18**, 79–81.

Warr, P.B. (1984). Job loss, unemployment and psychological well-being. In: *Role transitions,* (ed. V. Allen and E. Van de Vliert). Plenum Press, New York.

Warr, P.B. (1987). *Work, unemployment and mental health*. Oxford University Press, Oxford.

Warr, P.B. and Jackson, P.R. (1985). Factors influencing the psychological impact of prolonged unemployment and of re-employment. *Psychol. Med.* **15**, 795–807.

Warr, P. and Jackson, P. (1987). Adapting to the unemployed role: a longitudinal investigation. *Soc. Sci. Med.* **25**, 1219–24.

Westergaard, J., Noble, I. and Walker, A. (1989). *After redundancy: the experience of economic insecurity*. Polity Press, Cambridge.

White, M. (1983). *Long term unemployment and labour markets*. Policy Studies Institute, London.

White, M. (1994). *Against unemployment*. Policy Studies Institute, London.

Wilson, P. (1980). *Drinking in England and Wales*. HMSO, London.

Winefield, A.H., Tiggeman, M. and Goldney, R.D. (1988). Psychological concomitants of satisfactory employment and unemployment in young people. *Soc. Psychiatry Psychiat. Epidemiol.* **23**, 149–57.

Winefield, A.H., Tiggeman, M. and Goldney, R.D. (1991). The psychological impact of unemployment and unsatisfactory employment in young men and women: longitudinal and cross-sectional data. *Br. J. Psychol.* **82**, 473–80.

Zoccolillo, M., Pickles, A., Quinton, D. and Rutter, M. (1992). The outcome of childhood conduct disorder – implications for defining adult personality disorder and conduct disorders. *Psychol. Med.* **22**, 971–86.

Acknowledgements

Dr Bartley's research is supported by the Economic and Social Research Council, Grant number L128251001 and the Medical Research Council, Grant number G8802774.

Dr Ferrie's research was supported by the Economic and Social Research Council, Grant number R000235083, and is currently supported by Grant number L128251046.

Dr Montgomery's research was supported by the Economic and Social Research Council, Grant number L128251033.

6 Health and the psychosocial environment at work

Michael Marmot, Johannes Siegrist,
Tores Theorell and Amanda Feeney

6.1 Introduction

There has been a slow recognition that the importance of work for health goes beyond traditional occupational diseases (Schilling 1989). Indeed, it is likely that work makes a greater contribution to diseases and ill health not thought of as 'occupational'. Early research concentrated on the possible role of physical activity in the workplace (Morris et al. 1953). Other work, more in the spirit of traditional occupational health, has specified a number of physical and chemical exposures (e.g. lead, carbon disulphide, carbon monoxide, nitroglycerine, nitroglycol: Kristensen 1994). More recently the workplace has been seen as an appropriate setting for health promotion activities: providing the opportunity to influence life styles such as smoking, diet, and physical activity, and to conduct screening for disease risk (Breucker and Schroer 1996).

There is now evidence that psychosocial factors at work may play an important role in contributing to the social gradient in ill health. There have been several different approaches to measurement of work stress and, more recently, research has tended to focus on a few explicit theoretical concepts. Among these, the models of job demand–control (Karasek 1979; Karasek and Theorell 1990) and effort–reward imbalance (Siegrist et al. 1986; Siegrist 1996) have received special attention.

A number of different diseases have been related to psychosocial conditions in the workplace, most notably coronary heart disease (CHD), musculo-skeletal disorders, and mental illness. This chapter touches on two types of question: the relation between conditions at work and disease; and the contribution this relationship may make to variations in disease in society. Because variations in coronary heart disease have been studied extensively, we start and end with that disease, but as the chapter will endeavour to show, a number of other disease end-points are important.

6.2 Changes in the distribution of coronary heart disease

It is worth reviewing the changing distribution of CHD internationally to put into context the possible contribution of work stress to the development of ill health and disease. There have been two major changes in the epidemiology of CHD over recent years:

(1) a changing social class distribution of the disease (Marmot 1992), and

(2) a rise and fall in CHD in different countries (Uemura and Pisa 1988).

In many European countries, as in the USA, as CHD became a mass disease, it rose first in higher socio-economic groups and subsequently in lower, to the extent that the social distribution changed to the now familiar pattern of an inverse social gradient: higher rates as the social hierarchy is descended. More recently, the decline in CHD mortality both in the UK and the USA has been enjoyed to a greater extent by higher socio-economic groups, leading to a widening of the social gap (Wing et al. 1992). Concerns that the predominance of CHD in higher socio-economic groups may relate to the stress of their occupations go back at least to Osler (1910) who wrote that work and worry were major causes of the disease. The fact that CHD is now more common in lower socio-economic groups does not, by itself, refute the potential importance of work 'stress'. Research has moved on from the simplistic notion that high responsibility or dealing with multiple tasks represents work stress.

As discussed in Chapter 1, cardiovascular mortality has been declining in North America, Australia, and many countries of 'western' Europe, whereas it has been on the rise in the countries of central and eastern Europe and in the newly independent states of the former Soviet Union. Of the 6 year life expectancy gap between the countries of East and West in Europe, more than half is due to cardiovascular disease, and especially to CHD. This gap in life expectancy grew from around the late 1960s to the present (Bobak and Marmot 1996), corresponding to the time when cardiovascular disease was on the rise in the east and declining in the west. The concepts and data reviewed in this chapter may provide some explanation for the inverse social gradient in cardiovascular disease in the West and rising mortality in the East.

6.3 Explanations of the social distribution of coronary heart disease

There is now a widely validated body of knowledge on risk factors for CHD that relate to development of atherosclerosis, and a somewhat less secure body of knowledge relating to predisposition to thrombosis. The major risk factors are high levels of blood pressure and plasma total cholesterol and smoking.

Although smoking, in particular, shows a strong social gradient (Marmot et al. 1991), these risk factors account for no more than one third of the social gradient in cardiovascular disease (Marmot et al. 1978 1984). Similarly, smoking is high in many countries of central and eastern Europe and may relate to the high rates of cardiovascular disease (Bobak and Marmot 1996), but data from the international MONICA studies (MONICA 1994) show that international variations in smoking, high blood pressure, and raised plasma cholesterol account for less than half of the international variation in CHD mortality rates.

We are left then with two types of question. First, what accounts for the social and international variation in unhealthy behaviours such as atherogenic diet, smoking, and sedentary life style? Secondly, given that these factors appear to be inadequate explanations of social and international variations in cardiovascular mortality, what else could account for the observed differences? We have argued elsewhere that one must look for explanations in the nature of social and economic organization of societies (Marmot 1994). One particular feature is the nature of working life, both because what happens in the workplace may be important for health and because work and the operation of the labour market play a central role in the organization of social and economic life, which in turn are important in the social determinants of health. The evidence that supports the importance of work for cardiovascular and other diseases is presented below.

6.3.1 The changing nature of work

There are at least four important reasons for the centrality of work and occupation in advanced industrialized societies. First, having a job is a principal prerequisite for continuous income opportunities. Level of income determines a wide range of life chances. Secondly, training for a job and achievement of occupational status are the most important goals of primary and secondary socialization. It is through education, job training, and status acquisition that personal growth and development are realized, that a core social identity outside the family is acquired, and that intentional, goal-directed activity in human life is shaped. Thirdly, occupation defines a most important criterion of social stratification in advanced societies. Amount of esteem and social approval in interpersonal life largely depend on the type of job, professional training, and level of occupational achievement. Furthermore, type and quality of occupation, and especially the degree of self-direction at work, strongly influence personal attitudes and behavioural patterns in areas that are not directly related to work, such as leisure, family life, education, and political activity (Kohn and Schooler 1973). Finally, occupational settings produce the most pervasive and continuous demands during one's lifetime, and they absorb the largest amount of active time in adult life. Exposure to adverse job conditions carries the risk of ill health by virtue of the amount of time spent and the quality of demands faced at the workplace. At the same time, occupational settings provide unique opportunities to experience reward, esteem, success, and satisfaction. To understand the impact of working life on health in general, it is important to realize the profound changes that have taken place in the nature of work in established market economies. Among these are the following:

(1) fewer jobs are defined by physical demands, more by psychological and emotional demands;

(2) fewer jobs are available in mass production, more in the service sector;

(3) more jobs are concerned with information processing due to computerization and automation.

These changes in the nature of work have gone along with changes in the nature of the labour market. There has been increasing participation of women in the labour market, an increase in short-term and part-time working and, most importantly, an increase in job instability and structural unemployment. For instance, Hutton (1995) describes Britain as the 40–30–30 society: 40 per cent of the male population of working age have secure jobs, 30 per cent are not working, and 30 per cent are in insecure jobs. The 30 per cent not working may cause some surprise given that the official unemployment rate is around 8 per cent. The 30 per cent is made up of the official unemployed, those no longer seeking work, premature retirements, disabled, and others. If 30 per cent of the population are in insecure jobs, this must have effects on the rest of the working population who wonder if their job is next. This is a change. In Europe, until relatively recently there were national commitments to security of employment. Now, the rhetoric is labour market flexibility (Beatson 1995). The other side of flexibility is job insecurity.

The 30 per cent not working is not unique to Britain. In Finland, for example, the mean age of entry to the labour market is now 27 and mean age of exit is 53. When the Finnish social contract was nationally agreed, the assumption was that working life would last 40 years. If it lasts 26 years, on average, this has a profound importance for the costs of the welfare state. It also changes attitudes to work if a job for life is no longer a realistic expectation for large sections of the labour market. Research on work and health has to take this job insecurity into account, especially so as loss of job was shown to be associated with elevated risk of mortality in independent prospective studies both in Britain and in Finland (Morris et al. 1994; Martikainen and Valkonen 1996). This is dealt with in Chapter 5.

This changing nature of work and the labour market has occurred at the same time as there have been substantial increases in income inequalities in many countries (Joseph Rowntree Foundation 1995). Wilkinson (1992) has shown that, internationally, life expectancy is related more closely to income distribution than to overall wealth as measured by gross national product. This has now been documented in two independent studies for the states of the USA (Kaplan et al. 1996; Kawachi and Kennedy 1997). If inequality, rather than absolute level of deprivation, is an important driver of health differentials it may, as Wilkinson suggests in this book (Chapter 12) be a reflection of the quality of the social environment. It may also suggest that discontent related to unfavourable social comparison (relative social deprivation) and associated stress reactions may have important health consequences.

The scientific challenge, then, consists of identifying those stress-eliciting conditions related to the nature of work, the structure of salaries (income distribution), and labour market constraints that may account for differences in morbidity and mortality that are reported within and between populations.

6.3.2 The psychosocial work environment

Research on psychosocial work-related stress differs from traditional biomedical occupational health research by the fact that stressors cannot be identified by direct physical or chemical measurements. Rather, theoretical concepts are needed to analyse the nature of work in order to identify particular stressful job characteristics at a level of generalization that allows for their identification in a wide range of different occupations.

These theoretical concepts are operationalized using standardized methods of social and behavioural sciences (e.g. systematic observation, structured interviews, standardized questionnaires (so-called paper and pencil tests)). Therefore, measuring stressful working conditions provides a theoretical and methodological challenge. As mentioned, in theoretical terms, those components of working life need to be identified that produce intense, recurrent, and long-lasting stressful experience at least in a substantial proportion of those exposed. Moreover, researchers have to argue whether they restrict their formulations to particular job characteristics or whether they analyse stressful work experience in terms of an interaction of work characteristics and of coping characteristics of the working person.

At a methodological level, measures of work stress are expected to be reliable, sensitive to change, and valid. Two theoretical models – the demand control model and effort–reward imbalance model – fulfil these methodological criteria and identify stressful working conditions that are widely prevalent in advanced marked economies, such as changes in task profiles, work control, structure of salaries, and occupational stability. Over the past 10 years these two models have been tested in a number of studies, and a substantial body of knowledge has been generated, strengthening the assumption that stressful experiences at work are associated with elevated risk of CHD and other diseases.

6.3.3 The demand-control model

In the 1960s, research on job conditions and CHD had explored working demands and working hours (e.g. Hinkle et al. 1968). In the 1970s several research traditions found evidence for a favourable effect on mental health produced by skill development (Hackman and Lawler 1971) and autonomy at work (Gardell 1971; Kohn and Schooler 1973). It was Karasek's original contribution to formulate a two-dimensional concept of work stress, where a high level of psychological demands combined with a low level of decision latitude (low level of decision authority and low level of skill utilization) was predicted to increase the risk of stressful experience and subsequent physical illness (in particular CHD) (Karasek 1979). In 1981, Karasek first found evidence of a predictive role of high demand–low control conditions in CHD, using data on a representative Swedish sample (Karasek et al. 1981). Since then, a large number of prospective and cross-sectional studies on associations of stressful work, as defined by high demand and low control (job strain), with cardiovascular risk and disease have been conducted (for overviews see Karasek and Theorell 1990; Schnall and Landsbergis 1994; Kristensen 1995; Theorell and Karasek 1996; Hemingway and Marmot 1998). Several of these studies have focused on methodological considerations and have used new outcome measures, the majority of which have revealed positive findings.

Karasek's original hypothesis, that excessive psychological demands interact with lack of decision latitude in generating increased risk of cardiovascular disease, was supplemented by a second hypothesis which concerns the learning of new patterns of behaviour and skills on the basis of psychosocial job experience. According to this, learning for adults accrues over a lifetime of work experience. It may contribute to the worker's possibility to exert control over his or her working situation and thus have an impact on broader conditions of adult life. According to this hypothesis, the active situation is associated with the development of a feeling of mastery which inhibits the perception of strain during periods of overload, for instance. This makes it likely that the active job situation may stimulate healthy functioning. Epidemiological studies in Sweden indicated that the active job situation is associated with high rates of participation in socially active leisure and political activities (see Karasek and Theorell 1990), and, on the contrary, the daily residual strain arising in the strain situation gives rise to accumulated feelings of frustration which may inhibit learning attempts. It is obvious that some of the 'classic' high strain jobs are found in mass industry, especially under conditions of piece work and machine-paced assembly line work. Nevertheless, a number of strain jobs were also identified in the service sector. The concept therefore proves to be relevant in different employment sectors, and will remain important in the foreseeable future due to changing patterns of employment. For example, the rate of temporary employment is increasing in western Europe, particularly for those with low education. It is in these kinds of employment that lack of control will be a major problem. Even in those with a high education, the increasing demands for flexibility will create new decision latitude problems. The ever increasing demands for effectiveness from the workforce are raising the levels of psychological demands for all workers. This is particularly reflected in Swedish national welfare statistics.

More recently, the original demand–control concept was modified to include social support at work as a third dimension (Johnson and Hall 1988) and to assess work control in a life-course perspective, 'total job control exposure' (Johnson et al. 1990). Another important innovation concerns the exploration of health effects produced by intervention studies that are based on the theoretical concept, and several promising intervention studies have been reported recently (Karasek 1992; Theorell 1992; Orth-Gomer et al. 1994).

6.4   Evidence from studies

The importance of work-related psychosocial factors to the development of ill health and disease can be illustrated from the Whitehall studies of British civil servants. The finding of dramatic differences in mortality by grade of employment in the first Whitehall study, which could not be explained by conventional risk factors alone (Marmot, et al. 1984), led to the initiation of a second longitudinal study of civil servants – the Whitehall II study of 10 308 male and female civil servants. A major aim of this second study has been to investigate occupational and other social influences on health and disease in a white-collar, office-based population. In pursuing the work environment as providing possible explanations, we have examined characteristics of the demand–control model. One hypothesis is that the lower the grade of employment in the civil service, the lower the level of control over the job, the lower the use of skills, and the higher the level of monotony. These may be related to the higher rate of cardiovascular and other diseases in lower employment grades. Our initial analyses of the psychosocial work environment confirmed the above, with men and women in lower employment grades reporting lower levels of control, less varied work and use of skills, and a slower pace of work. Overall, fewer of the lower grades expressed themselves as satisfied with their work situation (Table 6.1) (Marmot et al. 1991).

The Whitehall II study has been studying psychosocial factors in relation to a range of health problems such as sickness absence, musculoskeletal and psychiatric disorder, and CHD. In analysing these health problems, the crucial task has been to separate the effects of work from those of other influences on health. In the analyses that follow we present data from the Whitehall II study examining the contribution of the psychosocial work

Table 6.1

Psychosocial work characteristics by grade of employment in the Whitehall II study of British civil servants (age-adjusted figures) (from Marmot et al. 1991)

	Sex	Employment grade[+]						Total sample	Test for trend
		1	2	3	4	5	6		
High control (%)	M	59.3	49.7	43.1	31.6	24.7	11.8	6877	***
	F	51.2	45.4	47.1	31.2	20.1	10.2	3341	***
Varied work (%)	M	70.5	52.1	41.9	27.1	18.2	3.9	6875	***
	F	71.2	55.2	40.5	31.7	14.0	4.7	3356	***
Fast pace (%)	M	58.0	43.6	34.7	27.9	20.8	15.8	6878	***
	F	60.9	50.3	43.7	31.1	29.7	18.0	3356	***
High satisfaction (%)	M	58.2	38.7	34.1	29.5	29.4	29.8	6865	***
	F	57.5	42.2	40.3	36.6	41.6	47.7	3337	ns

Grade categories: [+] grade 1, Unified Grades 1–6; grade 2, Unified Grade 7; grade 3, Senior Executive Officer and professional equivalents; grade 4, Higher Executive Officer and professional equivalents; grade 5, Executive Officer and professional equivalents; grade 6, Clerical Officer/Office Support.
P values: ns, $P > 0.10$; ***, $P \leq 0.001$.

environment to explaining the social gradient in sickness absence and CHD, controlling for other potential confounding factors.

6.4.1 Psychosocial work characteristics and sickness absence

We chose to analyse sickness absence as a measure of morbidity for a number of reasons. First, in the original Whitehall study, grade of employment was associated with mortality from a range of specific causes (Marmot et al. 1984). This suggested the possibility that, in addition to searching out the determinants of specific medical diagnoses, it was appropriate to search for determinants of general susceptibility to illness. Secondly, we take the view that ill health is important not only because it may hasten the time of death but because it interferes with social, psychological, and physical functioning during life. One way of looking at sickness absence is that it is a measure that integrates decrements in social, psychological, and physical functioning. Short spells of absence are more likely to represent decrements in psychological and social functioning, long spells are more likely to represent decrements in physical functioning or 'real illness'. Thirdly, sickness absence is a measure of great economic importance to employers. Studies of the determinants of sickness absence may therefore be of interest not only to those whose primary interest is in the aetiology of illness, but also to those interested in the health of the economy and of individual firms (Marmot and Feeney 1996).

There was a clear association between grade of employment and sickness absence. Men in the lowest grade had six times the absence rate of men in the highest grade for both short (<7 days) and long ($>=7$ days) spells of absence. Women showed a similar although slightly reduced gradient. As might be expected, the worse people rated their own health, the higher the sickness absence rates; sickness absence was also related to individual characteristics such as smoking, and to problems outside work, including financial problems and inadequate support (North et al. 1993).

Characteristics of the psychosocial work environment were also related to sickness absence. Men and women who rated their jobs as low on control, low on variety and use of skills, reported low support at work, and a slow pace of work had higher rates of short and long spells of sickness absence compared with those who rated their jobs high on these characteristics (North et al. 1993). Psychosocial work characteristics were also associated with sickness absence for psychiatric disorder and back pain. Low variety and use of skills and low support from colleagues and supervisors were associated with higher rates of short spells for psychiatric reasons in men and women (Stansfeld et al. 1997), and low control showed the most consistent effect, predicting both short and long spells of sickness absence for back pain in men and women (Hemingway et al. 1997).

One question we asked was how much of a contribution did work and other characteristics make to generating the social gradient in ill health as measured by sickness absence? Figure 6.1 shows long spells of sickness absence by grade, adjusted first for age and then for other predictors of sickness absence, including psychosocial work characteristics. This analysis suggested that about 25 per cent of the social gradient in men and about 35 per cent of the gradient in women is accounted for by these characteristics (North et al. 1993).

The above analysis relates to individual characteristics of the psychosocial work environment. We also examined the job strain model to see whether this predicted sickness absence in the Whitehall II study. We found partial support for the model, in that men who reported high levels of work demands and low levels of control had higher rates of short spells of sickness absence than those in other jobs; the results were similar for women, but were non-significant. Although predicting short spells, the job strain model did not predict long spells of sickness absence for either men or women. In examining psychosocial aspects of the work environment, it is important to reduce the problem of confounding. Employment grade is strongly related to several work, health, and personal characteristics, controlling for grade is therefore a way of controlling for many of the social and personal factors related to socio-economic status. We therefore examined the job-strain model stratified by employment grade, and after adjusting for grade found there was minimal support for the job-strain model in the whole study, but within the lower grades there was stronger support, with jobs characterized by high work demands and low control predicting sickness absence (North et al. 1996).

6.4.2 Psychosocial work characteristics and CHD

The design of the Whitehall II study is longitudinal and this has enabled us to assess the psychosocial work environment over a period of time and examine

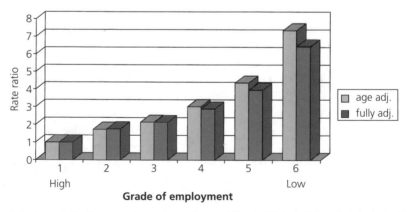

Fig. 6.1 Long spells of sickness absence by grade; men, Whitehall II study. Fully adjusted: age health behaviours, work characteristics, social circumstances outside work, ethnicity. (From North et al. 1993.)

its relationship to the development of new CHD. In addition to self-reported measures, we have also been able to use independent measures of the psycho-social work environment to address the question of whether job stress is influenced by subjective perceptions or by more objective appraisals of the work, or by both. Our results show that both men and women with low control, either self-reported or independently assessed, had a higher risk of newly reported CHD during a mean follow-up period of 5 years (Fig. 6.2). This association could not be explained by employment grade, negative affectivity, or classical coronary risk factors. We also examined the job strain model, but found that job demands and social supports and the interactions between work characteristics were not related to the risk of new CHD. Specific characteristics of our sample of white-collar workers may have contributed to this negative finding, high job demands were more common in higher employ-ment grades, and high job demands and high job control were positively associated, resulting in comparatively few high strain jobs (Bosma et al. 1997).

In addition to Whitehall II, other studies have looked at the association of characteristics of the work environment to heart disease. The Swedish case control study of over 2000 men and women in Stockholm (SHEEP) has investigated the role of psychosocial and other factors in the development of myocardial infarction. Men who reported high demands and low control in their job were at greater risk of developing a myocardial infarction. This relationship was more pronounced for manual workers (Hallqvist et al. 1998). An investigation of the psychosocial work environment in the 10 years

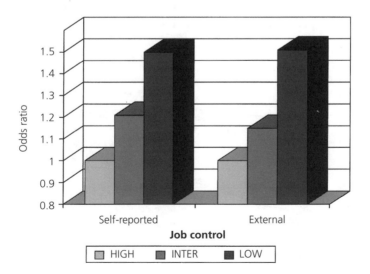

Fig. 6.2 Five-year CHD incidence by self-reported and external job control; men and women, Whitehall II study. (From Bosma et al. 1997.)

preceding myocardial infarction also showed that a decrease in the amount of control at work was associated with an increased risk of myocardial infarction; again this effect was stronger in manual workers and in men under 55 years of age (Fig. 6.3) (Theorell et al. 1998). Data from both the SHEEP and Whitehall II studies regarding loss of control and its possible effect on future risk of myocardial infarction illustrate that the increased risk does not develop rapidly after reported loss of control but increases gradually over time. Thus, there may be a possibility of preventing myocardial infarctions if individuals at risk can be identified within a specified time period.

The differing associations between aspects of the psychosocial work environment and CHD correspond to the review by Schnall and Landsbergis (1994), in which 17 out of 25 studies found significant associations between job control and cardiovascular outcome, whereas associations with job demands were significant in only 8 out of 23 studies. A further review of the role of psychosocial work characteristics and CHD has recently been conducted (Hemingway and Marmot 1998). This review used a quality filter to identify the best available evidence. The filter included:

(1) a prospective, population-based design;
(2) at least 500 participants (aetiological studies in healthy populations) or 100 participants (prognostic studies in CHD patient populations);
(3) instruments for exposure measurement used in two or more study populations; and
(4) fatal or validated non-fatal CHD as outcomes.

Table 6.2 shows that 6 of the 10 studies showed a positive association between aspects of the job strain model and CHD. The negative associations were possibly due to factors specific to the populations studied. For example, the

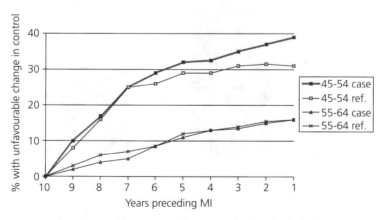

Fig. 6.3 Change in work control in years preceding myocardial infarction in the Swedish case control study – SHEEP. MI, myocardial infarction; % with unfavourable change in control = percentage in the least favourable quartile of change in control from 10 years to 1 year preceding MI. (From Theorell et al. 1998.)

Table 6.2 Psychosocial work characteristics and CHD (from Hemingway and Marmot, 1998)

Author, year, country	Total sample (% women)	Age at entry	Exposure	Follow-up (years)	Events: number	Events: type	Adjustments	Relative risk*	Summary†
Prospective aetiological studies									
Lacroix and Haynes (1984) USA	876 (37)	45–64	Job control/ demands (individual and ecological)	10	Not stated	Fatal CHD + non-fatal MI + coronary insufficiency + angina	Age, smoking, blood pressure, cholesterol	2.9* all women (clerical women RR=5.2) No association in men. Ecological exposure was associated with risk in men and women	+
Alfredsson et al. (1985) Sweden	958 096 (51)	20–64	Hectic work and few possibilities for learning (ecological)	1	1201	Non-fatal MI (hospitalization)	Age, 10 sociodemographic factors, smoking, heavy lifting	1.5*	+
Haan (1988) Finland	902 (33) factory workers	20–62	Job control, physical strain, variety (individual)	10	60	Fatal CHD + and non-fatal CHD	Age, smoking, blood pressure, cholesterol, alcohol, relative weight	4.95* for low control, low variety, high physical strain	++
Reed et al (1989) Hawaii (Japanese ancestry)	4737 (0)	45–65	Job control, demands, and their interaction (ecological)	18	359	Fatal CHD and non-fatal MI	Age	No effect of control, demands, or their interaction (ns trend for lower-strain men to have higher CHD)	0

Table 6.2 Psychosocial work characteristics and CHD (from Hemingway and Marmot, 1998) (cont.)

Author, year, country	Total sample (% women)	Age at entry	Exposure	Follow-up (years)	Events: number	Events: type	Adjustments	Relative risk*	Summary[†]
Netterstrom and Suadicani (1993) Denmark	2045 (0) bus drivers	21–64	Job variety, satisfaction	10	59	Fatal CHD	Age	2.1* *high* job variety and satisfaction associated with CHD risk	0
Suadicani et al. (1993) Denmark	1752 (0)	59 (mean)	Job influence, monotony, pace, satisfaction, ability to relax	3	46	Fatal CHD + non-fatal MI	None	Only inability to relax after work associated with CHD	0
Alterman et al. (1994) USA	1683 (0)	38–56	Job control, demands, and their interaction (ecological)	25	283	Fatal CHD	Age	1.4 for job strain	0
Bosma et al. (1997) UK	10 308 (33) civil servants	35–55	Job control, demands (individual, assessed twice 3 years apart, and ecological)	5	654	Angina + doctor-diagnosed ischaemia	Age, smoking, blood pressure, cholesterol, body mass index, employment grade	1.93* self-reported or externally assessed low job control predicted CHD	+

Study	Number (N)	Age	Exposures measured	Follow-up	Events	Outcome	Covariates	Results	Association
Lynch et al. (1997) Finland	1727 (0)	42–60	Job demands, resources, income	8.1	89	Fatal CHD + non-fatal MI	Age, behavioural, biological and psychosocial covariates	1.57* for the effect of high demands, low resources, and low income. 2.59 when adjustment made for age only	+
Steenland et al. (1997) USA	3575 (0)		Job control and demands (ecological)		519	Fatal CHD + non-fatal MI		1.41* for low control	+
Prognostic studies									
Hlatky et al. (1995) USA employed patients undergoing coronary angiography	1489 (24)	41–59	Job control, demands (individual)	5	112	Fatal CHD + non-fatal MI prevalence of coronary artery disease	Ejection fraction, extent of coronary atherosclerosis, myocardial ischaemia	0.96 for effect of job strain on events. Job strain was associated with normal coronary arteries	0
Hoffmann et al. (1995) Switzerland	222 (0) after first MI	30–60	Job work load, locus of control, social supports	1	19	All-cause mortality, reinfarction, severe symptoms or poor exercise capacity	Age, severity of MI, exercise	High workload and low external locus of control associated with outcome	+

* P value for relative risk < 0.05. †0 = no association; + = moderate (relative risk ≤2.0) association, ++ = strong (relative risk > 2.0) association.

studies by Reed et al. (1989) and Suadicani et al. (1993) studied men who were relatively old, particularly at the end of the follow-up period, when a large proportion had retired. The study by Hlatky et al. (1995) was not a representative sample and there may have been other selection factors in operation in determining who underwent coronary angiography. Finally, the bus drivers studied by Netterstrom and Suadicani (1993) may have had more reason than other workers to deny difficulties at work. Other studies using observational techniques instead of self-reports have confirmed this possibility (Greiner et al. 1997). It is likely that these results will influence the subsequent use and development of this theoretical model in future research studies. Improved measurement of the psychosocial work environment will lead to further methodological refinement of the model, and in particular for job demands, the issue of interaction within the job strain model warrants further investigation (Hallqvist et al. 1998).

6.5 Effort–reward imbalance model

At the beginning of this chapter we emphasized the growing importance of job insecurity in the current worldwide economy. 'Job control' in this perspective implies more than the original conceptualization, which was directed towards characteristics of work tasks. A related concept, the model of effort–reward imbalance, focuses more explicitly on links between work tasks and labour market dynamics. The model maintains that the work role defines a crucial link between self-regulatory needs of a person (e.g. self-esteem, self-efficacy) and the social opportunity structure. In particular, conferment of occupational status is associated with recurrent options of contributing and performing, of being rewarded or esteemed, and of belonging to some significant group (work colleagues). Yet, these potentially beneficial effects are contingent on a basic prerequisite of exchange in social life, that is, reciprocity. Effort at work is spent as part of a socially organized exchange process to which society at large contributes in terms of rewards. Rewards are distributed by three transmitter systems: money, esteem, and career opportunities, including job security. The model of effort–reward imbalance claims that lack of reciprocity between costs and gains (i.e. high cost/low gain conditions) defines a state of emotional distress which can lead to the arousal of the autonomic nervous system and associated strain reactions. For instance, having a demanding, but unstable job, and achieving at a high level without being offered any promotion prospects, are examples of high cost–low gain conditions at work. In terms of current developments of the labour market in a global economy, the emphasis on occupational rewards, including job security, reflects the growing importance of fragmented job careers, of job instability, underemployment, redundancy, and forced occupational mobility, including their financial consequences (Siegrist et al. 1986; Siegrist 1996). The model of effort–reward imbalance applies to a wide range of occupational settings, most markedly to groups that suffer from a growing segmentation of the labour market and to groups exposed to structural unemployment and rapid socio-economic change. Effort–reward imbalance is frequent among service occupations and professions, in particular the ones dealing with person-based interactions.

It is important to note that the two models mentioned, the demand–control and the effort–reward imbalance model, differ in the following respects. First, while the demand–control model puts its explicit focus on situational characteristics of the work environment, an explicit distinction is made between situational and person characteristics in the effort–reward imbalance model. It assumes that a combination of both sources of information provides a more accurate estimate of experienced stress at work than a restriction to one of these two sources. Secondly, as was mentioned, components of the effort–reward imbalance model (salaries, career opportunities/job security) are linked to more distant macroeconomic labour market conditions, while the former model's major focus is on workplace characteristics. Finally, in stress-theoretical terms, the range of control over one's environmental situation at work is the core dimension in the demand–control model, whereas in the second model, threats to, or violation of, legitimate rewards based on the assumption of reciprocity and fairness in social exchange represent the core dimension. Despite these differences, there is promise in studying the combined effects of the two models in future research.

6.5.1 Evidence from studies

Compared with the demand–control model, fewer studies have been conducted on the adverse health effect of effort–reward imbalance at work, but those that have suggest that the model provides a fruitful framework for examining work stress and its contribution to the development of disease. So far, six studies have reported findings with partial or full confirmation of the model's basic assumption. An overview of the studies is given in Table 6.3 which, unlike Table 6.2, includes other outcomes in addition to CHD, and obviously does not use a quality filter. Concerning the study design, three studies are prospective. These are the Whitehall II study mentioned above (Bosma et al. 1998); a German blue-collar study covering some 2000 person years (Siegrist et al. 1990), and a Swedish cohort study of some 5720 healthy employed men and women (Peter et al. 1998*a*). Two studies are cross-sectional: a study of 1337 male and female transport workers (Peter et al. 1998*b*), and a study of 179 male middle managers (Siegrist et al. 1997). Furthermore, a follow-up study of 106 coronary patients who underwent percutaneous transluminal coronary angioplasty was conducted to explore the role of effort–reward imbalance in predicting coronary restenosis

Table 6.3 Adverse health outcomes of effort-reward imbalance at work

Author, year, country	Total sample (% women)	Type of study	Exposure	Health measure	Adjustment	Relative risk	Summary
Bosma et al. (1998) UK	10 308 (33) civil servants	Prospective mean 5.3 years	High effort, low reward (proxy measures)	Angina, doctor-diagnosed ischaemia	Age, smoking, blood pressure, cholesterol, BMI, employment grade, negative affectivity, job control	2.15	+
Siegrist et al. (1990) Germany	416 (0) blue-collars	Prospective mean 6.5 years	High effort, low reward	Incident fatal or non-fatal coronary heart disease	Age, smoking, blood pressure, cholesterol, BMI	6.15	+
Peter et al. (1998a) Sweden	5720 (44)	Prospective (baseline data)	High effort, low reward (ratio and score overcommitment)	Hypertension, total cholesterol, LDL and HDL cholesterol	Age, smoking, BMI, physical exercise	1.62 for hypertension (ratio in men) 1.39 for LDL cholesterol (overcommitment in women)	+ (partial) + (partial)
Siegrist et al. (1997) Germany	179 middle managers	Cross-sectional	High effort, low reward	Hypertension, LDL cholesterol	Age, BMI, exercise, smoking, alcohol	5.77 3.57	+ +

Study	Sample	Design	Exposure	Outcome	Adjustments	Relative risk	Association
Stansfeld et al. (1998b) UK	10 308 (33) civil servants	Prospective mean 5.3 years	High effort, low reward (proxy measures)	New reports of psychiatric disorders	Age, employment grade, baseline mental health	2.57 for men 1.67 for women	+
				Subjective health functioning	Age, employment grade, baseline ill health, negative affectivity	All significant ranging from 1.44 to 2.33	+
Peter et al. (1998b) Germany	1337 (12) transport workers	Cross-sectional	High effort, low reward (proxy measures)	Level of reported symptoms	Reported health, physically demanding work, occupational hazards	Ranging from 1.99 to 3.06	+
Joksimovic et al. (1998) Germany	106 (0) coronary patients	Follow-up 1 year	High effort, low reward	Coronary restenosis, based on angiographic measures	Age, cholesterol, hypertension, smoking, multivessel disease	2.86	(partial)

* P value for relative risk < 0.05. †0 = no association; + = moderate (relative risk ≤2.0) association, ++ = strong (relative risk > 2.0) association.

(Joksimovic et al. 1998). In addition, a small-scale intervention study was performed to test the feasibility of a theory-based programme of stress reduction at work (Aust et al. 1997). In terms of health outcome measures, the majority of studies focused on cardiovascular risk factors or documented CHD. Other health indicators were psychiatric disorders, subjective health, reported symptoms, and sickness absence.

With regard to future incident CHD, effort–reward imbalance at work was associated with a two to sixfold elevated relative risk compared to those who were free from chronic work stress (Siegrist et al. 1990; Bosma et al. 1998). This excess risk could not be explained by established biomedical and behavioural risk factors as these variables were taken into account in multi-variate statistical analysis. Yet, additional evidence derived from cross-sectional investigations shows that chronic work stress in terms of effort–reward imbalance is associated with elevated risks of exhibiting high blood pressure, high level of atherogenic blood lipids, or, in one study, elevated fibrinogen. Depending on the sample size, population characteristics, and cardiovascular risk factor under study, respective odds ratios varied from 1.4 (Peter et al. 1998a) to 5.8 (Siegrist et al. 1997).

The adverse effects on health produced by high cost/low gain conditions at work are not restricted to cardiovascular health. In the Whitehall II study, the relative risk of exhibiting new psychiatric disorder, as assessed by the General Health Questionnaire, was 2.6 in men and 1.7 in women suffering from effort reward imbalance at work (Stansfeld et al. 1998b). Similarly, effort–reward imbalance predicted poor physical, psychological, and social functioning after adjustment for the potential confounding effects of age, employment grade, baseline ill health, and negative affectivity in the same data set (Stansfeld et al. 1998a). Another study found elevated reports of musculoskeletal and gastrointestinal symptoms, fatigue, and sleep disturbances among bus and subway drivers who suffered from effort–reward imbalance at work (Peter et al. 1998b). In the middle managers study mentioned above, conditions of low occupational reward only, in the absence of signs of high effort (indicative of a passive state of coping associated with withdrawal behaviour), predicted short-term and long-term sickness absence (Peter and Siegrist 1998). Finally, the probability of experiencing a coronary restenosis was significantly increased in those treated coronary patients who exhibited a high level of work-related overcommitment (high intrinsic effort at work) (Joksimovic et al. 1998). Moreover, in the subsample of coronary patients who were still economically active, the ratio between high effort and low reward at work predicted restenosis after adjusting for relevant clinical variables. In conclusion, the results presented above support the effort–reward imbalance model as a distinct work-related psychosocial risk condition that potentially can provide a scientifically grounded basis for health promotion measures at work.

6.5.2 Comparison of models in predicting future CHD

In the Whitehall II study, a first attempt to compare the two models with respect to the prediction of future reports of CHD has been made. The results show that both effort–reward imbalance and low job control were independently related to CHD outcomes. There was a two–fold higher risk of developing new CHD when each model was controlled for the other and for potential confounders (Figs. 6.4 and 6.5). These findings suggest the potential advantages in devising a job stress model that combines both personal and environmental factors to help explain differences in CHD and other diseases (Bosma et al. 1998).

6.6 East/West comparisons

We started this chapter reviewing the changes in the epidemiology of CHD, highlighting the rise and fall of CHD in different countries. The reasons for these differences are not clear, but are likely to be affected by adverse health behaviours such as poor diet, high levels of alcohol consumption, and increased rates of smoking. The availability of medical care and the effects of pollution are also likely to have contributed to this rise (Bobak and Marmot 1996). Another potential area for explanation is to investigate the role of psychosocial factors in explaining the mortality difference. A Czech case-control study found that low control at work and low levels of work demands were strongly related to the risk of myocardial infarction in men, independent of other risk factors (Bobak et al. 1998). The evidence linking potential explanations is scant, mainly because of lack of reliable and representative data. However, the above findings are consistent with research in Western populations and may provide a useful framework in which to

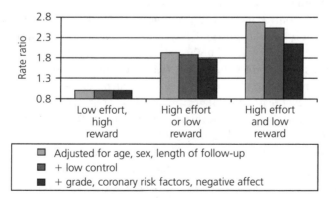

Fig. 6.4 Effort–reward imbalance and CHD incidence; men and women, Whitehall II study (from Bosma et al. 1998).

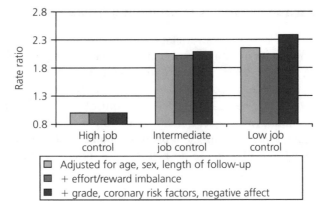

Fig. 6.5 Job control and CHD incidence; men and women, Whitehall II study (from Bosma et al. 1998).

understand and explain the causes of the social gradient in heart disease in eastern Europe.

6.7 Conclusion

In this chapter we have argued that two theoretical models hold particular promise in explaining at least part of the variation in CHD – a variation that may be attributed in part to work stress as defined by the demand–control and effort–reward imbalance models. High demand–low control conditions and high cost–low gain conditions at work are unequally distributed, both between and within societies, and potentially may provide a framework in which to understand the contribution of psychosocial factors at work to the development of disease.

The conceptual differences between the models have direct implications for the design of intervention measures to improve health. Whereas the emphasis of the demand–control model is on change of the task structure (such as job enlargement, job enrichment, and increasing the amount of support within the job, etc.), the reduction of high cost–low gain conditions includes action at three levels – the individual level (e.g. reduction of excessive need for control), the interpersonal level (e.g. improvement of esteem reward), and the structural level (e.g. adequate compensation for stressful work conditions by improved pay and related incentives, opportunities for job training, learning new skills, and increased job security).

Despite the central role of work in the above models, an exclusive focus on working life runs the risk of underestimating the true costs on health produced by other adverse stressful circumstances that can occur outside of work. This becomes dramatically clear if we consider the evidence on the health burden of long-term unemployment (Martikainen and Valkonen 1996).

The characteristics of family life and leisure activities are also of crucial importance in reducing the stresses and strains of working life. Conversely, stressful events in an individual's personal life, such as marital problems and lack of social support, can also exacerbate the burden of work-related stress and may increase a person's disposition towards developing disease. The study of the work–family interface points to the need to extend the framework of reference in stress research by taking into account the broader social determinants of health. These and other factors are the focus of specific chapters in this book.

References

Alfredsson, L., Spetz, C.L. and Theorell, T. (1985). Type of occupation and near-future hospitalization for myocardial infarction and some other diagnoses. *Int. J. Epidemiol.* **14**, 378–88.

Alterman, T., Shekelle, R.B., Vernon, S.W. and Burau, K.D. (1994). Decision latitude, psychologic demand, job strain, and coronary heart disease in the Western Electric study. *Am. J. Epidemiol.* **139**, 620–7.

Aust, B., Peter, R. and Siegrist, J. (1997). Stress management in bus drivers: a pilot study based on the model of effort-reward imbalance. *Int. J. Stress Manage.* **4**, 297–305.

Beatson, M. (1995). *Labour market flexibility.* Department of Employment, London.

Bobak, M. and Marmot, M.G. (1996). East–West mortality divide and its potential explanations: proposed research agenda. *BMJ* **312**, 421–5.

Bobak, M., Hertzman, C., Skodova, Z. and Marmot, M. (1998). Association between psychosocial factors at work and non-fatal myocardial infarction in a population based case-control study in Czech men. *Epidemiology* **9**, 43–7.

Bosma, H., Marmot, M.G., Hemingway, H., Nicholson, A., Brunner, E.J. and Stansfeld, S. (1997). Low job control and risk of coronary heart disease in the Whitehall II (prospective cohort) study. *BMJ* **314**, 558–65.

Bosma, H., Peter, R., Siegrist, J. and Marmot, M.G. (1998). Alternative job stress models and the risk of coronary heart disease. *Am. J. Publ. Hlth* **88**, 68–74.

Breucker, G.S. and Schroer, A. (ed.) (1996). *International experiences in workplace health promotion.* European Health Promotion, Series 6, WHO, Copenhagen.

Gardell, B. (1971). Alienation and mental health in the modern industrial environment. In: *Society, stress and disease. The psychosocial environment and psychomatic diseases,* (ed. L. Levi), pp. 148–80. Oxford University Press, London.

Greiner, B.A., Ragland, D.R., Krause, N., Syme, S.L. and Fisher, J.M. (1997). Objective measurement of occupational stress factors – an example with San Francisco urban transit operators. *J. Occupat. Hlth Psychol.* **4**, 325–42.

Haan, M.N. (1988). Job strain and ischaemic heart disease: an epidemiologic study of metal workers. *Ann. Clin. Res.* **20**, 143–5.

Hackman, J.R. and Lawler, E.E. (1971). Employee reactions to job character-istics. *J. Appl. Psychol.* **55**, 259–86.

Hallqvist, J., Diderichsen, F., Theorell, T., Reuterwall, C., Ahlbon, A. and the SHEEP study (1998). Is the effect of job strain on myocardial infarction due to interaction between high psychological demands and low decision latitude. Results from the Stockholm Heart Epidemiology Program (SHEEP). *Soc. Sci. Med.* **46** (11) 1405–15.

Hemingway, H. and Marmot, M. (1998). Psychosocial factors in the primary and secondary prevention of coronary heart disease: a systematic review. In: *Evidence based cardiology*, (ed. S. Yusuf, J. Cairns, J. Camm, E. Fallen and B. Gersch), pp. 269–85. BMJ Publishing Group, London.

Hemingway, H., Shipley, M., Stansfeld, S. and Marmot, M. (1997). Back pain sickness absence, psychosocial work characteristics and employment grade: a prospective study in office workers. *Scand. J. Work Environ. Hlth* **23**, 121–9.

Hinkle, L.E., Whitney, L.H., Lehman, E.W., et al. (1968). Occupation, educa-tion and coronary heart disease. *Science* **161**, 238–46.

Hlatky, M.A., Lam, L.C., Lee, K.L., et al. (1995). Job strain and the prevalence and outcome of coronary artery disease. *Circulation* **92**, 327–33.

Hoffmann, A., Pfiffner, D., Hornung, R. and Niederhauser, H. (1995). Psychosocial factors predict medical outcome following a first myocardial infarction. Working Group on Cardiac Rehabilitation of the Swiss Society of Cardiology. *Coron. Art. Dis.* **6**, 147–52.

Hutton, W. (1995). High risk. *Guardian,* 2–3.

Johnson, J.V. and Hall, E.M. (1988). Job strain, work place social support, and cardiovascular disease: a cross-sectional study of a random sample of the Swedish working population. *Am. J. Publ. Hlth* **78**, 1336–42.

Johnson, J.V., Stewart, W. and Fredlund, P. (1990). *Psychosocial job exposure matrix: an occupationally aggregated attribution system for work environ-ment exposure characteristics*, (221th edn). National Institute for Psycho-social Factors and Health, Stockholm.

Joksimovic, L., Siegrist, J., Peter, R., Meyer-Hammar, M., Klimek, W. and Heintzen, M. (1998). Psychosocial factors and restenosis after PTCA: the role of work-related overcommitment, submitted.

Joseph Rowntree Foundation (1995). *Inquiry into income and wealth chaired by Sir Peter Barclay*. Joseph Rowntree Foundation, York.

Kaplan, G.A., Pamuk, E.R., Lynch, J.W., Cohen, R.D. and Balfour, J.L. (1996). Inequality in income and mortality in the United States: analysis of mortality and potential pathways. *BMJ* **312**, 999–1003.

Karasek, R.A. (1979). Job demands, job decision latitude and mental strain: implications for job design. *Admin. Sci. Quart.* **24**, 285–308.

Karasek, R. (1992). Stress prevention through work reorganisation: a summary of 19 intervention studies. *Conditions of work digest*, Vol. 11, pp. 23–41. International Labour Office, Switzerland.

Karasek, R. and Theorell, T. (1990). *Healthy work: stress, productivity, and the reconstruction of working life.* Basic Books, New York.

Karasek, R., Baker, D., Marxer, F., Ahlbom, A. and Theorell, T. (1981). Job decision latitude, job demands and cardiovascular disease: a prospective study of Swedish men. *Am. J. Publ Hlth* **71**, 694–705.

Kawachi, I. and Kennedy, B.P. (1997). Health and social cohesion: why care about income inequality? *BMJ* **314**, 1037–40.

Kohn, M. and Schooler, C. (1973). Occupational experience and psychological functioning: An assessment of reciprocal effects. *Am. Sociol. Rev.* **38**, 97–118.

Kristensen, T.S. (1994). Cardiovascular diseases and work environment. In: *Encyclopedia of environmental control technology* (ed. P.N. Cherermisinoff), pp. 217–43. Gulf Publishing Company, Houston.

Kristensen, T.S. (1995). The demand-control-support model: methodological challenges for future research. *Stress Med.* **11**, 17–26.

Lacroix, A. and Haynes, S. (1984). Occupational exposure to high demand/low control work and coronary heart disease incidence in the Framingham cohort. *Am. J. Epidemiol.* **120**, 481.

Lynch, J., Krause, N., Kaplan, G.A., Tuomilehto, J. and Salonen, J.T. (1997). Workplace conditions, socioeconomic status, and the risk of mortality and acute myocardial infarction: the Kuopio Ischaemic Heart Disease Risk Factor Study. *Am. J. Publ. Hlth* **87**, 617–22.

Marmot, M.G. (1992). Coronary heart disease: rise and fall of a modern epidemic. In: *Coronary heart disease epidemiology* (ed. M.G. Marmot, and P. Elliott), pp. 3–19. Oxford University Press, Oxford.

Marmot, M.G. (1994). Social differentials in health within and between populations. *Daedalus* **123**, 197–216.

Marmot, M.G. and Feeney, A. (1996). Work and health: implications for individuals and society. In: *Health and social organisation*, (ed. D. Blane, E. Brunner and R. Wilkinson), pp. 235–54. Routledge, London.

Marmot, M.G., Adelstein, A.M., Robinson, N. and Rose, G. (1978). The changing social class distribution of heart disease. *BMJ* **2**, 1109–12.

Marmot, M.G., Shipley, M.J. and Rose, G. (1984). Inequalities in death – specific explanations of a general pattern. *Lancet* **i**, 1003–6.

Marmot, M.G., Davey Smith, G., Stansfeld, S.A., et al. (1991). Health inequalities among British Civil Servants: the Whitehall II study. *Lancet* **337**, 1387–93.

Martikainen, P.T. and Valkonen, T. (1996). Excess mortality of unemployed men and women during a period of rapidly increasing unemployment. *Lancet* **348**, 909–12.

MONICA (1994). The World Health Organisation MONICA Project. Ecological analyses of the association between mortality and major risk factors of cardiovascular diseases. *Int. J. Epidemiol.* **23**, 505–16.

Morris, J.K., Cook, D.G. and Shaper, A.G. (1994). Loss of employment and mortality. *BMJ* **308**, 1135–9.

Morris, J.N., Heady, J.A., Raffle, P.A.B., Roberts, C.G. and Parks, J.W. (1953). Coronary heart disease and physical activity of work. *Lancet* **II** 1053–7.

Netterstrom, B. and Suadicani, P. (1993). Self-assessed job satisfaction and ischaemic heart disease mortality: a 10 year follow-up of urban bus drivers. *Int. J. Epidemiol.* **22**, 51–6.

North, F., Syme, S.L., Feeney, A., Head, J., Shipley, M.J. and Marmot, M.G. (1993). Explaining socioeconomic differences in sickness absence: the Whitehall II study. *BMJ* **306**, 361–6.

North, F.M., Syme, S.L., Feeney, A., Shipley, M. and Marmot, M. (1996). Psychosocial work environment and sickness absence among British civil servants: the Whitehall II Study. *Am. J. Publ. Hlth* **86**, 332–40.

Orth-Gomer, K., Eriksson, I., Moser, V., Theorell, T. and Fredlund, P. (1994). Lipid lowering through work stress reduction. *Int. J. Behav. Med.* **3**, 204–14.

Osler, W. (1910). The Lumleian Lectures on angina pectoris. *Lancet* **i**, 839–44.

Peter, R. and Siegrist, J. (1998). Chronic work stress, sickness absence and hypertension in middle managers: general or specific sociological explanations. *Soc. Sci. Med.* **45**, 1111–20.

Peter, R., Alfredsson, L., Hammar, N., Siegrist, J., Theorell, T. and Westerholm, P. (1998*a*). High effort, low reward and cardiovascular risk factors in employed Swedish men and women – baseline results from the WOLF study. *J. Epidemiol. Commun. Hlth* **52**, 540–7.

Peter, R., Geissler, H. and Siegrist, J. (1998*b*). Associations of effort–reward imbalance at work and reported symptoms in different groups of male and female public transport workers. *Stress Med.* **14**, 175–82.

Reed, D.M., Lacroix, A.Z., Karasek, R.A., Miller, D. and MacLean, C.A. (1989). Occupational strain and the incidence of coronary heart disease. *Am. J. Epidemiol.* **129**, 495–502.

Schilling, R.S.F. (1989). Health protection and promotion at work. *Br. J. Indust Med.* **46**, 683–8.

Schnall, P.L. and Landsbergis, P.A. (1994). Job strain and cardiovascular disease. *Ann. Rev. Publ. Hlth* **15**, 381–411.

Siegrist, J. (1996). Adverse health effects of high-effort/low-reward conditions. *J. Occupat. Hlth Psychol.* **1**, 27–41.

Siegrist, J., Siegrist, K. and Weber, I. (1986). Sociological concepts in the etiology of chronic disease: the case of ischaemic heart disease. *Soc. Sci. Med.* **22**, 247–53.

Siegrist, J., Peter, R., Junge, A., Cremer, P. and Seidel, D. (1990). Low status control, high effort at work and ischemic heart disease: prospective evidence from blue-collar men. *Soc. Sci. Med.* **31**, 1127–34.

Siegrist, J., Peter, R., Cremer, P. and Seidel, D. (1997). Chronic work stress is associated with atherogenic lipids and elevated fibrinogen in middle-aged men. *J. Int. Med.* **242**, 149–56.

Stansfeld, S.A., Fuhrer, R., Head, J., Ferrie, J. and Shipley, M. (1997). Work and psychiatric disorder in the Whitehall II study. *J. Psychosom. Res.* **43**, 73–81.

Stansfeld, S., Bosma, H., Hemingway, H. and Marmot, M. (1998*a*). Psychosocial work characteristics and social support as predictors of SF-36 functioning: the Whitehall II study. *Psychosom. Med.* **60**, 247–55.

Stansfeld, S., Bosma, H., Hemingway, H. and Marmot, M. (1998*b*). Work characteristics predict psychiatric disorder: prospective results from the Whitehall II study. *Occupat. Environ. Med.*, in press.

Steenland, K., Johnson, J. and Nowlin, S. (1997). A follow-up study of job strain and heart disease among males in the NHANES1 population. *Am. J. Indust. Med.* **31**, 256–60.

Suadicani, P., Hein, H.O. and Gynetelberg, F. (1993). Are social inequalities associated with the risk ischaemic heart disease a result of psychosocial working conditions? *Atherosclerosis* **101**, 165–75.

Theorell, T. (1992). Health promotion in the workplace. In: *Health promotion research. Towards a new social epidemiology*, (ed. B. Badura and I. Kickbusch), pp. 251–66. WHO, Copenhagen.

Theorell, T. and Karasek, R.A. (1996). Current issues relating to psychosocial job strain and cardiovascular disease research. *J. Occupat Hlth Psychol.* **1**, 9–26.

Theorell, T., Tsutsumi, T., Hallqvist, J., et al. (1998). Decision latitude, job strain, and myocardial infarction: a study of working men in Stockholm. *Am. J. Publ. Hlth* **88**, 382–8.

Uemura, K. and Pisa, Z. (1988). Trends in cardiovascular disease mortality in industrialised countries since 1950. *World Hlth Statist. Quart.* **41**, 155–78.

Wilkinson, R.G. (1992). Income distribution and life expectancy. *BMJ* **304**, 165–8.

Wing, S., Casper, M. and Riggan, W. (1992). Geographic and socioeconomic variation in the onset of decline of coronary heart disease mortality in white woman. *Am. J. Publ. Hlth* **82**, 204–9.

Acknowledgements

The Whitehall II study has been supported by various grants including from the Medical Research Council, British Heart Foundation, Health & Safety Executive, National Heart Lung & Blood Institute, National Institute for Aging, John D and Catherine T MacArthur Foundation Research Networks on Successful Midlife Development and Socio-economic Status and Health.

7   Transport and health

Mark McCarthy

7.1   Background

Epidemiology, the study of health and disease in populations, is quite a new science. Much of the early work on infectious diseases, the leading cause of death and disease until recent times, led to effective control through public policies of sanitation, quarantine, and immunization. Chronic disease epidemiology developed in the mid-twentieth century, and the new paradigm of 'risk factors' emphasized individual responsibility and the opportunities for health promotion through changing behaviour. More recently, however, the importance of public policy in sustaining or damaging health has been re-established. It is the intention of this chapter to show that transport is a crucial contributor to health and disease in contemporary European countries, and that major changes are needed in public policy to reverse existing trends.

The new paradigm in thinking about transport and health has been to shift the debate from 'safety' to health benefits (Adams 1985; Davis 1993). 'Safety' has been used by public authorities to create transport systems that are sometimes harmful to health. For example, a law introduced in Victoria, Australia requiring cyclists to wear helmets led to fewer people cycling – and therefore not getting the health benefit that cycling provides (Whitelegg and Davis 1992). Another example of the difference between 'safety' and health has been the use of the financial 'costs' attributed to loss of life in accidents as a justification for further road building. Such calculations are flawed, however: new roads generate more cars and more journeys by a means of transport that is more dangerous than its alternatives (buses and trains).

Many older epidemiologists learned their basic statistics from textbooks that described the Poisson distribution (of infrequent random events) using Bortkiewicz's example of the number of people kicked to death by horses – infrequent in distribution over time, although when added together (e.g. for a whole year) remarkably consistent. If we substitute the modern people transporter, the car, for the horse in Bortkiewicz's example, we have very similar results – deaths are infrequent and scattered over time according to a Poisson distribution. The unexpectedness of the event, and its possible avoidance, led to the term 'accident'; but epidemiologists, noting the recurrent nature of these 'accidents', have found associations (environmental, for example opportunities for speeding, or individual, for example drunk driving) which increase the likelihood of an accident happening. (In the literature, there is often argument whether the term used should, instead, be 'injury', emphasizing the actual rather than chance nature of the event. However the term 'accident' will be retained here, as it has a commonplace meaning and there may be confusion for 'injury' between the event itself and the physical effects.)

7.2 Sustainable development – a global perspective

Essential to debate on transport and health is the concept of 'sustainable development'. The United Nations 'Earth Summit' in Rio de Janiero in 1992 focused world opinion on protecting the Earth's resources, biosystems, and societies for present and future generations. The Earth Summit report mentioned 'health' more than 200 times (World Health Organization 1997), and the World Health Organization and other agencies have reaffirmed the relationship between sustainable development and health.

Sustainable development acknowledges that economic development will continue in all parts of the world, and, along with population increase, there will be pressure on scarce resources. One particular focus is the use of energy. The 1997 Kyoto United Nations conference set international agreements for controlling carbon dioxide, produced from fossil fuels, which is a 'greenhouse gas' with the potential to create global warming. Although oil is needed for much industrial production in developing countries, advanced economies do not rely so much on industrial products as on 'services'; and, in both business and leisure, the use of transport – especially the car – has been growing. Predictions that transfer the existing patterns of car use of Western countries to all the people in developing countries show that the car is quite unsustainable – from the energy perspective – as a means of global transport. (The same will apply to oil-fuelled air travel if current trends persist.) Western economies are using cars at a far greater level of CO_2 production per capita than is acceptable globally, and will have to cut down their car use. Sustainable development provides a critical perspective on transport patterns.

Oil is a dominant economic presence in the world economy. The 1991 gulf war involving NATO, against Iraq, was launched to protect Western sources of oil. Development of Russia and the central Asian republics is giving pre-eminence to oil extraction and transport to the West. Much oil is used for motor vehicles, and the market is continually growing. In the *World disasters report* for 1998, the International Federation of Red Cross and Red Crescent Societies (1998) warn that, annually, motor vehicles kill more than half a million people a year, and injure more than 15 million. It is predicted that road crashes will be the third greatest cause of death and disability, worldwide, by the year 2020, just behind clinical depression and heart disease but ahead of respiratory infections, tuberculosis, and HIV.

7.3 Patterns of travel

Travel can be by different modes of transport, depending on the distances to be travelled – walking, cycling, buses, cars, trains, boats, and aircraft. International comparative data are available only for the main modes. In recent decades in western Europe the number of journeys by bus and rail have remained stable or diminished, whereas travel by car and air have increased. By contrast, in countries of central and eastern Europe, and the newly independent states, bus travel has remained an important component of travel while car use has expanded only slowly (Fig. 7.1).

There are also considerable international differences in the dependency of cities on cars. Table 7.1 shows use of petrol in the early 1990s in three European cities compared with the USA and Australia (with greater car use) and Far Eastern countries (with less car use).

The national travel survey in the UK divides journeys according to their different reasons (Fig. 7.2). Work thus forms the minority of journeys, although business has much further distances travelled per journey, and leisure and 'other personal' have shorter distances. Rail and cycling are the most frequent means of commuting, local buses are most frequently used for shopping, and walking is the most frequent means of transport for leisure. But length of journey is also closely related to mode of transport: for journeys over 12 km, cars are, by far, the most used means of transport.

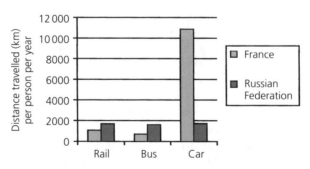

Fig. 7.1 Travel in eastern and western Europe: average distance (km) travelled/person/year in France and Russia by mode of transport (data from early 1990s). (Source: Economic Commission for Europe 1994.)

Table 7.1

Petrol use and vehicle speeds in selected cities
(source: Newman and Kenworthy 1989)

Cities	Petrol used/year (MJ per person)	Average traffic speed (km/h)	Average bus speed (km/h)
Houston	74 510	51	22
Boston	54 185	39	18
Adelaide	28 791	43	21
Hamburg	16 671	30	22
London	12 426	31	18
Amsterdam	9 171	39	18
Tokyo	8 488	21	12
Singapore	6 003	30	15

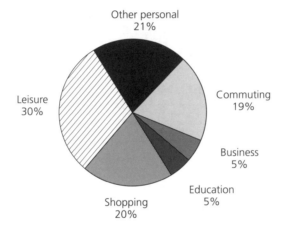

Fig. 7.2 Proportions of journeys by type in the United Kingdom 1992–94 (source UK National Travel Survey 1992/94 in British Medical Association (1997) p. 10).

Travel patterns are related to income. Table 7.2 shows that people in low-income families in the UK make more journeys by walking and more by bus than people in high-income families, while high-income families make many more journeys by car. Similarly, people in households with a bicycle only (6 per cent nationally) made 9.6 journeys per week by walking and 2.4 in a car or van. In contrast, people in families with one car made 5.8 journeys by walking and 12.9 by car or van.

Table 7.2
Travel by selected income groups: number of journeys per week (source: UK National Travel Survey 1991/93, from Potter (1997) table 6.5)

	£3000–£5900	£25 000–£34 999	All households
Walk	7.3	4.3	5.9
Bicycle	0.2	0.3	0.4
Car/van driver	2.6	11.5	7.4
Car/van passenger	2.6	5.4	4.3
Bus	2.1	1.0	1.4
Rail	0.1	0.4	0.3
Other	0.6	0.4	0.6
Total	15.5	22.8	20.3

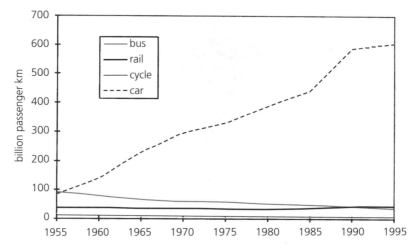

Fig. 7.3 Transport in Great Britain, 1995–95 by mode: billion passenger kilometres (source: Department of Environment, Transport and Regions 1997).

7.4 Trends

The dominant trend of transport in recent decades has been the rapid rise in motor vehicle travel, with a parallel decline in travel by public transport and cycling. Figure 7.3, for the UK, shows the great increase in travel by cars and vans, while bus and coach travel and cycling have diminished and rail travel has remained approximately steady.

There have been similar increases in road traffic in other European countries, but some have made greater recovery in rail transport: for example, passenger kilometres increased by 50 per cent in France, from 40.9 billion in 1970 to 63.9 billion in 1990 (Eurostat 1993).

Part of this change has been through an increase in the length of journeys: for example, in the UK, based on the National Travel Survey which started in the 1970s, the number of journeys increased over 20 years by 10 per cent, whereas the average length of journeys increased by 44 per cent – through more longer journeys (Table 7.3).

For freight, also, there has been an increase in both volume (measured as weight) and distance. Road transport volume doubled in the period 1952–94, but the distance carried increased four fold. In the same period, rail volume diminished (Table 7.4).

7.5 Health impacts of transport

It is possible to consider the health effects of transport both as the resulting health status (usually diseases) and through causal mechanisms. The health impacts in broad disease groups will be described here first, and the mechanisms then considered in relation to actions that can be taken.

Table 7.3
Average journeys and distances travelled per person per year, Great Britain, 1972–73 and 1992–94 (source: UK National Travel Survey, reproduced from Potter (1997) table 3.1)

	Journeys	Distance (km)
1972–73	956	7 189
1992–94	1053	10 367

Table 7.4
Changes in freight transport by mode, UK, 1952 and 1994 (source: Transport Statistics Great Britain, from Potter (1997) table 1.6)

	1952	1994	Index of change (1952 = 1.00)
Volume: million tonnes			
road	861	1689	1.96
rail	289	97	0.33
Distance: million tonne km			
road	31	144	4.64
rail	37	13	0.35

7.5.1 Heart disease

Probably the most important contribution of transport to health is through encouraging exercise – either walking or cycling – which protects against heart disease. Coronary heart disease is the leading cause of death in European Union countries (European Commission 1996) – more frequent than cancer – and contributes to both premature adult deaths (people under 65) and deaths at older ages. The many factors contributing to heart disease are not fully known, and include early life experiences (differences in heart disease mortality between people brought up in different towns) and genetic factors. But there is strong epidemiological evidence that regular exercise, a balanced diet, and not smoking are crucial to cardiac health.

Walking, the most accessible form of regular moderate physical exercise, is beneficial for adults of young and middle age, and also for older people. Regular exercise probably has both short-term effects of cardiovascular 'fitness' and long-term cumulative protective effects – by limiting development of obesity, strengthening the heart muscle and reducing blood pressure, and metabolic effects, including improving cholesterol and fibrinogen levels, and insulin sensitivity (Morris and Hardman 1997).

Two major studies showing the protective effects of exercise are shown in Fig. 7.4 and Table 7.5. Beneficial exercise may be undertaken in bouts of continuous moderate activity, for example, daily 30-minute periods, or accumulated during the day in shorter periods. In other words, it is not necessary to create 'special' exercise, but instead exercise can be incorporated within a day's activities, including travel, gardening, leisure, and social visits.

The British Medical Association (1992) report on the health benefits of cycling was prompted by doctors who were concerned whether they should

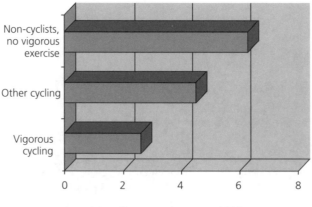

Heart attack rate per 1000

Fig. 7.4 Heart attack rates in male cyclists and non-cyclists aged 45–64 followed over a 10-year period, UK, 1976–86 (source: Morris 1990).

Table 7.5
Risk of death over 4 years of older men (age range 56–75) related to regular daily walking (source: Wanamethee et al. 1998)

Regular daily walking (min/day)	Age-adjusted relative risk (men 60+)
0	1.00
<20	0.99
21–40	0.85
41–60	0.76
60+	0.52

recommend their patients to cycle, because of the perceived risks to cyclists on the roads. The beneficial effects of cycling to reduce heart disease, hypertension, and obesity were clearly described. Indeed, the report estimated that the benefits of cycling outweighed the risks many times (Hillman 1993).

A further benefit of exercise comes in limiting progression of osteoporosis (loss of bone density that develops in older people, especially women, and leads typically to hip and arm fractures). Regular exercise and weight-bearing ensure continued bone strength, and is probably more beneficial, on a population level, than current expensive drug treatments for osteoporosis.

7.5.2 Mental health

Exercise is recognized to have mental health benefits (Morris and Hardman 1997) through stimulating thought and protecting from depression – there is probably a direct physiological causal path. A rather more complex relationship to mental health is the effect of traffic through 'community severance' – the separation of geographical parts of a community because of traffic flows. Studies in the USA and Europe (British Medical Association 1997, pp. 38–43) have shown that streets with less traffic (speed and volume) have a better quality of life (measured, for example, by counts of street activities, open windows, flower boxes, and other signs of personal care), and are perceived by families to be more friendly and free from danger. In San Francisco, people living in three streets in a single neighbourhood with different intensities of traffic were shown to have a marked gradient in social contacts (Fig. 7.5). With heavy traffic density there is a relative fall in land values, the houses are less desirable, and the streets are perceived as more stressful, especially for children and elderly people. Sir Richard Rogers has argued persuasively for 'compact cities' that strengthen community ties, and have their centres of commercial and social activity located at public transport nodes (Rogers 1997, pp. 32–40).

Good social networks are important for children and elderly people, and social support influences both mental health and also overall death rates

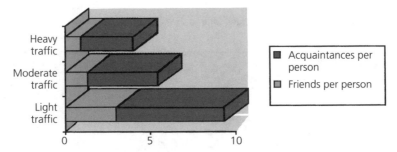

Fig. 7.5 Social contacts with level of street traffic, San Francisco (source: British Medical Association (1997) p. 41).

(House et al. 1988; see also Chapter 8 in this volume). Thus, in the USA, the Alameda County Study compared death rates at 8 years' follow-up in a sample divided into four groups of high to low social contacts (Table 7.6). There were clear gradients in the protective effect of high social contacts. While motor journeys can help link some people who live at a distance from each other, the effect is largely borne by other people who live close to the traffic routes. The underlying social phenomenon of dispersed social contacts assisted by car transport may thus be damaging health.

The link between traffic noise and mental health has been difficult to demonstrate (Berglund and Lindvall 1995). Cars are the most widespread noise nuisance, but trains and aircraft are also significant causes. The effects of aircraft noise have been used to argue for resiting airports and limiting flights during sleeping hours. The unpleasant effects of both airport and trunk road noise are demonstrated through lower house prices.

7.5.3 Respiratory disease

There is widespread concern about air quality, partly because we can each of us readily detect unpleasant-smelling air, and partly because air respects few boundaries so that pollution from one neighbourhood can affect another, even over very long distances (for example, tall industrial chimneys creating 'acid rain', which crosses international boundaries). However, the relationship of transport to respiratory diseases is complex, and sometimes perhaps overstated (Anderson 1997; Schwartz 1997).

It has been estimated that most people in towns spend 90 per cent of their lives indoors, and about 5 per cent in the open air and 5 per cent on transport. The major effects on respiratory diseases are from indoor air: coal fires are associated with respiratory diseases in childhood, while central heating and damp walls, creating environments suitable for house dust mites and mould, increase allergic asthma. In external air, the smogs of the nineteenth- and early twentieth-century cities, caused by heavy industry, have almost dis-

Table 7.6
Levels of social contact compared with proportions in each group dead after 8 years, males and females initially aged 50–59 (source: Berkman and Syme 1979)

Social contact level	Males % dead	Females % dead
I highest	9.6	7.3
II	12.1	4.9
III	18.2	8.0
IV lowest	30.8	15.3

appeared in western Europe because of new heating fuels (oil and gas) and central heating. Instead, the new, increasing, air pollution is from motor vehicles. For example, in the UK black smoke emissions from households fell between 1970 and 1992 from 780 000 to 140 000 tonnes/year, while over the same period black smoke from road transport (mainly freight) increased from 75 000 to 170 000 tonnes/year. Large cities such as Athens and San Francisco, where there is bright sunlight and little wind during the summer, are especially prone to severe air pollution. In London 80 per cent of black smoke is from vehicles (British Medical Association 1997, p. 32).

The health effects of vehicle air pollution can be separated into three parts: directly poisonous emissions such as benzene, a known carcinogen; greenhouse gases, especially carbon dioxide, affecting the global climate; and small particulates (measured as black smoke), especially produced by diesel vehicles. They also act in two different ways: by long-term action, as 'background' pollution, and through acute episodes (McMichael 1997). It is the latter, especially as photochemical smog, that catches public awareness, and has led governments, for example, to advise car drivers to leave their cars at home for the day. A UK scientific committee (British Medical Association 1997, p. 36) did not find a causal link between asthma and outdoor air pollution. While acute smog episodes may temporarily increase asthma rates, the effects are on people with previous respiratory disease – suggesting the need for policies much more complete than temporary car restriction.

7.5.4 Accidents

Thinking about accidents and injuries needs to be clearheaded: there are a number of pitfalls worth considering. Data on deaths are more reliable than on injuries because of more complete recording; however, countries use different approaches in applying coding rules, so that differences between countries should be interpreted with caution. Traveller injury rates vary by mode of transport, but there are different ways of presenting these data. Using distance travelled, long-distance modes including rail and air appear the most safe, with motor cyclists the highest risk. For individuals, however, it is probably the rate per journey that matters. Risks per journey emphasize the hazards of car travel.

Countries show persistent differences in road traffic accident death rates that relate, in part, to cultural and technical characteristics. All countries appear to follow Smeed's law (Adams 1985) in starting with high accident rates per driver, falling as drivers become more experienced. Death rates in Ireland, Spain, Greece, and Portugal are the highest in the European Union (Fig 7.6). Death rates are also higher in Germany, where there are no speed limits on motorways, and in France, where there is a high per capita intake of alcohol (although consumption is falling, European Commission 1996, Fig. 4.1.4) than in the Netherlands and UK.

However, safety is not represented by accident rates because it is mediated by human action and exposure (Adams 1988). Motorways are not safe to cross as a pedestrian, but pedestrian deaths on motorways are very few because pedestrians recognize that they are very unsafe. Cyclist death rates per head of population are higher in the Netherlands than in most other European countries but, as there are also many more journeys made by bicycle in the Netherlands, the risk per journey is lower.

Speed is an important factor in road accidents. There is an exponential rise in risk to pedestrians with increasing traffic speed (Finch et al. 1994). At 30 km/h only 5 per cent of pedestrians involved in road accidents are killed, and most injuries are slight. At 40 km/h 45 per cent of pedestrians are killed, while in crashes at more than 50 km/h up to 85 per cent of pedestrians struck by a car are killed. It is estimated that, in the UK, about 30 per cent of all road deaths are caused directly by speeding (British Medical Association 1997, p. 30).

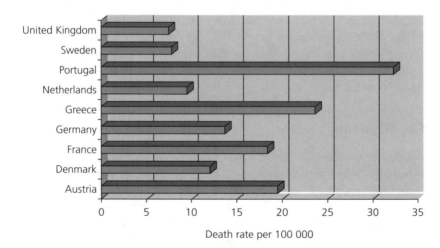

Fig. 7.6 Road traffic accident death rates in adults (age 15+) in selected European countries, 1994.

Different road users have different accident profiles: the cause of an accident should not be attributed to the victim. It is car driving that is 'unsafe' (it causes injuries because of velocity), while cycling is much safer (rarely causing deaths either to car drivers or cyclists). Much effort has been put into 'improving' roads to reduce accidents: however, the net effect, linked with higher car technical performance, has been increasing car speeds, fuller roads, and greater perceived risk for those not using cars. Few people would regard town roads in the 1990s as safer than in the 1950s, even if the accident rate per kilometre travelled is lower. 'Safety' improvements (for other road users) have been translated into 'performance' improvements (for car drivers).

Road injuries occur to people of all ages, but there are different exposures by age. Pedestrian road deaths are highest in children and old people; young adults are particularly at risk as drivers and passengers of cars and motor-bikes. Middle-aged male car drivers are at greater risk because of high exposure. Cyclists are at risk at all ages – studies in cycling countries show deaths from motor vehicle accidents in elderly cyclists. Internationally, these rates differ country by country according to exposure, environment, and cultural habits. Child pedestrian deaths (age 0–14 years), for example, vary from 0.5 per 100 000 in Finland to 2.0 per 100 000 (four times as frequent) in the United Kingdom (Jarvis et al. 1995).

Accidents characteristically show a social class gradient – in the UK, deaths from road traffic accidents to children from the poorest families (social class V) are more than four times greater than those in the richest (social class I) families (Jarvis et al. 1995). In the USA, accident rates for drivers from deprived areas are also higher than for those from rich areas (Abdalla et al. 1997).

7.6 Interventions

The focus of interventions proposed here is strategic and mainly within the responsibilities of national or municipal departments of transport. There is a relative lack of research to support these proposals. In contrast, however, broad motivational and behavioural changes (such as health education campaigns) are not proposed as these have been of very limited success (Towner et al. 1993; British Medical Association 1997, p. 31).

In line with the argument of this chapter, the foremost health policies for transport should be to give the highest priority to walking, cycling, and public transport – forms of travel that are health promoting, of low risk and fulfil sustainability objectives. However, up to the present, cycling and walking have often appeared, at best, to be an afterthought in transport policies. Even, for example, a report on sustainable cities by the European Community proposes policies first for 'traffic demand management' and improving public transport, and only after these is attention given to cycling and walking

(Expert Group on the urban environment 1996). The greatest concern of the Commission of the European Community and the United Nation's Economic Commission for Europe (1993) has been to support road transport, followed by rail and then waterways. Similarly, European international transport statistics (United Nations 1994) simply do not include walking and cycling.

On grounds of health and environmental sustainability, it is crucial to promote walking and cycling, and public transport, as the main modes of travel for urban journeys. But promotion of these is difficult. They are not perceived by business as necessary for goods transport – although, of course, much individual economic consumption (shopping, eating, using services) is achieved through pedestrian journeys. Increasing affluence, 'convenience', and commercial forces are all leading to greater use of motor vehicles. However, policy support for walking and cycling have been developing in some European cities in the past three decades.

7.6.1 Policies for walking

(1) Changing thinking. In the past, pedestrians in towns have been physically separated from motor traffic, restrained by barriers, detoured into underpasses, on the questionable grounds that this will improve 'safety'. Transport planning must prioritize pedestrians over cars in transport decisions, especially when crossing roads at junctions.

(2) Increasing access. Priority should be given to good interchange between pedestrians and public transport, with frequent access points.

(3) Improving quality. Walking should be an enjoyable environmental experience, with a good sense of safety. This can be encouraged by 'greening' towns, widening footways, narrowing roads, placing street furniture (traffic signs, barriers) in roads rather than on footways, ensuring good lighting, reducing traffic volumes and road parking to increase the pleasantness of journeys.

(4) Creating clearly linked pedestrian networks for important routes; for example, for shopping, to schools, libraries, and hospitals.

(5) Ensuring that there are good local facilities for all neighbourhoods within convenient walking/cycling distance.

7.6.2 Policies for cycling

(1) Changing thinking. Cycling must be seen as *the* normal means of travelling short to middle-length distances in towns, backed by local authority and police support (including ensuring that their own staff use bicycles regularly). Special attention to promote cycling is needed in cities with hills.

(2) Provision must be made for all potential cycle journeys – it is estimated that cycling could replace at least half of all present car trips (Friends of the Earth 1992, p. 32).

(3) Until car traffic has been severely reduced and on-street parking abolished, there should be separate cycle lanes on all roads, as there are (already) pavements.

(4) Cycle parking facilities should be widespread, well designed (for safety) and prioritized for interchange with public transport

Many examples of good practice in promoting cycling exist in the Netherlands, Denmark, and Finland, and also in cities in other European countries, for example Ferrara in Italy, York in England, Sandnes in Norway (Box 7.1).

Box 7.1 **Examples of good practice for cycling in European cities (source: Expert Group on the Urban Environment 1996 , p. 187; Friends of the Earth 1992, p. 32)**

- Erlangen, Germany, has developed a network for cycling with signalling and parking facilities, and cycle priority routes. Over a 20-year period, cycling has risen from 14 per cent to 29 per cent of journeys. The city plans to reduce private car trips from 40 per cent to 30 per cent of the total by the year 2000.

- Groningen, the Netherlands, has created cycle paths near main shopping areas, improved its bus services, and restricted car parking. The level of cycling, 50 per cent, is one of the highest in Europe.

7.6.3 Improving public transport

Public transport is the key to middle- and long-distance travel. Group travel saves energy and is both economical and more sustainable. People who rarely travel by public transport on land are willing to use large passenger aeroplanes.

Debate about public transport sometimes gets caught in disagreement on the level of subsidies. There are few grounds for subsidies that retain inefficient practices and arguments in favour of prices reflecting true costs, especially environmental costs. However, direct subsidies of public transport may be an efficient way of redressing income and access inequalities. It is necessary to invest in, and maintain, public transport to ensure a strong alternative to individual car travel. It is more important for central and local governments to maintain good services (through contracts and subsidies) than it is for the public authority actually to operate the service – although some public authorities do provide excellent services.

Policies for public transport include:

(1) integration of all modes of public transport between each other (e.g. with transferable tickets) and with walking and cycling (e.g. cycle parking);

(2) good facilities for cycles on buses and trains;

(3) frequent and reliable services;

(4) routes that serve suburbs and rural areas: this may involve good inter-connections rather than many long routes going through the city centre;

(5) innovation and responsiveness to consumer concerns.

7.6.4 Policies for vehicle restraint

It is now recognized at the level of the European Community that, rather than the relentless increase in vehicle transport of the twentieth century, during the twenty-first century there will need to be a major reversal of this trend (Expert Group on the Urban Environment 1996, p. 178). Traffic reduction is the necessary basic policy – the means of achievement vary from country to country and at different levels. Perhaps most important is that national, regional, and local authorities set targets for traffic reduction, and then assess the effectiveness of their policies against these targets.

Historical trends for transport growth in European countries in the twentieth century, except during wars, have been for annual increases in car ownership and use, and a shift from rail to road transport of goods. The trends have been interpreted by planners as requiring more roads to be built – a process mockingly called 'predict and provide' by critics. But there are almost always advocates of road building – the construction companies, the landowners, the people living in a town that will be 'bypassed', and the motoring organizations. Instead, the new approach to sustainable transport must actively seek to restrain car journeys and road transport.

Car use declines when people choose a nearer destination (shorter car trips), switch from car to an alternative mode (walking, cycling, or public transport), or decide not to travel (alternative modes of communication). Car reduction policies will need all three choices to be completely effective.

Strategies for reducing traffic have to be comprehensive:

(1) reducing traffic in one area must not lead to its diversion into another area;

(2) all members of society must contribute (including, for example, politicians, professionals, and executives);

(3) incentives for change are needed – change must not depend just on goodwill from a minority;

(4) traffic reduction should be integrated with other priorities – increasing cycling and walking, improving public transport and urban environments,

reducing 'car-dependent' urban facilities (for example, those using car parking, such as supermarkets and large leisure facilities).

Some of the strategies currently used for traffic reduction include:

(1) traffic calming: for example, chicanes that narrow streets, road 'humps' and raised tables at intersections and crossways, moving 'street furniture'(parking meters and notices, road signs) off pavements and into the road;

(2) closing roads: roads that are pedestrianized, and culs-de-sac, can reduce vehicles, but can retain the same number of journeys by other means of transport if planned effectively;

(3) bans and permit schemes: closing areas of cities to traffic, requiring vehicles to have at least three passengers, limiting the total number of vehicles licensed (e.g. in Singapore);

(4) substantial taxation of vehicles: on parking spaces (public and private), on licences, on buying and selling vehicles, on fuel.

Some cities have remained entirely car-free in their historic centres – Venice and Fez (in Morocco) are two important examples; others have reduced the use of cars substantially in their ancient streets (e.g. Rome). Even cities built during the days of carriages and trams (e.g. Zurich) have achieved major reductions in vehicle use through integrated policies of limiting car access while promoting walking and cycling and good public transport.

Pedestrianizing city centres is now a normal policy in many cities to stem the otherwise inexorable increase of traffic and consequent traffic jams; but car reduction is a much larger concern. It must address the increasing car ownership across a wider range of the population – retired people, young people in their first job, parents with young families. Cars are exceedingly cheap to buy and run because their costs to other people are not properly paid. The marginal cost of commuting or leisure trips can be significantly less than that of public transport when there is more than one person in the car. Raising the price of car travel to reflect environmental costs can be achieved by road pricing (e.g. car mileage meters) and capital taxes (Singapore levies a high tax on buying a new car unless an old car is concurrently destroyed).

Car reduction must also address the increasing use of cars across outer parts of cities, or as transport in from the countryside to the town. The predictions of car use over the next decades are not for more city-centre traffic, but for more rural driving. Having saturated the city centres, cars are now increasing in the emptier suburban and rural roads, assisted by peri-urban road building. More than ever before, rich people want to live in the countryside and use cars for access to towns and rural facilities. There is a further challenge – that the rural car owner claims more 'need' for a car because public transport is less available than in towns because it is less economic. But the number of people who work in farming is falling across

Europe: people are making choices to live in the countryside (and work in the town) because of its physical and social environmental advantages. Land-use planning, which is under the direct control of central and local governments, is crucial in reversing the trend to rural commuting and expanding 'dormitory' villages.

Changes in the transport of goods are also needed. Some of these are national policies; for example, governments should concern themselves to maintain local production of natural local products (where skills and/or resources exist) and resist the commercial trends of globalization, where transport costs are significant. International trade in buses, for example, makes little sense if a country has a sufficiently developed home market for local production; on the other hand, electronic goods and services (e.g. through the Internet) are tradable with less environmental damage. Local governments need to pay special attention to local distribution of goods. A study of cyclists' deaths in London (Gilbert and McCarthy 1994) showed that more than half were killed by heavy (more than 3 tonne) lorries. Leiden is introducing a system of transferring goods from large vehicles to small vans for city distribution: it is estimated that 70 per cent of the goods and 80 per cent of the journeys can be converted in this way (Expert Group on the Urban Environment 1996, p. 183).

7.7 The politics of change

The three integrated policies needed for transport and health are therefore: promoting walking and cycling, improving public transport, and reducing motor vehicle transport (both passenger and goods).

In the oil 'crisis' of the 1970s, the cartel of oil-producing countries raised their prices dramatically and generated the first major understanding of the international dependence on oil. Many countries introduced energy-saving regulations, including, for example, 80 km/h speed limits on main roads and improved insulation in housing. However, as the oil supply stabilized, road speed limits were raised again: neither health nor environmental arguments were as strong as the pressure from road-user organizations to allow increased speeds.

The forces working politically for private transport have been described collectively as 'the road lobby' (Hamer 1987). The lobby includes motoring organizations (with millions of members subscribing to receive insurance and emergency services); road construction companies (some of the richest public building contracts have been for motorway construction); car manufacturers (most European countries build and sell cars at home and abroad); oil companies (with points of sale across the country); and advertisers, working to portfolios for all the previous groups. That many journeys are made by foot is not reflected in the relative lobbying power of pedestrians against the road lobby. Getting a bypass built around 'his' or 'her' town can be a major local success for a Member of Parliament. Improving facilities for cyclists gains few votes.

The difficulty of implementing change is described in detail in a study of the northern Danish city of Aalborg (Flyvbjerg 1998). This town was one of the first to take traffic restriction seriously, and sought to implement an inner-city scheme of improved bus services, partial pedestrianization, and improved cycle access. The study describes how these objectives of the city planners were thwarted by local coalitions – especially the Chamber of Commerce (worried about any change in journeys to local shops), the police (preferring car users to bus passengers or cyclists), and the local press (using the scheme to attack the political majority). Despite acclaim of the scheme by the Danish professional planning association, the actual results were modest: indeed, over a 10-year period, car traffic had increased.

However, Aalborg was a pioneer. The innovative ideas of that time have now become more commonplace, and have been shown to be successful in a number of towns and cities. At the same time as Aalborg, Copenhagen, the capital of Denmark, introduced city policies to limit cars that were far more successful, and travel in Copenhagen now, by bus, metro, or cycle, is one of the pleasantest of experiences. A city council that is convinced of its course can have a considerable impact. Car Free Cities (Eurocities 1998) is a group of local authorities across Europe sharing experience on traffic-reduction policies and practice. Through publications and conferences they are developing and demonstrating integrated local transport policies and promotion of walking and cycling.

Changing attitudes towards transport across Europe were shown by a 'Eurobarometer' survey of the (then) 12 countries of the European Community. Respondents were asked to rate their perceptions of urban car traffic. Responses for 'unbearable' ranged from 14 per cent in Denmark and 18 per cent in the Netherlands to over 40 per cent in Italy and Greece, with the European mean as 22 per cent (European Commission 1996, Fig. 4.2.6). There is also strong support, a Europe-wide average of 71 per cent, for actions to limit car traffic in town centres. On the other hand, European public opinion was against road pricing: 65 per cent said it would be ineffective in limiting car use (International Research Associates 1991).

It is only a first step to describe the problem from the health perspective. Cars may be seen as the fourth addiction (after smoking, alcohol, and drugs) (McCarthy 1993), with very strong consumer convenience, pleasure, and identification. People strongly believe in 'their' right to use 'their' car, and these attitudes pervade most groups of society, and both public and private organizations. Thus, four groups of actions are needed for change:

(1) Information and attitude change. Understanding of the health impact of transport must be disseminated much more widely, both within the

professional health field and to the general public. In the UK, organizations such as Transport 2000 (a non-governmental organization (NGO) supported financially by the public transport unions) and the British Medical Association (the national medical group, influenced on transport policy by public-health physicians) have made important contributions through publications and press statements. Similar organizations in other countries may be important allies in developing national influence. Crucially, in the workplace (both manufacturing and service industries, both private and public sector) the link of transport and health needs to be recognized and integrated with policies for sustainable development.

(2) National governments. National ministries of transport, that typically have a very close relationship with the 'road lobby' and industry, need to have greater understanding of the health benefits of transport through closer contact with health agencies. Equally, Ministries of Health need to improve their understanding of transport and health. The WHO International Ministerial Conference on Environment and Health in London in 1999, at which transport and health is a major topic, provides a defining moment for these ministries. Regular inter-ministerial meetings can identify the opportunities for policy development: the first steps are a re-evaluation of policies for road transport, and setting targets and policies for traffic reduction.

(3) Local governments. It is evident across Europe that, while national governments can set agendas through legislation and financial incentives, implementation depends crucially on local authorities. Action involves broad structural plans that will enhance walking and cycling as well as reducing vehicle use (for passengers and goods); annual investments that create new opportunities for walking and cycling; substantial improvements in public transport; incentives to reduce car use, such as increased parking costs, decreasing access for cross-town and out-of town car journeys; and strengthening of local shopping and facilities to support these changes. Schemes that reduce goods carried by large vehicles are also necessary.

(4) Local action. The local authority's public-health department is responsible for maintaining the health of the local population by all means available. It has an important contribution, particularly because it is able to support concerns of minority groups (for example, children and older people affected by increasing traffic), as well as putting health arguments forward at the political level.

The public-health department in Camden and Islington Health Authority, an area of inner London, worked with the two local authorities on transport and health issues (McCarthy 1997). Actions included:

◆ holding a seminar on transport and health with local politicians;

- holding a public meeting about traffic at one of the worst traffic intersections;
- holding discussions with officers of the local authority and the central government planning authority;
- seeking funding for a transport and health traffic project to measure road danger;
- supporting a 'walk to school week' with local schools;
- responding to the local authorities' road 'safety' and cycling development plans;
- describing use of transport within the National Health Service locally and by local government staff;
- including discussion on transport and health in the annual Public Health Report;
- producing a specialist report on transport and health for the whole of London.

7.8 Conclusions

The policies and priorities for transport of most Western governments do not match the needs for health. The solid facts are that walking and cycling benefit health, while motor vehicles damage health. Thus, walking and cycling need to be prioritized in transport planning; compact cities that minimize vehicle journeys need to be prioritized in economic and land-use planning; public transport must be significantly improved, while car travel is reduced; and leadership is needed from politicians, industry, and 'civil society' (non-government organizations including unions, community groups, interest associations, etc.). The 'road lobby', so powerful in the twentieth century, must be recognized as harming societies in the same way that commercial interests for smoking, tobacco, and (illicit) drugs are now recognized.

7.9 Acknowledgements

In the UK a small group of academics and professionals from the fields of health and transport and local government met together from the mid 1980s as the 'Transport and Health Study Group'. Through quarterly meetings and annual conferences, the group developed a wide understanding of the issues, and in 1988 wrote a seminal document *Health on the move – policies for health promoting transport* (Transport and Health Study Group 1991). Much of the content of this chapter derives from ideas first brought together formally in *Health on the move*; from important contributors to the field, including John Adams (1985), Adrian Davies (British Medical Association 1997), Bob Davis

(1993), Mayer Hillman (British Medical Association 1992), and John Whitelegg (Hillman et al. 1990); and from public-health colleagues, Stephen Watkins and Steve Morton.

References

Abdalla, I., Barker, D. and Raeside, R. (1997). Road accident characteristics and socio-economic deprivation. *Traff. Engin. Control* **38**, 672–6.

Adams, J. (1985). *Risk and freedom: the record of road safety regulation.* Transport Publishing Projects, Cardiff.

Adams, J. (1988). Risk homeostasis and the purpose of safety regulation. *Ergonomics* **31**, 407–28.

Anderson, R. (1997). Health effects of air pollution from traffic: discussion. In: *Health at the crossroads: transport policy and urban health*, (ed. T. Fletcher and A.J. McMichael), pp. 82–5. John Wiley and Sons, London.

Berglund, B. and Lindvall, T. (ed.) (1995). *Community noise.* Centre for Sensory Research, Department of Psychology, Stockholm University, Stockholm.

Berkman, L. and Syme, L. (1979). Social networks, host resistance and mortality: a nine year follow-up study of Alameda County residents. *Am. J. Epidemiol.* **109**, 186–204.

British Medical Association (1992). *Cycling towards health.* British Medical Association, London.

British Medical Association (1997). *Road transport and health.* British Medical Association, London.

Davis, R. (1993). *Death on the streets: cars and the mythology of road safety.* Leading Edge Press, Hawes, North Yorshire, UK.

Department of the Environment, Transport and Regions (1997). *Transport statistics in Great Britain, 1997.* HMSO, London.

Economic Commission for Europe (1994). *Annual bulletin of transport statistics for Europe.* United Nations, Geneva.

Eurocities (1998). *Car free cities magazine.* Eurocities, Brussels. (cfc@ eurocities.be)

European Commission (1996). *The state of health in the European Community.* Office for Official Publications of the European Union, Luxembourg.

Eurostat (1993). *Transport annual statistics 1970–1990.* Statistical Office of the European Communities, Luxembourg.

Expert Group on the Urban Environment (1996). *European sustainable cities.* European Commission Directorate General XI, Brussels.

Finch, D., Kompfner, P. and Maycock, G. (1994). *Speed, speed limits and accidents.* Transport Research Laboratory, Crowthorne.

Flyvbjerg, B. (1998). *Rationality and power: democracy in practice.* University of Chicago Press, London.

Friends of the Earth (1992). *Less traffic, better towns.* Friends of the Earth, London.

Gilbert, K. and McCarthy, M. (1994). Cycling deaths in London 1985–92: the hazards of traffic. *BMJ* **308**, 1534–7.

Hamer, M. (1987). *Wheels within wheels: a study of the road lobby.* Routledge and Kegan Paul, London.

Hillman, M. (1993). Cycling and the promotion of health. *Policy Studies* **14**, 49–58.

Hillman, M., Adams, J. and Whitelegg, J. (1990). *One false move . . . a study of children's independent mobility.* Policy Studies Institute, London.

House, J.S., Landis, K.R. and Umberson, D. (1988). Social relationships and health. *Science* **241**, 540–4

International Federation of Red Cross and Red Crescent Societies (1998). *World disasters report.* International Federation of Red Cross and Red Crescent Societies, Geneva.

International Research Associates (1991). *European attitudes towards urban traffic problems and public transport.* INRA (Europe), Brussels.

Jarvis, S., Towner, E. and Walsh, S. (1995). Accidents. In: *The health of our children,* (ed. B. Botting for the Office of Population Censuses and Surveys). HMSO, London.

McCarthy, M. (1993). Cycle helmets – the case against. *BMJ* **305**, 881–2.

McCarthy, M. (1997). Transport, health and policies in London. *London J.* **22**, 176–81.

McMichael, A.J. (1997). Transport and health: assessing the risks. In: *Health at the crossroads: transport policy and urban health* (ed. T. Fletcher and A.J. McMichael), pp. 9–26. John Wiley and Sons, London.

Morris, J.N. (1990). Exercise in leisure time: coronary attack and death rates. *Br. Heart J.* **63**, 325–34.

Morris, J.N. and Hardman, A.E. (1997). Walking to health. *Sports Med.* **23**, 306–32.

Newman, P.W. and Kenworthy, J.R. (1989). *Cities and automobile dependence.* Gower Publishing, Aldershott.

Potter, S. (1997). *Vital travel statistics.* Landor Publishing, London.

Rogers, R. (1997). *Cities for a small planet.* Faber and Faber, London.

Schwartz, J. (1997). Health effects of air pollution from traffic: ozone and particulate matter. In: Health at the crossroads: transport policy and urban health (ed. T. Fletcher and A.J. McMichael), pp. 61–82. John Wiley and Sons, London.

Towner, E.M.L., Dowsell, T., Jarvis, S.N. (1993). *Reducing childhood accidents: the effectiveness of health promotion interventions.* Health Education Authority, London.

Transport and Health Study Group (1991). *Health on the move.* Public Health Alliance, Birmingham.

United Nations Economic Commission for Europe (1993). *Transport information.* Economic Commission for Europe, Geneva.

United Nations (1994). *Annual bulletin of transport statistics for Europe.* Economic Commission for Europe, Geneva.

Wanamethee, S.G., Shaper, A.G. and Walker, M. (1998). Changes in physical activity, mortality and incidence of coronary heart disease in older men. *Lancet* **351**, 1603–8.

Whitelegg, J. and Davis, R. (1992). Cycle helmets [letter]. *BMJ* **305**, 504.

World Health Organisation (1997). *Sustainable development and health: principles and a framework for action for European cities and towns.* World Health Organisation Regional Office for Europe, Copenhagen.

8 Social support and social cohesion

Stephen A. Stansfeld

8.1 Introduction

The evidence that social support is beneficial to health and that social isolation leads to ill health is now considerable. Social support has a positive effect on many different aspects of both physical and mental health. Yet the exact nature of the positive influence of social support on health remains elusive. As a concept, social support is used in many different ways and, in order to evaluate the evidence that social support influences health, it is important to be clear about its definition.

Social support has been defined as 'resources provided by other persons' (Cohen and Syme 1985). It has been seen as 'information leading the subject to believe that he is cared for and loved, is esteemed and valued and belongs to a social network of communication and mutual obligation' (Cobb 1976). Much of the theoretical work on social support is derived from the study of attachment and separation in early life (Bowlby 1969), in other words the effects of loss of relationships. Personal relationships are diverse in nature and have behavioural, cognitive, and affective components. The behavioural aspects include episodes of social interaction whose quality and content need to be assessed as part of social support. The cognitive aspects include the type of exchanges and rewards implicit in support transactions and how these are perceived by the participants.

8.2 Measurement of support

One of the most important distinctions is between social networks and the functional aspects of support, that is the quality and type of support that is provided by the network member. Social networks refer to the social contacts of a group of persons. Such contact can be described in terms of number of contacts and frequency of contacts (Table 8.1). These measures can be further refined by separating them into the number of contacts from the primary group, or group of persons to whom the subject is most attached, and from more distant contacts, less likely to provide meaningful support. Other useful

Table 8.1 Measures of social support and social networks

Social networks	Contacts
	Number of contacts
	Frequency of contacts
	Density of network
Social support	Types of support
	Emotional
	Informational
	Self-appraisal
	Instrumental or practical
	Negative interaction

measures include 'density' of the network, where it is estimated how much each network member is in contact with each other – this gives some idea of how integrated network members are. The great advantage of network measures to research on social relations is that they are relatively easy to measure, easy for respondents to recall reliably in surveys, and fairly easily verifiable by an external assessment. Such measures are also probably less susceptible to reporting socially desirable responses. These measures can provide an index of social integration, how much the individual is part of a community of mutual obligation and exchange – thus linking the needs of the individual with those of wider society. However, the major disadvantage of network measures is that they do not provide any indication of the quality of the interaction taking place in social contacts. Although sources of support may be identified, the type of support is not. This means that whereas a gross lack of social support, such as social isolation, may be identified, a more finely graded appreciation of social support transactions is not available.

A much greater richness of analysis may be achieved by examining the quality of support as well as the social network. In general, types of support may be divided into 'emotional' and 'practical', or 'instrumental', support. In some studies other aspects of support have been identified which may be allied to emotional support. These include 'informational' support, where support sources provide information which may help the respondent in problem solving. A further important component of emotional support is related to self-appraisal, providing support that boosts self-esteem and encourages positive self-appraisal. Practical support is manifest in many forms, including practical help and financial support.

In assessing the impact of support on health it is important also to acknowledge the source of the support, as the impact of, say, emotional support from different sources may have a different meaning, dependent on closeness of that source to the respondent. In recent years social support research has recognized that close relationships can have negative, as well as positive, aspects. There is increasing evidence to suggest that these negative aspects of close relationships may have a very powerful effect on ill health (Coyne and Downey 1991), perhaps rather greater than the positive effect on health.

There are methodological differences in the way questions about support are asked. The 'availability' of support is tapped by questions that ask the respondent whether there is someone available to provide support should the respondent need it. This has the advantage of assessing how supported people feel but is somewhat abstract. 'Perceived' support indicates how much support the respondent feels and reports they have been given. The advantage of this measure is that it may indicate more accurately how much support the person has actually received. However, in cross-sectional studies of health causation there is a risk that it may be measuring support elicited as a result of ill health rather than support, or the lack of it, leading to ill health.

It is easy, but misleading, to view social support as unidirectional. Social support involves both interactions and transactions between people. Hence, what a person gives in a relationship may also be important for their health as well as what they receive from someone else – so-called 'reciprocity'. Reciprocity may have implications for the maintenance of good social relations. For instance, relations in which there is a mutual balance of give and take may be easier to sustain than those where there is an imbalance. However, there are likely to be structural prerogatives which guide these patterns of reciprocity. For example, the relationships between parents and young children will involve greater provision of practical support by parents. Both biological and social structural conditions shape the expectation of reciprocity in today's society, where social roles are much less fixed. The expectations of reciprocity in social relationships are also much less clearly defined and may lead to conflict where occupational and domestic roles collide.

8.3 Social support and personality

One difficulty in evaluating the evidence for social support on health is in distinguishing between the health-giving effects of the content of transactions in social relations from the inherent ability to develop and maintain relationships. It is likely that the ability to develop positive social relations is dependent on satisfactory early relationships with both mother and father (Fig. 8.1). Conversely, unhappy or disruptive early relationships may lead to patterns of anxious attachment, or dissociation from attachments, which may persist into adult life. These disturbed patterns of early relationships may in themselves be related to ill health, either through the development of abnormal or excessive responses to stress or through the adoption of unhealthy behaviours such as excessive eating, drinking, or smoking as a partial substitution for satisfactory emotional relationships. Thus it may be that part of

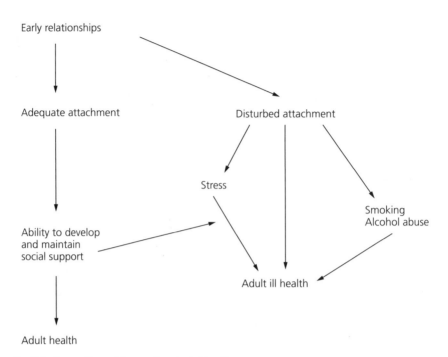

Fig. 8.1 Personality, social support, and adult health.

the explanation for the relationship between social support and health is related to underlying personality factors which determine whether relationships are established. It is also likely that underlying personality factors influence the ability to maintain, nurture, and develop relationships. Of course, that personality factors could contribute to the relationship between social support and health does not rule out the likelihood that social interactions themselves can promote health. Indeed, it is likely that the effects of social support on health include both the aspects of personality, which encourage the development and maintenance of relationships, as well as the health-giving effects of those interactions and transactions. Indeed, it is almost a prerequisite for social support to occur in any effective long-term manner that the personality characteristics are available to develop and sustain it. Curiously, it is the negative aspects of personality which provide this evidence, for there are some aspects of personality which work against the development of positive social relations. For instance, hostility, which has been shown in several studies to be predictive of future coronary heart disease (Barefoot et al. 1995), tends to have an inverse relationship with measures of social support.

8.4 Mechanisms for the action of social support on health

Two types of mechanisms have been described for the action of social support on health. The first mechanism is that of direct effects of support on health. According to this mechanism, positive effects of support, or the lack of support resulting from social isolation, have direct effects on people's health. The second mechanism operates through the so-called buffering effect. According to this mechanism, support does not have any direct effect on health but helps to moderate the impact of acute and chronic stressors on health (Fig. 8.2). It has long been recognized that the experience of a stressor, such as an acute life event, leads to ill health in some people but not others. It is hypothesized that this is explained by the causal impact of the life event on the development of illness being moderated by protective factors such as support, although it is more likely that 'vulnerability factors', such as lack of support, predispose the person to the development of ill health following the experience of a life event. There is evidence for both direct and buffering mechanisms.

How does a largely psychologically perceived set of processes, such as social relations, directly influence bodily physiology? There are a number of pathways through which social support may affect health. For instance, direct effects on health may be mediated through health-related behaviours. Support from others may encourage healthier behaviours, such as reducing fat in the diet, taking exercise, or giving up smoking. But this seems to explain only part

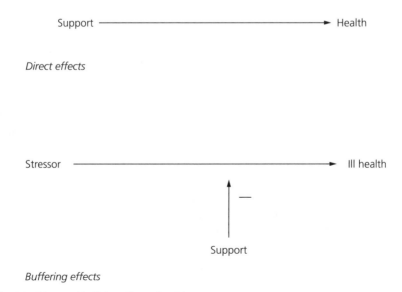

Support —————————————————→ Health

Direct effects

Stressor —————————————————→ Ill health

Support

Buffering effects

Fig. 8.2 Direct and buffering effects of social support.

of the direct effect of support on health, and support from other people may only be health inducing if they practice healthy behaviours themselves. If your spouse continues to smoke, it is less likely that you will be able to give up smoking than if he or she does not smoke. Direct effects of support on health may also result from support increasing perceptions of control over the environment, and giving an assurance of self-worth, which in turn may improve well-being and immunity to disease.

There are several ways in which the buffering effects of social support may act. First, discussion of a potential threat with a supportive person may help to reappraise the threat implicit in a stressor, perhaps thus making it more manageable or even avoiding it. Secondly, practical aid or emotional consolation may help to moderate the impact of the stressor and help the person deal with the consequences of the stressor, which might otherwise be damaging for health.

8.5 Hormonal pathways for the effects of support

Environmental stressors may have direct effects on bodily systems. Acute stressors may stimulate the adrenal system, resulting in the classic 'fight-or-flight response' in which adrenal medullary hormones, such as adrenaline and noradrenaline, are secreted to prepare bodily metabolic systems for action by increasing levels of lipids and glucose (see Chapter 2). While this may be adaptive in the short term, if stressors are excessive or prolonged, the body may be subjected to undue strain, and the cumulative strain on the body, the ups and downs of physiological responses (so-called allostatic load) may lead to illness. Similarly, stimulation of the hypothalamic–pituitary–adrenal (HPA) axis will lead to raised cortisol secretion, often also found in severe depressive illness, and may cause suppression of immune functioning and thus increase the susceptibility to infection. Social relationships may act to modulate or damp down neuroendocrine reactivity (Seeman and McEwen 1996). This may be the mechanism for a common pathway for the effects of both social status and social support on health, as is illustrated by studies of primates. Dominant male primates in stable social situations have lower levels of adrenocorticotrophic hormone (secreted by the pituitary gland to stimulate the production of cortisol by the adrenal gland) and cortisol (Sapolsky 1989), and hence seems to show less stress response. Interestingly, however, dominant social status in an unstable social environment, associated with greater competition and hostility – the antithesis of a supportive environment – is associated in male primates with raised cortisol, sympathetic nervous system activity, and the development of atherosclerosis – the precursor of coronary heart disease (Williams et al. 1991). Similarly, social isolation in primates contributes to increased activity of the HPA axis and the development of atherosclerosis. It was interesting that this biochemical response was attenuated by the presence of other adult primates.

There have also been a small number of human studies which have found that high levels of social support have been associated with lower heart rate, lower blood pressure, and lower levels of cortisol, adrenaline, and nor-adrenaline (Seeman et al. 1994). Hence it is possible that social support has a direct effect on the neurohumoral responses of the body to environmental stress.

8.6 Social support and mortality

What is the evidence that social support affects health? This section will examine the effects of social support on health. The evidence suggests that social support influences both mental and physical health. Perhaps the most striking evidence for the effect of social support on health, which is also some of the earliest evidence, relates to the effect of social support on mortality. The evidence that social networks influence mortality has come from a number of large prospective community studies. One of the earliest reports was that of the Alameda County Study, in which a social network index was constructed of marital status, number of contacts with friends and relatives, church and group membership. Low scores on this index were related to 1.9–3 times greater mortality over a 9-year period (Berkman and Syme 1979). Those with the fewest social connections had the highest mortality rate. A major strength of this study was to adjust for potential confounding factors, such as health-related behaviour, and particularly prior ill health, which might lead to a reduction in social contacts and give a spurious relationship between social networks and subsequent ill health. These early findings have been confirmed in a number of subsequent studies of community-based samples, including the Tecumseh Study (House et al. 1982), and in older people in the Durham County Study (Blazer 1982). Although in the Evans County, Georgia Study (Schoenbach et al. 1986) social network interaction was only found to have a protective effect on morbidity in white males. In Europe, studies from Sweden and Finland have provided further evidence for the positive effects of social integration on mortality. Social integration has been related to longevity in a Swedish cohort study of 50-year-old men (Welin et al. 1985) and lack of social ties was associated with considerably high risk in the North Karelia Study (Kaplan et al. 1988). Similarly, by linking social network interactions and Swedish National mortality data in 17 433 Swedish men and women, and comparing the lowest with the highest network group, an increased total mortality risk of 3.3 was found. This was reduced to a relative risk of 1.34 after adjustment for smoking, exercise, and chronic illness (Orth-Gomér and Johnson 1987).

Most studies of social support and mortality have measured social networks but not the functional aspects of support. Kaplan et al. (1994) reported from the Kuopio Study in eastern Finland that among 2682 men followed up for just under 6 years, those at increased risk of death reported few persons to whom they gave, or from whom they received, support, and a low quality of social relationships. Lack of participation in organizations, few friends, and not currently being married were also associated with greater overall mortality risk. These findings were not confounded by baseline health status, smoking, alcohol intake, coffee consumption, physical activity, body mass index, or income.

Functional aspects of social support are likely to have a stronger association with mortality than social networks because they capture more of the social interaction, as is shown in the results of the Kuopio Study as opposed to the Swedish National Study (Orth-Gomér and Johnson 1987). Frequency of interaction and use of emotional support when troubled were not associated with mortality risk in the Kuopio Study, although use of instrumental or practical support when troubled was associated with increased risk. It may be the case that the heavy use of instrumental support is associated with existing illness, loss of functioning in everyday activities, and hence additional need of support. Overall, Kaplan et al. (1994) argue that social support does not appear to be a proxy for baseline health status, in fact, associations between social support and mortality appeared to be stronger in the healthy subgroup at baseline.

One question which remains to be answered conclusively is whether social support has a non-specific protective effect across all causes of death. This has implications for the type of biological mechanism underlying its effects and would be in keeping with support showing an effect on general susceptibility to disease. Most studies in Western populations have examined cardiovascular mortality, unsurprisingly in view of its importance as a cause of death in both men and women, and have consistently found an effect. In a study of 32 624 US male health professionals, Kawachi et al. (1996) confirmed that social isolation was related to increased cardiovascular disease mortality, and deaths from accident and suicide, but was not related to other causes of death, namely cancer, although the study yielded fairly few cases of cancer. A previous study had found a link between social isolation and smoking-related cancers (Reynolds and Kaplan 1990) but this was not confirmed by Kawachi and co-workers.

Different studies have tended to use different measures of social networks and the findings have not been uniform across all the studies. Nevertheless, the general pattern of an association between social integration and lower mortality remains. Certain of these studies have suggested that the protective effect of social networks seems to be greater in men than women but, as Seeman (1996) has pointed out, many of the middle-aged women in these samples have not reached the period of highest risk and hence the smaller number of events among women may have reduced the power of these studies to detect differences in risk by level of social integration. In comparative analysis of men and women aged 65 years or older in the National Institute on Ageing's established populations for epidemiological study of the elderly, social integration was found to be significantly associated with a lower 5-year mortality risk for both women and men.

8.7   Social support and physical morbidity

In terms of physical illness and morbidity, the relationship between social support and cardiovascular disease – particularly coronary heart disease and stroke – has been studied most. Social isolation has been linked to stroke incidence in a large study of US male health professionals (Kawachi et al. 1996). A longitudinal community-based study from Sweden, examining men aged 50, found a significant protective effect of social integration on the incidence of non-fatal myocardial infarction in those found to be free of heart disease at baseline (Welin et al. 1985). One other study (Vogt et al. 1992) has also found a protective effect of social integration, measured by range of different ties, on the 15-year incidence of myocardial infarction, but not all measures of social network based on network size or frequency of contacts showed this association (Kawachi et al. 1996), and other studies, such as the Japanese American Study in Hawaii, did not find a relationship between social ties (marital status and ties with children and parents, social activities, and co-workers and group memberships) and the incidence of coronary heart disease (Reed et al. 1983). The lack of consistent association between social support and incidence of CHD might be explained by the results of an Israeli study which reported that high levels of family problems were related to an increased risk of developing angina (Medalie and Goldbourt 1976). As Seeman (1996) points out, 'greater social integration, to the extent that it is accompanied by greater interpersonal conflict or other interpersonal problems, may not be uniformly associated with health benefits, including reduced risk of heart disease (or other health outcomes)'.

There have been several studies of patients undergoing coronary angiography to examine the association between social support and severity of progression of coronary atherosclerosis. In general, social network membership does not seem to have been related to degree of atherosclerosis (Seeman and Syme 1987). However, a significant inverse association was found between levels of instrumental support provided by others and atherosclerosis. A significant inverse association has been found between levels of emotional support and the extent of atherosclerosis, particularly among those patients classified as showing the type A behaviour pattern (Blumental et al. 1987). Thus although more structural features of social integration, as indicated by social network measures, do not appear to be associated with disease severity, more qualitative features, such as levels of social support, do exhibit a negative association with disease severity and are in favour of a role for social support in the development of coronary heart disease. However, the results of angiography studies need to be viewed cautiously because of the possibility of selection bias in such samples, on the basis of how people are referred for angiography.

8.8   Social support and prognosis

Social support may not only have a protective effect in preventing or decreasing the risk of development of illness but may also be helpful for people who have to adjust to, or cope with, the stress of a chronic illness.

The association between social support and the prognosis of post-myocardial infarction patients is strong and consistent. Ruberman et al. (1984) were the first to report that more socially isolated men were at increased risk of death post-myocardial infarction. This has been confirmed in several subsequent studies. Williams et al. (1992) found that individuals who were not married and had no confidant had significantly poorer survival post-myocardial infarction over a 5-year follow-up period. Berkman et al. (1992) suggested that low levels of emotional support may be the reason why social isolation conveys greater mortality risk in post-myocardial infarction patients. In her study emotional support was measured prior to the myocardial infarction, as all subjects were part of a longitudinal study in New Haven. Diagnosis of myocardial infarction was identified through hospital monitoring and chart review for all cohort members. In analyses adjusting for age, the severity of the myocardial infarction and other morbidity, subjects who reported no sources of emotional support experienced a nearly threefold higher mortality rate at 6 months than those reporting one or more sources of support. It is possible that the effects of lack of social support on mortality post-myocardial infarction are mediated through the development of depression. Depression, and especially recurrent depression, has been associated with increased mortality risk post-myocardial infarction (Lespérance et al. 1996). It is possible that depression could increase the risk of sudden death from ventricular arrhythmias via increased sympathetic activation influencing a susceptible, damaged heart (Cameron 1996). A randomized control study (Frasure-Smith and Prince 1985) suggested that monthly supportive and educational interventions by a nurse-therapist to patients post-myocardial infarction who were identified by questionnaire to be under stress was associated with greater longevity than in subjects who did not receive this intervention. In addition, stress scores were also reduced in the intervention group. However, in a subsequent intervention this favourable response was not replicated and, if anything, women fared less well in the intervention group (Frasure-Smith et al. 1997). Results examining social support and stroke have been fairly similar in pattern. Amongst subjects who experienced a stroke, those who were more socially isolated exhibited significantly worse functional status 6 months post-stroke, as measured by impairment of activities of daily living and more frequent nursing home placement. Other studies have also found that levels of emotional support post-stroke are predictive of better recovery, suggesting that greater available emotional support may be one reason why social integration predicts better outcome post-stroke.

Less dramatically, but no less importantly, social support has been shown to be helpful in dealing with chronic disabling and painful diseases such as rheumatoid arthritis, preventing the onset of secondary depression and limiting disability (Fitzpatrick et al. 1991). In this way social support may not only be contributing practical help to people who are restricted in activities of everyday living, but also providing crucial emotional support to maintain morale in the face of chronic illness. It is also possible that emotional support has a beneficial effect on the immune system in chronic illness. Social support has also been shown to be influential in some studies of cancer survival. Group therapy in melanoma patients was associated with increased survival time and reduced psychological distress (Kiecolt-Glaser and Glaser 1995). It may be that social support is operating here to strengthen the immune response to the illness. This certainly seems to be the case in AIDS, where the bereavement of an AIDS patient is associated with a fall in the CD4 lymphocyte count while increases in social support have been associated with an improvement in this index of immune function (Kiecolt-Glaser and Glaser 1995).

8.9 Social support and mental health

The fact that social support influences psychiatric disorder has been known since the nineteenth century, when Durkheim (1951) showed that social isolation was associated with higher rates of suicide. It has also long been known that bereaved adults experience high and unexpected levels of illness and mortality in the year following the death of their spouse (Parkes et al. 1969). Bereaved persons without a network of friends or relatives to whom they could turn for consolation were also at greater risk of developing lasting psychiatric problems.

Cross-sectional studies show a clear negative association between levels of support and psychiatric disorder, largely depression, although it is not clear that this is necessarily aetiological (Paykel 1994). The association appears in both community and patient samples, and in both men and women. There is, however, a consensus that emotional support buffers the effects of life events on minor psychiatric disorder (Aneshensel and Stone 1982; Kessler and McLeod 1985). A similar effect has also been found in studies examining chronic as well as acute stressors (Brown and Harris 1978). Alloway and Bebbington (1987), in a cautious review of buffering studies in minor affective disorder, suggest that, overall, Brown's vulnerability model of low emotional support as a risk factor for depression in women experiencing life events does receive appreciable support.

There have been fewer longitudinal studies of social support where questions of causation can be better addressed. Several community studies have been completely prospective, identifying deficiencies in social support prior to the onset of psychiatric disorder and relating this to the onset of disorder. Two studies found a buffering or interactive effect (Brown et al. 1986; Bolton and Oatley 1987) and a third (Henderson 1981) found some evidence for direct effects. The study by Brown et al. (1986) found little predictive effect on mental health of 17 measures of emotional support, measured at baseline in an inner-city sample of married mothers. However, they did find a greater risk of depression in women who received little 'crisis support', that is little support when it was needed to cope with a life event. A negative response from a partner in a crisis was also associated with a greater subsequent risk of depression. On the other hand, among single mothers, report of a close relationship at baseline was protective against the development of depression following a subsequent life event. They also found that women who reported the availability of adequate emotional support at baseline, but who were subsequently 'let down' and found support was not forthcoming when they needed it, were at much greater risk of developing depression.

In Henderson's community study in Canberra (1981), a modest negative association was found between the availability of attachment and social integration, on the one hand, and neurotic symptoms on the other. However, measures of perceived adequacy of support showed a much stronger negative relationship with neurotic symptoms: perceived adequacy of close relationships was important for women, while that of more diffuse relationships was important for men. This was interpreted as indicating that those who view their social relationships as inadequate were substantially more at risk of developing neurotic symptoms. There is debate as to whether this reflects mainly the relationship between aspects of personality and psychiatric disorder, or whether it indicates the quality of the social support provided. A North American study in 1982 also measured perceived adequacy of emotional and tangible support, and found that they predicted depressive symptoms at follow-up interview in 1985 in a sample of non-institutionalized elderly persons (Oxman et al. 1992). A further longitudinal study of British, middle-aged civil servants (Whitehall II Study) showed a protective effect on mental health of emotional support from the closest person in men (Stansfeld et al. 1998b) and from the primary group in women (Fuhrer et al., 1999), which was not abolished by adjusting for either hostility, as a measure of personality or psychiatric disorder at baseline. Moreover, this study showed prospectively that negative aspects of close relationships were associated with greater risk of future psychiatric disorder up to 5 years later. In certain psychiatric conditions, such as schizophrenia, critical comments, hostility, and overinvolvement from the patient's primary group are related to a higher risk of psychotic relapse (Bebbington and Kuipers 1994). This risk may be reduced by adequate medication, curtailing contact between the person and his or her primary group and, more positively, by reducing the high 'expressed emotion' in the primary group, using educational and therapeutic techniques.

A few studies have followed up clinical samples of depressed patients to assess the effect of support on outcome of depression. Brugha et al. (1990) found that the number of primary-group members named and contacted, and satisfaction with support, predicted recovery in women. In men, negative interaction with the primary group, and marriage were associated with recovery.

A study of women who had been 'in care' during childhood (Quinton et al. 1984) shows how social support in adulthood may exert a beneficial effect on parenting problems, marital difficulties, and psychiatric disorder. Many of these women returned from care to a discordant home environment from which they then tried to escape by early marriage. But their marital relationships also often turned out badly and resulted in these women becoming more vulnerable to further difficulties. Nevertheless, a third of those studied showed good parenting ability themselves. This seemed to relate to both positive school experiences, including examination success, and good relationships with peers, but also to the later presence of a supportive marital relationship, which prevented subsequent parenting difficulties and depression from occurring.

Provision of adequate support at various critical stages in the life cycle when support is required, where its lack may lead to depression, may be a good prevention strategy in mental illness. In particular, support for mothers with young children can help prevent social isolation from other adults, and patterns of socialization in many societies encourage this. Although prevention of life events that may lead to depression is not generally feasible, there are opportunities for prompt intervention in crises, which may prevent the development of psychiatric disorder from understandable distress (Paykel 1994). Voluntary agencies providing support to bereaved persons may be included in this type of intervention, although there has been little systematic study of the efficacy of these interventions.

8.10   Social support and sickness absence

We found that negative aspects of close relationships, material problems in terms of financial, household, and neighbourhood problems, and social support at work were important predictors of sickness absence for psychiatric disorder in the Whitehall II Study, an occupational cohort study of civil servants (Fig. 8.3; Stansfeld et al. 1997). However, effects vary by gender and length of spell of sickness absence. The most marked finding relating to sickness absence was for negative aspects of close relationships. High levels of negative aspects of close relationships were followed by increased rates of long

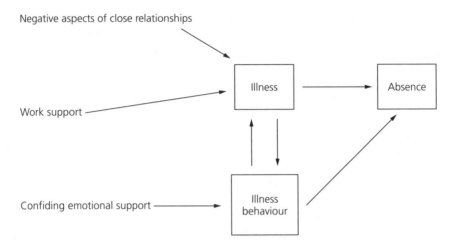

Fig. 8.3 Mechanisms for the influence of direct effects of support on illness behaviour and absence.

spells of psychiatric sickness absence (spells greater than 7 days' duration) in men; while for women intermediate levels of negative aspects of close relationships were followed by increased rates of short spells (spells less than 7 days' duration) of sickness absence.

Negative aspects of close relationships are not synonymous with a lack of positive aspects of support, and have been recognized increasingly as risk factors for mental ill health (Coyne and Downey 1991; Lakey et al. 1994). Negative aspects of close relationships also predicted higher rates of sickness absence for physical illness (Rael et al. 1995). There might be two possible explanations: either negative aspects of close relationships are part of the cause of illness, or negative aspects of close relationships encourage taking sick leave in the presence of illness. It is more likely to be the former for two reasons: the association was also present in other analyses where negative aspects of close relationships predicted psychiatric disorder scores on a screening questionnaire for anxiety and depression. Secondly, after adjusting for baseline psychiatric disorder score, that is to say adjusting for illness, rather than illness behaviour, the association between negative aspects of close relationships and sickness absence was consistently diminished.

In women, medium and high levels of emotional support from the closest person were associated with higher risk of long spells of sickness absence. This is in keeping with findings for sickness absence for physical illness (Rael et al. 1995). This association was surprising in the light of findings that emotional support is protective against the development of depression in those exposed to life events (Brown and Harris 1978). However, the apparent contradiction could be explained if this were an effect on illness behaviour rather than illness. In this case confiding/emotional support from the closest person may encourage empowerment, security, and perceptions of control in the employee, which legitimise taking leave from work when he/she is depressed or anxious (Stansfeld et al. 1997).

We also found that social support at work was protective against short spells of sickness absence for both men and women. Work support, as defined here, included support from colleagues, support from supervisors, and consistency and clarity of information from supervisors. Work support was also protective for those with high levels of negative aspects of close relationships, suggesting that support at work may help people cope with interpersonal stressors from home and thus not take time off in short spells of absence. It was notable that the protective effect of work support on short spells of absence was much stronger than that of non-work support, which shows very few effects other than for negative aspects of close relationships.

8.11 Gender differences

Studies of cardiovascular morbidity and mortality suggest that being married is more beneficial to health for men than for women, and that women benefit as much from relationships with friends or relatives. Our own research suggests that for middle-aged civil servants the most important support is provided for men by their spouse, whereas for women there is a greater likelihood of support being provided by their immediate close network. We found that emotional support from the closest person was a predictor of good mental health in men but not in women (Stansfeld et al. 1998*b*). On the other hand, for women there was a beneficial effect of emotional support on mental health when support from up to four close persons was included (Fuhrer et al. 1999).

8.12 Society, social integration, and health

Social support operates at both an individual and a societal level. Social integration may have a positive effect on the whole community. Social cohesion, the existence of mutual trust and respect between different sections of society, contributes to the way in which people and their health are cherished. There is increasing evidence that communities with high levels of social cohesion have better health than those with low levels of social cohesion. Social cohesion means cohesive community relationships with high levels of participation in communal activities and public affairs, and high levels of membership of community groups. This often goes together with an egalitarian ethos in local politics. Various pieces of evidence support the link between social cohesion and health (Wilkinson 1996). Cities with stronger civic communities have lower infant mortality. In Russia, during periods of immense social upheaval in the 1970s and 1980s there were greatly increased levels of mortality. It was striking that this was especially the case amongst divorced men, who might be expected to be more socially isolated.

The inhabitants of the Pennsylvanian town of Roseto in the United States, settled by Italians who emigrated from the town of the same name in Italy, seemed to retain the low levels of coronary heart disease that their relatives in Italy enjoyed, as long as they kept their traditional family-oriented social structure. But as people became assimilated into the surrounding American culture, where the individual rather than the family and community was considered to be the dominant unit, the incidence of coronary heart disease rose. It seemed unlikely that the rise in coronary heart disease could be attributed to the conventional cardiac risk factors, as diet had improved and levels of smoking had fallen. It was the case that the inhabitants of Roseto had become more sedentary, but this did not seem to be enough to explain the large increase in coronary heart disease, which could be attributed to the loss of social cohesion. Societies in which there are high levels of income inequality and diminished social cohesion have higher levels of crime and violence and higher mortality rates (Kawachi and Kennedy 1997).

8.13   Social class and social support

Could the effect of social inequalities on health, such as those caused by income inequality, be partly mediated through an influence of social class on social support and thence on health? If this is the case, there should be evidence of social class gradients in social support. Much work has gone into defining patterns of social network interaction in different communities, but relatively little work has attempted to relate macro-social variables, such as social class, to social support. The evidence that individuals of lower socio-economic status (SES) have relationships of lower quality is scattered and contradictory. The evidence for social networks is more consistent. Fischer (1982) found higher income and education to be associated with larger networks, more contact with network members, and more voluntary associations. Turner and Marino (1994), in a study of 1394 adults in metropolitan Toronto, found that higher levels of perceived social support (measured by a global score of support from spouses, relatives, friends, and co-workers) was related to higher socio-economic status. We have found similar results in the Whitehall II Study (Stansfeld et al. 1998c). Perceived social support was measured by asking respondents to nominate up to four close persons; respondents then had to rate the amount of three types of support (confiding/emotional, practical, and negative aspects of close relationships) given by each of these persons. Confiding/emotional support from the person mentioned as closest was highest for both men and women in higher employment grades. Practical support was highest for men in the higher employment grades, although this effect was not found for women. Conversely, negative aspects of close relationships tended to be more common in those of lower employment grade for men, while there was no clear gradient for women. Unlike the Toronto study, among civil servants there were more contacts with friends among those of higher employment grade and more contact with relatives among those in lower employment grades. This is likely to reflect greater mobility amongst those of higher SES, and perhaps also greater opportunities for making friends. On the other hand, those in lower employment grades may have restricted opportunities for mobility and may be more closely in touch with their families of origin. Thus there is some evidence for a differential distribution of social support by social class but, in general, it does not seem to be a major influence in explaining employment grade differences in depression (Stansfeld et al. 1998c) or sickness absence (Rael et al. 1995).

8.14 Social support and the physical environment

Apart from the macro-social environment encapsulated by social cohesion, the arrangement of the physical built environment can also influence social support and hence health. The physical environment can, to some extent, determine the opportunities for social support among residents of a particular area. In this context social support from neighbours is especially important. That the relationship between support and the physical environment is influential is indicated by the fact that the quality of relationships with neighbours largely explains reports of residents' satisfaction with the area in which they live. Moreover, residents who are more involved in the local community tend to be happier where they live, regardless of the physical quality of their homes (Halpern 1995).

Various factors tend to increase friendliness between neighbours. Areas that have high social homogeneity tend to increase neighbourliness, although there is a danger of such areas becoming so different from adjacent areas that ghettos may develop. More intimate physical settings for housing such as cul-de-sac roads are related to a greater likelihood of making friends and neighbours and to generally higher levels of friendliness, as was found by Willmott in his studies of Dagenham in East London (Willmott 1963). The relationship of these physical factors to ill health is indirect and not always easy to trace. However, some findings are fairly consistent. For instance, the low group density of a minority group in any population relates to worse mental health (Halpern 1993). This may be because of the relative isolation felt by people of a minority group in areas where they are genuinely in a minority and have few of their own community around them. Studies have looked at perceptions of helpfulness of neighbours and health and have found a negative association between helpfulness and symptom levels. In fact,

Halpern (1995) suggests that the associations between the objective character-istics of the residential environment and symptoms may be mediated through the rated helpfulness of neighbours.

It has been recognized that the design of buildings, and groups of buildings, their layout and the way in which buildings relate to each other, may help to encourage or discourage neighbourliness and hence may have effects on health. Buildings or housing estates that have little opportunity for informal social contact tend to be disliked by their residents. Yancey (1971) emphasized the importance of 'semi-private space' where people could make informal social contacts in a non-threatening communal setting. Thus shared space, specifically allocated to local residents, will encourage the development of potentially supportive relationships. Studies of residential living have suggested that bedrooms arranged as small clusters around a common area tend to be associated with greater social interaction than bedrooms arranged along corridors (Baum and Valins 1977). These studies illustrate a common theme that people generally prefer to have control over their social inter-actions. Frequent interactions with strangers not of the participants' choosing may paradoxically lead to social withdrawal and a feeling of intrusion on privacy, rather than the reverse. Similarly, there may be adverse social effects on health which derive from physical living conditions. It has been suggested that the adverse effects of crowding on psychological health in a study of inner-city Indian households was related to the breakdown of social support systems (Evans and Palsane 1989). Thus, the design of the physical environ-ment can have an impact on social integration and social support and, through this, may influence health.

8.15 Intervening to improve social cohesion and health

Another factor that needs to be taken into consideration is the fear of violence and crime. This fear may inhibit social interaction and tend to increase mistrust. Several studies have tested interventions in terms of making unsafe housing estates more safe, with a consequent improvement in health. A land-mark study was described by Halpern (1995), who assessed the refurbishment of a housing estate called Eastlake. This relatively conventional estate of two-storey row houses in a British new town had become very unpopular and was developing a reputation as a high-crime area. Apart from signs of a run-down area, such as graffiti, broken windows, and dismantled cars, the estate was characterized by a strong sense of distrust related to a network of alleyways through which strangers could easily gain access to the estate. At the time of initial intervention there was close consultation between the planners and the residents. Interventions to improve the estate included the introduction of measures to slow traffic on the estate, provision of more convenient parking, the fencing in of 'ambiguous semi-private space', and the closing of alleyways. Internally, house windows were replaced and kitchens and bathrooms were refitted. At the same time the facilities for children in a play area were improved and access to this was also improved. As a result of this intervention residents' concern about safety from traffic and about the danger of personal attack and car theft reduced considerably from baseline interview to follow-up interview after the intervention. At baseline only 41 per cent of residents described the estate as 'safe or very safe' but by the time this work was all completed this had risen to 81 per cent of residents. At the same time, residents' perception of the friendliness of the area greatly increased. What was most striking was that the mental health of the residents improved in terms of a fall in measures of anxiety and depression and an improvement in terms of self-esteem on simple self-report questionnaire scales between the baseline and the final follow-up of the study. This simple but striking study illustrates how important the interaction between the physical and social environment is in terms of determining mental health. It certainly seems plausible that it might have similar effects on physical health.

In a follow-up study in Oslo, 503 persons were re-interviewed over a period of 10 years with the same questionnaire (Dalgard and Tambs 1997). Only one satellite town to Oslo showed marked social changes over time. At baseline there were high levels of mental ill health and the town was characterized by a relative 'lack of services, recreational possibilities and other facilities, economic problems and qualitative poor social networks'. During the 10-year follow-up period there were reported significant improvements in playgrounds, shops, kindergartens, youth activities, and 'in general' in the satellite town compared to the other areas studied. There was also an improvement in social support which was not statistically significant. These improvements in the social environment, which seem to include greater opportunities for social interaction, were associated with an improvement in mental health in those who continued to live there. Although there was no direct evidence that social support was the major factor in the mental health improvements, decreased environmental stress associated with the social changes seems a plausible explanation. As in the Eastlake study and Leighton's (1965) follow-up study of Stirling County in rural Nova Scotia, 'increased trust and interaction between the residents, as well as increased feelings of community cohesion and empowerment, seemed to be of crucial importance for the improvement in mental health. Obviously this is related to the social organization as well as to the physical characteristics of the neighbourhood' (Dalgard and Tambs 1997).

8.16 Conclusions

Social support has a wide spectrum of action on health, from influencing mortality at one end through physical morbidity to psychological morbidity at the other end. Social support is a very personal matter and yet research shows that it is influenced by social structural imperatives and becomes more than the sum of the individual links of networks in terms of social cohesion. At the level of society, social cohesion can have a powerful effect on health which transcends that available from individual social relationships. This has implications for improving the health of communities. In terms of improving the general health of the population, it is important to recognize that many economic and fiscal policies may influence the social cohesion of a society. Those policies that increase income inequalities are likely also to increase health inequalities. On a slightly smaller scale, the design of the built environment may also influence possibilities for social interaction which may subsequently influence health.

At a more specific level, it can be important to identify particular groups who might be at risk of illness through social isolation. There have been several projects to increase support for young women with children who may be at risk of depression. It may also be important to target parents with the aim of improving parenting skills and hence giving children a better start in life. This has been especially effective in the Home Start Programme for high-risk children. Another possibility is to target support services for particular stressful life events that frequently occur throughout the life cycle, including school change, job entry, unemployment, bereavement, and retirement.

It does not seem likely that social networks can be artificially induced and remain long lasting. However, conversely, it seems very possible that interventions at a population level could reduce social support and impair health. Policy makers need to be aware of the costs and benefits of their policies in social terms across a wide range of different policies, from economics and town-planning, to health services distribution. Finally, there is considerable scope for giving support to those with existing illness, especially myocardial infarction and stroke, and chronic illnesses such rheumatoid arthritis and depression, who may very well benefit from continuing support.

References

Alloway, R. and Bebbington, P. (1987). The buffer theory of social support: a review of the literature. *Psychol. Med.* **17**, 91–108.

Aneshensel, C.S. and Stone, J.D. (1982). Stress and depression: a test of the buffering model of social support. *Arch. Gen. Psychiat.* **39**, 1392–6.

Barefoot, J.C., Larsen, S., von der Lieth, L. and Schroll, M. (1995). Hostility, incidence of acute myocardial infarction, and mortality in a sample of older Danish men and women. *Am. J. Epidemiol.* **142**, 477–84.

Baum, A. and Valins, S. (1977). *Architecture and social behaviour: psychosocial studies of social density.* Laurence Erlbaum Associates, Hillsdale, NJ.

Bebbington, P. and Kuipers, L. (1994). The clinical utility of expressed emotion in schizophrenia. *Acta Psychiat. Scand.* **89**, 46–53.

Berkman, L.F. and Syme, S.L. (1979). Social networks, host resistance, and mortality: a nine-year follow-up study of Alameda County residents. *Am. J. Epidemiol.* **109**, 186–203.

Berkman, L.F., Leo-Summers, L. and Horwitz, R.I. (1992). Emotional support and survival after myocardial infarction: a prospective, population-based study of the elderly. *Ann. Int. Med.* **117**, 1003–9.

Blazer, D.G. (1982). Social support and mortality in an elderly community population. *Am. J. Epidemiol.* **115**, 684–94.

Blumental, J.A., Burg, M.M., Barefoot, J., Williams, R.B., Haney, T. and Zimet, G. (1987). Social support, type A behaviour, and coronary artery disease. *Psychosom. Med.* **49**, 341–54.

Bolton, W. and Oatley, K. (1987). A longitudinal study of social support and depression in unemployed men. *Psychol. Med.* **17**, 453–60.

Bowlby, J. (1969). *Attachment and loss.* Vol. 1 *Attachment.* Hogarth Press, Institute of Psycho-Analysis, London.

Brown, G.W. and Harris, T. (1978). *The social origins of depression.* Tavistock Publications, London.

Brown, G.W., Andrews, B., Harris R., Adler, Z. and Bridge, L. (1986). Social support, self-esteem and depression. *Psychol. Med.* **16**, 813–31.

Brugha, T.S., Bebbington, P.E., MacCarthy B., Sturt, E., Wykes, T. and Potter, J. (1990). Gender, social support and recovery from depressive disorders: a prospective clinical study. *Psychol. Med.* **20**, 147–56.

Cameron, O. (1996). Depression increases post-MI mortality: how? *Psychosom. Med.* **58**, 111–12.

Cobb, S. (1976). Social support as a moderator of life stress. *Psychosom. Med.* **38**, 300–13.

Cohen, S. and Syme, S.L. (ed.) (1985). *Social support and health.* Academic Press, London.

Coyne, J.C. and Downey, G. (1991). Social factors and psychopathology: stress, social support, and coping processes. *Ann. Rev. Psychol.* **42**, 401–5.

Dalgard, O.S. and Tambs, K. (1997). Urban environment and mental health: a longitudinal study. *Br. J. Psychiat.* **171**, 530–6.

Durkheim, E. (1897). *Suicide.* Reprinted in 1951 by The Free Press, New York.

Evans, G.W. and Palsane, M.N. (1989). Residential density and psychological health: the mediating effects of social support. *J. Person. Soc. Psychol.* **6**, 994–9.

Fischer, C.S. (1982). *To dwell among friends.* University of Chicago Press, Chicago.

Fitzpatrick, R., Newman, S., Archer, R. and Shipley, M. (1991). Social support, disability and depression: a longitudinal study of rheumatoid arthritis. *Soc. Sci. Med.* **33**, 605–11.

Frasure-Smith, N. and Prince, R. (1985). The ischemic heart disease life stress monitoring program: impact and mortality. *Psychosom. Med.* **47**, 431–45.

Frasure-Smith, N., Lespérance, F., Prince, R.H., et al. (1997). Randomised trial of home-based psychosocial nursing intervention for the patients recovering from myocardial infarction. *Lancet* **350**, 473–9.

Fuhrer, R., Stansfeld, S.A., Hudry-Chemali, J. and Shipley, M.J. (1999). Gender, social relations and mental health: prospective findings from an occupational cohort (Whitehall II Study). *Soc. Sci. Med.*, **48**, 77–87.

Halpern, D.S. (1993). Minorities and mental health. *Soc. Sci. Med.* **36**, 597–607.

Halpern, D. (1995). *Mental health and the built environment. More than bricks and mortar?* Taylor and Francis, London.

Henderson, A.S. (1981). Social relationships, adversity and neurosis: an analysis of prospective observations. *Br. J. Psychiat.* **138**, 391–8.

House, J.S., Robbins, C. and Metzner, H.L. (1982). The association of social relationships and activities with mortality: prospective evidence from the Tecumseh Community Health Study. *Am. J. Epidemiol.* **116**, 123–40.

Kaplan, G.A., Salonen J.T., Cohen R.D., Brand, R.J., Syme, L. and Puska, P. (1988). Social connections and mortality from all causes and cardio-vascular disease: prospective evidence from eastern Finland. *Am. J. Epidemiol.* **128**, 370–80.

Kaplan, G.A., Wilson, T.W., Cohen, R.D., Kauhanen, J., Wu, M. and Salonen, J.T. (1994). Social functioning and overall mortality: prospective evidence from the Kuopio ischemic heart disease risk factor study. *Epidemiology* **5**, 495–500.

Kawachi, I. and Kennedy, B.P. (1997). Health and social cohesion: why care about income inequality? *BMJ* **314**, 1037–40.

Kawachi, I., Colditz, G.A., Ascherio, A., et al. (1996). A prospective study of social networks in relation to total mortality and cardiovascular disease in men in the USA. *J. Epidemiol. Commun. Hlth* **50**, 245–51.

Kessler, R.C. and McLeod, J.D. (1985). Social support and mental health in community samples. In: *Social support and health,* (ed. S. Cohen and S.L. Syme), pp. 219–40. Academic Press, Orlando, FL.

Kiecolt-Glaser, J. and Glaser, R. (1995). Psychoneuroimmunology and health consequences: data and shared mechanisms. *Psychosom. Med.* **57**, 269–74.

Lakey, B., Tardiff, R.A. and Drew, J.B. (1994). Negative social interactions: assessment and relations to social support, cognition, and psychological distress. *J. Soc. Clin. Psychol.* **13**, 63–85.

Leighton, A.H. (1965). Poverty and social change. *Sci. Am.* **212**, 21–7.

Lespérance, F., Frasure-Smith, N. and Talajic, M. (1996). Major depression before and after myocardial infarction: its nature and consequences. *Psychosom. Med.* **58**, 99–110.

Medalie, J.H. and Goldbourt, U. (1976). Angina pectoris among 10,000 men: II. Psychosocial and other risk factors as evidenced by a multivariate analysis of a five-year incidence study. *Am. J. Med.* **60**, 910–21.

Orth-Gomér, K. and Johnson, J.V. (1987). Social network interaction and mortality. A six year follow-up study of a random sample of the Swedish population. *J. Chronic Dis.* **40**, 949–57.

Oxman, T.E., Berkman, L.F., Kasl, S., Freeman, D.H. and Barrett, J. (1992). Social support and depressive symptoms in the elderly. *Am. J. Epidemiol.* **135**, 356–68.

Parkes, C.M., Benjamin, B. and Fitzgerald, R.G. (1969). Broken hearts: a statistical study of increased mortality among widowers. *BMJ* **1**, 740–3.

Paykel, E.S. (1994). Life events, social support and depression. *Acta Psychiat. Scand. Suppl.* **377**, 50–8.

Quinton, D., Rutter, M. and Liddle, C. (1984). Institutional rearing, parenting difficulties and marital support. *Psychol. Med.* **14**, 107–24.

Rael, E.G.S., Stansfeld, S.A., Shipley, M. et al. (1995). Sickness absence in the Whitehall II Study, London: the role of social support and material problems. *J. Epidemiol. Comm. Hlth* **49**, 474–81.

Reed, D., McGee D., Yano K. and Feinleib M. (1983). Social networks and coronary heart disease among Japanese men in Hawaii. *Am. J. Epidemiol.* **117**, 384–96.

Reynolds, P. and Kaplan, G.A. (1990). Social connections and risk for cancer: prospective evidence from the Alameda County Study. *Behav. Med.* **16**, 101–10.

Ruberman, W., Weinblatt, E., Goldberg, J.D. and Chaudhary, B.S. (1984). Psychosocial influences on mortality after myocardial infarction. *N. Engl. J. Med.* **311**, 552–9.

Sapolsky, R.M. (1989). Hypercortisolism among socially subordinate wild baboons originates at the CNS level. *Arch. Gen. Psychiat.* **46**, 1047–51.

Seeman, T.E. (1996). Social ties and health: the benefits of social integration. *Ann. Epidemiol.* **6**, 442–51.

Seeman, T. and McEwen, B.S. (1996). Impact of social environment characteristics on neuroendocrine regulation. *Psychosom. Med.* **58**, 459–71.

Seeman, T.E. and Syme, S.L. (1987). Social networks and coronary artery disease: a comparative analysis of network structural and support characteristics. *Psychosom. Med.* **49**, 331–40.

Seeman, T.E., Berkman, L.F., Blazer, D. and Rowe, J.W. (1994). Social ties and support as modifiers of neuroendocrine function. MacArthur Studies of Successful Aging. *Ann. Behav. Med.* **16**, 95–106.

Schoenbach, V., Kaplan, B.H., Fredman, L. and Kleinbaum, D.G. (1986). Social ties and mortality in Evans Country, Georgia. *Am. J. Epidemiol.* **123**, 577–91.

Stansfeld, S.A., Rael, E.G.A., Head, J., et al. (1997). Social support and psychiatric sickness absence: a prospective study of British civil servants. *Psychol. Med.* **27**, 35–48.

Stansfeld, A.S., Bosma, H., Hemingway, H. and Marmot, M.G. (1998*a*). Psychosocial work characteristics and social support as predictors of SF36 health functioning: the Whitehall II Study. *Psychosom. Med.* **60**, 247–55.

Stansfeld, S.A, Fuhrer, R. and Shipley, M. (1998*b*). Types of social support as predictors of psychiatric morbidity in a cohort of British Civil Servants (Whitehall II Study). *Psychol. Med.* **28**, 881–92.

Stansfield, S.A, Head, J., Marmot, M.G. (1998*c*). Explaining social class differences in depression and well being. *Social Psychiatric and Psychiatric Epidemiology*, **33**, 1–9.

Turner, R.J. and Marino, F. (1994). Social support and social structure: a descriptive epidemiology of a central stress mediator. *J. Hlth Soc. Behav.* **35**, 193–212.

Vogt, T.M., Mullooly, J.P., Ernst, D., Pope, C.R., Hollis, J.F. (1992). Social networks as predictors of ischemic heart disease, cancer, stroke and hypertension: incidence, survival and mortality. *J. Clin. Epidemiol.,* **45**, 659–66.

Welin, L., Tibblin G., Tibblin, B., et al. (1985). Prospective study of social influences on mortality: the study of men born in 1913 and 1923. *Lancet* **1**, 915–18.

Wilkinson, R.G. (1996). *Unhealthy societies: from inequality to well-being.* Routledge, London.

Williams, J.K., Vita, J.A., Manuck, S.B. (1991). Psychosocial factors impair vascular responses of coronary arteries. *Circulation* **84**, 2146–53.

Williams, R.B., Barefoot, J.C., Califf, R.M., et al. (1992). Prognostic importance of social and economic resources among medically treated patients with angiographically documented coronary artery disease. *JAMA* **267**, 520–4.

Willmott, P. (1963). *The evolution of a community.* Routledge and Keegan Paul, London.

Yancey, W. (1971). Architecture, interaction, and social control: the case of a large-scale public housing project. *Environ. Behav.* **3**, 3–21.

Acknowledgements

Dr Stansfeld's research is supported by the Department of Health in analyses of social support and mental health in the Whitehall II Study.

9 Food is a political issue

Aileen Robertson, Eric Brunner, and Aubrey Sheiham

9.1 Introduction

This chapter explores the causes of food-related ill health. We argue that these causes are located at the national and international levels, and that the 'cure' for food-related ill health at this population level must be sought by government and the food industry, as well as by individual action. The links between diet and a range of diseases are incontrovertible and there is a consensus among scientists not connected with industry (Cannon 1998). This chapter refers to some of the serious diseases and conditions associated with diet. Diseases such as coronary heart disease, diabetes, high blood pressure, cancers, dental caries, and obesity. Important conditions such as low birth-weight, which will influence the life course and diseases in later life, are related to diet. Foodborne diseases are increasing and are the most widespread health problems in Europe. An analysis of the determinants of the trends in such diseases and the international agreements to harmonize the regulations of food hygiene standards is followed by suggestions on what governments should do to improve food safety.

Then we outline the main determinants of why people eat what they do. Economics is a major determinant of availability of food. Food trade, globalization, and the growth of the agri-food sector with its greater potential for developing automated technologies have profound affects on availability of foods, employment, and sustainable agriculture. Local food production and manufacture by small firms, which are unable to compete with international corporations, is threatened in the rush towards free trade. We discuss the Common Agricultural Policy and suggest directions for its improvement.

These macro-economic changes, with their impact effects on national and local production and manufacture of foods, and the important role of advertising, have serious effects on food culture. Food choice depends a great deal on tradition and culture. Trends in breast feeding and marketing of breast-milk substitutes are analysed to illustrate the change of food culture. The new food culture is heavily influenced by supermarkets.

With the growing rates of unemployment and poverty in Europe, food poverty is of increasing concern. Indeed, the term 'food deserts', which refers to sections of cities and towns where affordable food is not available to poor people, has entered the language used in government reports.

What can be done to promote health by improving access to good food produced and sold? 'Do we want food to come to the people or the people to go to the food?' (T. Lang, personal communication). Local production and small-scale agriculture can provide a solution in some circumstances. More importantly, agreed nutrition recommendations and dietary guidelines are needed to assist policy makers and individuals to move to food-policy targets. The food chain from plough to plate needs scrutiny to ensure that healthy food choices are the easy ones and unhealthy choices more difficult.

Food is about:

(1) Politics: because global trends may threaten food security and traditional culture.

(2) Economics: because food production, processing, and marketing contribute around 30 per cent of gross domestic product (GDP) in most countries.

(3) Socio-economic change: because of urbanization and movement away from agricultural employment; these, and other factors, affect the availability of, and access to employment and consumption of food.

(4) Environment: because food is grown, transported, stored, processed, packaged, and wasted. Sustainability from the farm to the kitchen could save much energy.

(5) Science and technology: because new developments are changing the food supply. Genetically modified foods, pre-cooked meals, dietary supplements, and zero-calorie fats challenge traditional values about diet.

Food is also about health (WHO 1990). There is a global epidemic of diet-related non-communicable disease, while at the same time undernutrition afflicts some 1 billion of the world's population.

WHO's Health for All policy recommends that member states focus on the 'determinants of health', and two of the main determinants of health, and consequently ill health, are food and nutrition. Traditionally, nutrition is linked to problems such as the deficiency of nutrients, such as energy, protein, vitamins, or minerals. However, the relationship between food, nutrition, and health is more than just a matter of nutrients. Food and health are affected by globalization, macro-economics, social values, and culture.

In the future, public health needs to consider the many ways that *food determines health*, in a global perspective, rather than just considering which diseases are directly related to the nutrients that have characterized our daily diets. In Europe, for instance, where deficiency of neither protein nor energy is a public-health problem, policy makers must consider the policy implications of the lack of essential foods such as vegetables and fruits, and address some of the implications of promoting healthy and sustainable food production and consumption at local, national, and global levels.

9.2 Epidemiology of diet-related disease

Good nutrition is essential for good health. Government policies that aim to promote health therefore need to include the provision of safe, adequate, and affordable food for the whole population. Diet-related diseases can be grouped into two categories: those due to undernutrition, such as iodine deficiency, and those due to overnutrition, such as cardiovascular disease. These problems exist side by side in the WHO European Region but, as Fig. 9.1 shows, cardiovascular disease is the overwhelming cause of premature mortality, followed by cancer.

Approximately one-half of all premature deaths in Europe are diet-related and thus many are preventable. For the European Union it has been estimated that around 150 000 deaths/year could be avoided if death rates for cardio-vascular disease (CVD) and cancer were reduced, respectively, to those of France and Mediterranean countries (Abel-Smith et al. 1995). The link between the traditional Mediterranean diet and low mortality from these diseases is well known.

In addition to coronary heart disease and stroke, about one-third of cancers are diet-related (Anonymous 1997*b*). Research is continuing in order to clarify

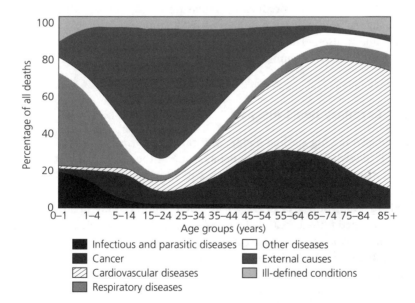

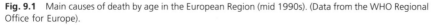

Fig. 9.1 Main causes of death by age in the European Region (mid 1990s). (Data from the WHO Regional Office for Europe).

the links between diet and common cancers. Epidemiology has shown dietary contributions to risks of diabetes, gallstones, dental caries, some gastro-intestinal disorders, and osteoporosis. The recent large rise in prevalence of obesity in many countries is a further indication that the modern diet is less than optimal. Obesity is related to many of the diseases listed above, and to diabetes in particular.

There are several distinctive features of the modern food supply which lead to high rates of CVD, cancer, and other non-communicable diseases. First, there has been rapid industrialization of agriculture. This has increased food security and helped to reduce undernutrition and periodic famine. Childhood growth and nutritional status has generally improved and, as a result, resistance to infectious disease is greater. Secondly, modern production has increased the availability of refined, energy-dense foods rich in animal fat and sugars, but which may be lacking in dietary fibre, vitamins, and minerals. Third, food retailing and marketing tend to encourage the purchase of certain processed and long shelf-life foods. Together, these developments have promoted food habits that have undesir-able health effects.

Dietary and nutritional recommendations at national and international level aim to improve public health (WHO 1990; Cannon 1998). The recom-mendations are based on evidence that alterations in diet will help to prevent the most important health problems in developed countries, namely CVD and cancer. Broadly similar changes in diet are required to prevent most nutrition related diseases, with an emphasis on lowering intakes of saturated fatty acids (by reducing animal and dairy fat intake), salt, and refined sugars, and increasing intakes of fresh fruit and vegetables, unrefined cereals, and pulses. The latter changes are intended to raise intakes of antioxidants, many vitamins, and dietary fibre.

9.2.1 Coronary heart disease

The evidence linking specific dietary saturated and *trans* fatty acids to heart disease is overwhelming. A new understanding of the mechanisms that under-lie heart disease highlights the importance of vitamins and flavonoids found in vegetables and fruit in minimizing heart disease by several mechanisms (Steinberg 1992; Bobak et al. 1998). A seven-country study highlighted that a high saturated fat/red meat diet, combined with low vegetable consumption, contributes to the cause of heart disease (Keys 1970).

Heart disease accounts for some 1.4 million deaths in EU each year (out of a population of 340 million). In the UK, 2 million people have evidence of heart disease and 66 million working days are lost each year through heart disease, at a cost of around £1420 million to health services and £3 billion in lost production (Abel-Smith et al. 1995).

9.2.2 Cerebrovascular disease

The incidence of stroke is especially high in the countries of central and eastern Europe (CCEE) and the newly independent states of Europe (NIS) and the risk is strongly linked to high blood pressure, obesity, and excess salt consumption. Disability following strokes is a major burden on families and health services.

9.2.3 Non-insulin-dependent diabetes mellitus

Over 1 per cent of the European population has diabetes, with prevalence increasing markedly in older age groups. Diabetes accelerates coronary heart disease and peripheral vascular disease and is closely related to weight gain in adult life. During the war in Sarajevo (1992–95), probably due to substantial weight loss, WHO observed a 30 per cent reduction in the need for oral hypoglycaemic agents and insulin, and an improvement in diabetic control (Kulenovic et al. 1996).

9.2.4 High blood pressure

Raised blood pressure is caused mainly by obesity and high salt intake. During the war in Sarajevo, WHO observed practically no need for hypotensive medication since, in most diabetics, blood pressure had returned to normal, most probably due to major dietary changes during the war (Kulenovic et al. 1996).

9.2.5 Cancers

Estimates suggest that 30–40 per cent of cancers are preventable by feasible dietary means. Relatively new data provide strong support for a protective role of vegetables and fruit with fibre-containing starchy foods. Smokers who have a particularly poor diet, limited in vegetables and fruit, are at higher risk of cancer than smokers consuming high levels of vegetables and fruit (Anonymous 1997*b*).

9.2.6 Overweight and obesity

Overweight affects around half of the middle-aged adults in the whole European Region, with the highest prevalence in NIS. A high-fat, energy-dense diet is the main cause of this pan-European problem, together with reduced levels of physical activity. In European countries, around 8 per cent of total health service costs have been estimated to be spent on the effects of obesity, as much as health programmes for cancer and AIDS.

While being mildly overweight is not a significant health problem, obesity (body mass index (BMI) greater than 30) does pose a risk to health; for example, by raising blood pressure and risk of stroke. The prevalence of obesity ranges from around 8 per cent in men to 22 per cent in women in the eastern parts of the region (Table 9.1).

The location of body fat is also an important factor in health risks, particularly for coronary heart disease. Abdominal fat mass can vary dramatically within a narrow range of total body fat or BMI. Excess fat in the abdomen (stomach area) is a greater risk than excess fat on the hips and thighs. Indeed, men have, on average, twice the amount of abdominal fat than that which is generally found in pre-menopausal women (Larsson et al. 1992). Extra fat in the abdomen is linked to high blood pressure, diabetes, early heart disease, and certain types of cancer, and in most surveys conducted in western Europe and North America, this body fat pattern is linked with lower social position (Brunner 1997; Brunner et al. 1998).

9.2.7 Dental caries

Dental caries is the most common disease in industrialized countries. In the UK dental disease is the fifth most expensive disease to treat, more expensive than all neoplasms and genitourinary diseases. The data linking sugar, and in particular sucrose, intake to the occurrence of dental caries is unequivocal. Dental caries is a sugar-induced disease. The acids formed by the degeneration of sugars demineralize teeth.

Table 9.1
Mean body mass index and percentage of obese men and women in Russia, the Baltic countries, Kazakstan, England, Finland and the Netherlands

Country	BMI, males		BMI, females	
	Mean BMI	Proportion obese (BMI >30)	Mean BMI	Proportion obese (BMI >30)
Russia[a]	24.9	8.5	26.9	22
Lithuania[b]	25.8	11	25.9	18
Latvia[b]	25.5	9.5	25.8	17
Estonia[b]	25.1	8	23.3	8
Kazakstan[c]	24.2	8	25.8	20
Finland[d]	25.4	11	24.1	10
The Netherlands[d]	25.7	12	24.8	14
England[e]	26.3	16	26	18

[a] Russian longtitudinal monitoring survey (1993);
[b] Baltic National surveys (1997), co-ordinated by WHO;
[c] UNDP and Institute of Nutrition Kazakstan (1996);
[d] National surveys carried out during the nineties;
[e] Health Survey for England (1998).

The justification for a reduction of sugar, and in particular sucrose, consumption is that there is considerable evidence that reducing the sugar level of the diet would be beneficial, and it is most unlikely that lowering the sugar content of the diet to below 10 per cent of total energy from sugars would be harmful.

9.2.8 Socio-economic status

Social class differences in health are seen at all ages, with lower socio-economic groups having greater incidence of premature and low birthweight babies, heart disease, stroke, and some cancers in adults. Risk factors, including lack of breast feeding, smoking, physical inactivity, overweight and central obesity, hypertension, and poor diet, are clustered in the lower socio-economic groups. The diet of low-income groups in the UK provides low-cost energy from foods such as meat products but lacks vegetables and fruit. This type of diet is lower in essential nutrients such as calcium, iron, magnesium, folate, and vitamin C. Although the exact contribution of diet to the generation of inequalities in health is uncertain, there is scope for substantial health gain if a diet rich in unrefined cereals, vegetables, fruit, fish, and quality vegetable oils could be more accessible to poor people (Davey Smith et al. 1997; James et al. 1997).

9.2.9 Health of older people

Older people have high levels of cardiovascular disease, diabetes, cancers, osteoporosis, arthritis, and dental problems. High levels of physical inactivity lead to low food intake and therefore constipation from inadequate fibre intake. In addition, the elderly are at risk of micronutrient deficiency if their diets lack vegetables and fruit.

By the year 2020 one-fifth of the EU population, some 50 million, will be over 65 years old. Nearly 10 per cent of those over 65 need long-term care or regular support: in the UK, 47 per cent of health expenditure is currently on those over 65. Prevention of disease and promotion of well-being through nutrition policies is particularly important in this age group.

9.2.10 Infant and child health

Poor infant feeding practices and their consequences are one of the world's major problems and a serious obstacle to social and economic development. Being to a great extent a man-made problem, it must be considered a reproach to our science and technology and our social and economic structures, and a blot on our so-called development achievements.

(WHO and UNICEF statement on infant health in 1979).

High levels of infant and young child mortality (Fig. 9.2) are due to increased risk of infection combined with reduced immunity. Increased levels of exclusive breast feeding until around 6 months, timely introduction of appropriate complementary foods, and changes in the parts of the health sector dealing with ante- and postnatal care could significantly improve the health and well-being of infants and their mothers.

The extent to which adult health is determined by nutritional factors *in utero* and in infancy has been the subject of much debate since Barker observed that low birthweight and weight at 1 year are associated with adult disease (Barker 1993). One of the explanations for these findings is that nutritional deficiencies at critical periods of fetal and infant growth may induce organ impairment and permanent changes in physiological function.

A low birthweight baby has an increased risk of early death and, if the baby survives, an increased risk of suffering disability and disease during childhood and adult life. The growing fetus receives nutrients from the mother – either from her dietary intake or from her body store. Although not the only risk factor, poor maternal nutrition can impair fetal development, increase maternal mortality, and retard growth in infancy.

If the mother has a history of poor nutrition, her nutrient stores will be low, reducing the ability of the fetus to gain adequate access to nutrients. If the

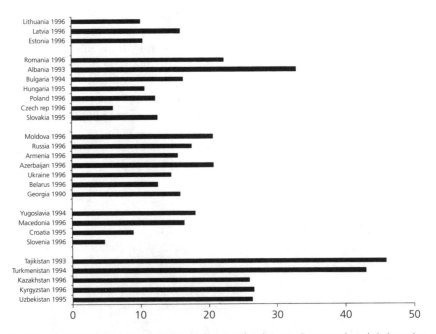

Fig. 9.2 Infant mortality rates per 1000 live births, central and eastern Europe and newly independent states. The Health for All European target is that 10–20 deaths/1000 should be reduced to less than 10, and greater than 20 deaths/1000 should be reduced to 15.

mother's diet during pregnancy is also nutrient deficient, this will further increase the risk of inadequate nutrition for the growing fetus. There is a high requirement for the nutrients essential for body growth from the time of conception, especially among vulnerable women who are at higher risk because of poor socio-economic circumstances or medical conditions.

It is difficult to overstate the impact of poor nutrition before and during pregnancy. Failure to provide a nutritionally adequate diet has both social and economic consequences for both parents, babies, and society as a whole. Yet, research over many decades demonstrates that most countries do not invest sufficiently in nutrition to ensure infant and child health of the next generation.

Infant mortality in the European Region is highest in the Central Asian Republics (Fig. 9.2), where infants experience upper respiratory tract infections, diarrhoeal diseases, vaccine-preventable diseases such as tuberculosis, and nutritional deficiencies. Seven out of 10 child deaths are due to these illnesses and often to a combination of them. Among children under 5 years of age, respiratory infection, including pneumonia, is responsible for between one-third and a half of infant deaths. In Kazakstan, diarrhoea and respiratory infection, including flu and pneumonia, are responsible for some 40 per cent of the mortality in children under 5 years old.

The highest mortality risks are associated with diarrhoea, respiratory infection, and other infections when infants are not exclusively breast fed (Fig. 9.3). Only 1 per cent of exclusively breast-fed infants had diarrhoea, compared with 17 per cent of bottle-fed infants (Popkin et al. 1990). Similarly, considering infants aged from 8 days to 12 months in Brazil, the breast-fed infants had only a 1 per cent risk of dying from pneumonia, compared with a 4 per cent risk in bottle-fed infants (Victora et al. 1997). Wheezing, vomiting, runny nose, colic and abdominal pain, asthma, constipation, eczema, and rashes are all associated with lack of breast feeding.

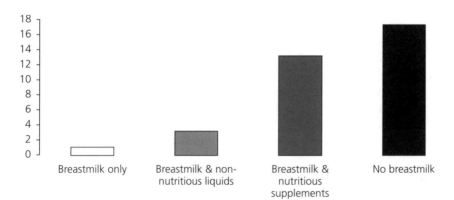

Fig. 9.3 Risk of diarrhoea by feeding method, Philippines, infants aged 0–2 months (from Popkin et al. 1990).

In western Europe, breast feeding for 13 weeks reduces the incidence of gastrointestinal and respiratory illness during the first year of life (Howie et al. 1990). Exclusive breast feeding, for at least 15 weeks, is associated with a significant reduction in respiratory illness (17 per cent compared with 32 per cent in bottle-fed infants), less risk of high blood pressure, childhood obesity, and wheezing at the age of 7 years. The associations showed the protective dose response effect of the period of exclusive breast feeding (Wilson et al. 1998).

In the UK, 64 per cent of infants are breast fed initially, with only 19 per cent still being breast fed at 4 months of age. Additionally, 90 per cent of infants start eating solid foods before the age of four months. With this large difference between recommendation and practice, robust evidence is needed to support the implementation of successful breast-feeding policies. Fortunately, many policies are now effective. In Scotland, breast-feeding rates have increased from 36 per cent in 1990 to 42 per cent in 1997 at around the seventh day after birth.

In Scandinavian countries, especially Norway and Sweden, rates of breast feeding are very high over 80 per cent at 3 months. Although levels seem very high in other countries, such as Bosnia, infants are not usually exclusively breast fed. There is still a widespread and mistaken belief by both health professionals and the public that stress reduces the ability to breast feed. There is also a mistaken belief that the administration of water, tea, glucose solutions, and milk-based formulas is needed during the early months of life.

9.2.11 Micronutrient deficiency

Two major nutritional problems in the European region are iodine deficiency disorders (IDD) and anaemia (which may, be related to dietary deficiency of micronutrients, such as iron and folate). More investigations need to be carried out into the causes of the low levels of haemoglobin found in some parts of the region.

IDD is the major cause of preventable mental retardation and it is estimated that around 16 per cent of the European population are affected. Iodine deficiency is prevalent throughout Europe and only six countries have no IDD (Finland, Iceland, Norway, Sweden, Switzerland, and the UK). Iodine deficiency is re-emerging in some countries in Europe, and in countries such as Albania, Tajikistan, and Uzebekistan severe deficiency exists. In most other countries mild to moderate forms of iodine deficiency exist and it is especially important that people living in the vicinity of nuclear reactors, such as Chernobyl, are fully protected by being saturated with iodine in case of nuclear fall-outs.

9.2.12 Food safety

Foodborne diseases are among the most widespread health problems in Europe. In rich and poor countries alike they impose substantial health burdens, ranging in severity from mild indispositions to fatal illnesses. The emergence of new foodborne diseases is an ominous trend and appears to be exacerbated by globalization and increased industrialization of the food industry.

There is an increase in foodborne diseases in many countries and the emergence of newly identified pathogens, such as *Salmonella* DT 104, *Campylobacter jejuni, Listeria monocytogenes, Escherichia coli* 157: H7, *Aeromonas hydrophila, Vibrio cholerae* 0139, *Cryptosporidium,* and bovine spongiform encephalopathy (BSE), has hit industrialized countries. In 1995 it was estimated that each year around 130 million Europeans (15 per cent of the total population of the WHO European Region) are affected by episodes of foodborne diseases.

Salmonella outbreaks are one of the main causes of epidemics in Europe. The incidence rates of salmonellosis vary tremendously, but in most countries the incidence in 1992 exceeded the figures in 1985, with the highest increases in Austria, Germany, the Czech Republic, Denmark, and the UK. In Denmark there was a ten fold increase in the number of registered cases infected with salmonella over the past 20 years: from around 500 people in the 1950s and 1970s to 5000 in 1997. Clearly, this is not an acceptable situation when neighbouring countries such as Sweden have food which is practically free of salmonella.

The causes of the increased incidence are not always well understood, especially in western parts of the region. Changes in food production since the war has meant that the food chain is longer than before. Food is now subjected to a variety of processes which make it safer (e.g. pasteurization) but paradoxically more vulnerable to bacteria, toxins, and contamination: in 1989 there was a food scare after it emerged that apples were commonly sprayed with the Alar, a fungicide thought to cause cancer; in 1998 over 2 million cans of fizzy soft drinks were recalled after traces of cancer-causing benzene were found in carbon dioxide supplies. Changes in population habits, such as the increased consumption of meals outside the home, as well as the extent of national and international trade in food have made foodborne disease an important health issue.

Global trade will make it more difficult to respond to and contain food-borne diseases within national borders. Traditional food control systems may no longer be adequate to respond to these new and dynamic situations. In addition, chemical contamination, toxic materials, pesticides, veterinary drugs, and other agrochemicals require constant surveillance to ensure their safe use. The use of food additives can improve the quality of the food supply but appropriate controls are necessary to ensure their proper use, and there is increasing consumer concern about antibiotic resistance, genetically modified foods, and excessive use of weed killers.

More and more food is moving across country borders due to a combination of social, economic, and technological trends. The growth rates of food movement are phenomenal. For example, Chile and Thailand exported 36 times and 1178 per cent more food, respectively, in 1990 than in 1970 (FAO 1997). On the import side, Spain's imports increased by 947 per cent and France imported 717 per cent more food over the same period. Yet these figures could have been even greater if imports had not been rejected because they did not conform to the food standards of the recipient country. However, pressure from global trade authorities is growing to abolish or harmonize national standards, which are seen as barriers to trade.

The FAO/WHO Codex Alimentarius Commission (Codex) was established in 1962 to protect the health of the consumer and, at the same time, to ensure fair practices in food trade. Member states have been asked to accept the standards elaborated by Codex, but it was left to governments to decide whether or not they will implement them. In 1995, the World Trade Organization (WTO) was established and at the same time countries agreed, for the first time, to abolish national regulations and reduce tariff barriers for many food products in order to facilitate the free trade in food commodities. Economists believe that these national regulations and barriers to trade undermine the promotion of international trade, especially if applied in an arbitrary or discriminatory way.

To address some of these contradictions and lack of harmonization, the WTO Agreement on the Application of Sanitary and Phytosanitary Measures (SPS Agreement) was drawn up by Codex to ensure that countries apply measures to protect human and animal health (sanitary measures) and plant health (phytosanitary measures). The SPS Agreement incorporates the safety aspects of foods being traded. Another important standard is the Agreement on Technical Barriers to Trade (TBT Agreement). This complements the SPS Agreement since it covers technical requirements and standards, such as labelling, that are not covered in the SPS Agreement. Many countries will have to strengthen their national food control systems in order to comply with the provisions of the Codex agreements.

9.3　Strategies for prevention

9.3.1　High risk or whole population?

Despite advances in medicine, many cancers remain incurable and heart disease continues to kill many adults prematurely. Around one-half of heart attack victims have no warning symptoms, and half of these die before reaching hospital. Prevention is therefore the only effective way to tackle these problems. The late Geoffrey Rose highlighted the need to consider the population as a whole when devising prevention strategies (Rose 1992). While it might seem logical to identify the individuals most likely to develop disease, and to give them special treatment, he demonstrated that such a 'high-risk' approach cannot succeed.

The identification of individuals at high disease risk through screening programmes can only be useful if certain criteria are met. Tests must be sensitive and specific, meaning that the majority of individuals who would develop the disease, and those who will not, must be correctly identified. Effective treatment must be available for those shown to be at high risk. The screening programmes must reach the whole population. Taking each of these points in turn, it is evident that a high-risk approach will often be inferior to a whole-population approach. Screening tests of sufficient accuracy to make a substantial impact on death rates from cancers, apart from those of the cervix and, arguably, the breast, do not exist.

For heart disease, a high blood cholesterol level does identify individuals at highest risk, but epidemiology has shown that heart disease risk, and the distribution of blood cholesterol levels, is raised throughout the populations of industrialized countries. Cholesterol tests thus cannot identify the majority of those who will die of the disease. For the minority, effective cholesterol-lowering treatment has recently become available: the statin drugs lower blood cholesterol by some 20 per cent, and trials show a dramatic reduction in heart attacks as a result. However, statins are costly, and hundreds of millions of dollars would be added to national drugs bills if commonly used. Finally, universal screening is expensive and probably not feasible in many countries, even if tests and treatments were available.

Whole-population or 'mass intervention' policies therefore can utilize scarce resources to maximum benefit. Whole-population food and nutrition polices are justified in most of Europe because heart disease and cancer rates are high in comparison to other countries and because public-health gains will be the largest if the whole population improves its diet. In southern Europe and developing countries such policies could prevent the emergence of an epidemic of diet-related disease, by avoiding the structural problems now being tackled in northern countries.

9.3.2 Health education: necessary but not sufficient

It is sometimes assumed that, just by providing people with information, individuals will be able to change their unhealthy life style. Although it is important to increase knowledge about health in the general population, information and health education alone often are not enough to change behaviour. Smoking rates, for example, have declined faster in higher socio-economic groups in many countries, and vulnerable groups have increased their smoking. Social and personal experience tend to have a more powerful influence on health-related behaviour than health education messages. Thus, efforts to provide information to the individual need to be accompanied by appropriate policy and environmental changes.

Messages aimed at the individual may have an indirect impact on public health, by maintaining support for public-health policies. For example, health education and information distributed through the mass media can be a strong advocacy tool and can help to support social and public policy initiatives. Understanding of health can be strengthened through education, but ultimately the environment where people live and work can have a much greater influence on encouraging change to healthy life styles. Changes in our social, cultural, living, and work environments are needed in order to make the healthy choices the easiest choices.

If social exclusion is to be reduced and equity improved, new approaches have to found. One approach that appears to hold promise involves the participation of the community in identifying and solving their own problems. Rather than just providing information and then blaming the individual if he or she does not change, permanent, large-scale behavioural change is best achieved by changing community policies. The emphasis should be on community mobilization and organization. Comprehensive community programmes, such as the North Karelia project (1995), can have a positive effect on health choices, including the use of alcohol, tobacco, healthy eating, and physical activity. Such programmes lead to favourable changes in the health of the whole population.

9.4 Food industrialization and food poverty

9.4.1 Food trade

Increasing affluence in many areas, including Europe, North America, and the Far East, has led to the market place becoming both more competitive and more global. At the same time, there have been moves to reduce barriers to trade by harmonization of many regulations, including those relating to food. These efforts have tended to develop on a regional basis, with the EU representing one example. The creation of the WTO signals the drive toward market harmonization at the global level.

The implications of globalization for the food trade and health are beginning to be understood. Globalization is leading to complex interdependence of economies across national borders, including the food sector. For example, foreign and multinational firms dominated a list of the 10 largest operators in the Hungarian agri-food sector in 1997. Only two Hungarian firms appeared in the list, both of which were meat product producers, and the rest were international corporations based outside Hungary. One of the consequences is that events, decisions, and activities in one part of the world can have a significant impact on communities in a distant part of the globe, potentially taking control out of the hands of the local population.

Globalization gives rise to increasing convergence of structures and attitudes between countries. The market economy and consumerism are becoming the norm. Furthermore, the integration of political, economic, and social activities across borders is accelerating, with increased free trade, international financial markets, and transnational corporations. The food industry, as a key part of the manufacturing and service sectors, is greatly influenced by these global economic trends and the international trade alliances which have been formed.

A necessary prerequisite of globalization is the development of technology and quality control systems, which are usually highly automated and expensive. These systems lead to increased research and development costs for food firms in order to compete globally. Therefore, economic growth will only be achieved by those firms, usually the transnational corporations, who can afford to invest in globalized standardization.

Such companies, armed with the technological capability and quality certificates, will be highly competitive in the global market. In contrast, small firms with weak technological capabilities will be disadvantaged and unable to compete. The danger is that regulations will become so complex that only large producers and retailers will be successful, and small enterprises will be forced out of business. The battle for the world market looks increasingly fierce and it seems that only very large-scale businesses will be able to afford to improve product quality and consistently satisfy the demand for competitively priced food.

In theory, transnational food trade could improve national food control and so improve public-health protection. However, food trade may also have an adverse impact on public health, especially if countries become largely dependent on imported food and lose their ability to produce food locally. One of the authors (AR) witnessed this phenomenon during the autumn of 1998, after economic collapse in Russia. Many of the food shops and supermarkets were empty in cities in north-western Russia and east of the Ural mountains because importers were no longer importing food to Russia. At the same time, local producers were going out of business because of the break down of the economic infrastructure. The local foods which were for sale were not always being sold in a safe way. For example, unpasteurized milk was being sold directly to the public on street corners from the large milk tankers in which the milk had been collected from the farm. Policy makers should consider how to promote safe local food production, since this will provide a vital insurance policy against any potential adverse effects of globalization and economic collapse.

An issue for many countries will be how to protect their national and local food products, and the associated employment, without interfering with free trade. For example EU agriculture is still subsidized and so non-EU countries, who comply with the rules of free trade, may be extremely vulnerable to cheap, imported food from the EU. For example, in the Czech Republic in 1997, half the apples consumed by the Czechs were imports from the EU. As a result a very high proportion of Czech-grown apples were destroyed or sold for apple juice at low prices. In order to protect local producers the Czech government introduced a levy of 95 per cent on imported apples above a quota of 24 000 tons a year. The EU then threatened to suspend preferential tariffs on meat, poultry, and fruit juice from the Czech Republic, and so in May 1998 the Czech Republic decided to abolish the quota on EU apples.

Similarly, around half of the chickens and 30 per cent of meat consumed in the Russian Federation is imported (Economic Research Service 1997; personal communication, Russian Institute of Nutrition). Imports are essential during times of hardship and economic transition, but in the long term food and agricultural polices should promote sustainable local production. Russian meat producers have called for urgent measures to protect their market, because in the period from January 1997 to January 1998 all imported goods into Russia increased by 25 per cent whereas agricultural imports increased by 43 per cent.

9.4.2 Infant health, breast feeding, and marketing of breast-milk substitutes

While the health service in Kazakstan is desperately trying to promote breast feeding and discourage bottle feeding, a large infant food company is planning to build a new factory. The International Code of Marketing of Breast Milk Substitutes (1981) (Box 9.1) and subsequent resolutions of the World Health Assembly (the policy-setting body of WHO) were established to try to counteract the harmful affects of aggressive marketing and to protect the practice of breast feeding.

Most WHO member states have agreed to adopt the international code as national legislation. In 1991, the Commission of the European Communities adopted Directive 91/321/EEC. The directive addresses only the marketing of infant formulae and follow-up milks, while the code covers all breast-milk substitutes, including feeding bottles and teats, and has stricter marketing and labelling provisions. By June 1994, all EU countries should have incorporated the directive into national legislation. Since they are also WHO member states, they should consider harmonizing this legislation with the code and subsequent resolutions, since this would not contravene the European rules.

A study carried out recently in four countries, (Taylor 1998) including Poland, showed that companies that produce breast-milk substitutes continue to violate the international code. Violations of the code were detected in all of the countries studied. Across the four countries, 8–50 per cent of health facilities had received free samples which were not being used for research or professional evaluation, and 2–18 per cent of health workers had received gifts from companies involved in the manufacturing or distribution of breast-milk substitutes. Information that violated the code had been received by 15–56 per cent of health facilities.

Policy makers can be reassured that passing a law based on the code will have economic benefits for households, employers, and the country: savings in foreign exchange on the purchase and distribution of commercial breast-milk substitute, savings on health care from preventable acute and chronic illness in infants, and savings in ecological damage avoided by reduced production, distribution, and disposal of breast-milk substitute containers and bottles.

In 1997 families from the former Yugoslavia spent approximately 70 per cent of their income on the purchase of breast-milk substitutes in the first 6 months if they did not breast feed. The same survey showed that only 30 per cent of the infants were breast fed at 4 months. If this figure could be increased to 70 per cent it was calculated that almost US$450 million could be saved, while 99 000 respiratory infections and 33 000 ear infections could be averted each year. Can we afford that infants pay such a high price to be bottle fed?

WHO estimates that reversing the decline in breast feeding could save the lives of 1.5 million infants every year, yet some baby food companies continue to market artificial foods in ways that undermine breast feeding. Policy makers should strive to incorporate all the articles of the code and subsequent resolutions into national legislation. Enforcement of the law should be carried out with the help of regular monitoring and legal action when violations are found.

9.4.3 Common Agricultural Policy

After the Second World War the main aim in Europe was to increase the supply of food, especially animal products, e.g. meat and milk. This was

---

Box 9.1 **Summary of the International Code**

1. No advertising of any breast-milk substitutes to the public.
2. No free samples to mothers.
3. No promotion of products in healthcare facilities, including no free samples.
4. No company mothercraft nurses or nutritionists to advise or teach.
5. No gifts or personal samples to health workers.
6. No words or pictures idealizing artificial feeding, including pictures of infants, on the labels of products.
7. Information to health workers should be scientific and factual.
8. All information on artificial infant feeding, including labels, should explain the benefits of breast feeding and the costs and hazards associated with artificial feeding.
9. Unsuitable products, e.g. sweetened condensed milk, should not be promoted for babies.
10. All products should be of a high quality and take account of the climatic and storage conditions of the country where they are used.

achieved through the development of the Common Agricultural Policy (CAP) which provides subsidies to farmers in Europe. Many economists are concerned about the impact when more countries join the EU because the CAP is not sustainable. The CAP spends almost half the EU budget, and in 1995 it cost EU taxpayers 39 billion ECU. Only 20 per cent of the farmers get the majority (80 per cent) of the EU subsidies, which means that the rich farmers get richer and the majority, the small, less wealthy farmers, are forced out of business. This has already happened in western Europe, with only around 2 per cent of the population in some EU countries employed in agriculture. It could be a disaster for both rural and urban health if countries in central and eastern Europe went down the same path as EU countries.

This post-war food policy was in some ways too successful, and for the past 25 years Europe has had surplus stocks of butter, meat, and milk.

Lessons learned over the past decades suggest that future food policies should ensure that cereal and potato production is geared to supply more than 50 per cent of energy requirements, and that vegetable (in addition to potatoes) and fruit production should be geared to supply *more than* 400 g/day/person (WHO 1990). Without a food policy that guarantees food security in the form of cereals, potatoes, vegetables, and fruit, it is difficult to see how targets for a healthy diet can be achieved (WHO 1990).

CAP subsidies result in the production of fruits which either are not harvested or are destroyed by dumping in massive pits. From 1992 to 1994 almost 50 per cent of French apples, Spanish and Greek oranges, plus nearly all Spanish lemons were destroyed. Of the Italian and Dutch tomato crops, 60 and 20 per cent, respectively, were destroyed. This waste of resources and destruction of food is irrational, not only because the amount of vegetables and fruit available in some European countries is insufficient to meet the WHO dietary recommendations (Fig. 9.4), but also because the damage to the environment and producer communities is devastating.

9.4.4 Food trends within Europe

Loss of food culture

Food choice depends a great deal on tradition and culture. Traditionally 'agri-culture' was a major economic activity as well as the main source of food. Since the 1950s food productivity has been switching to 'agri-business'. During the twenty-first century it is likely that we will see yet another food industrial revolution as biotechnology develops. Most people eat for enjoyment, and satisfy their hunger by eating the foods they like and that are available at accessible prices. Family and friends play a major role in the way people select food and plan meals. However, advertising and the media are playing an increasingly dominant role, especially in relation to children.

The role of children as opinion leaders, in influencing what their families

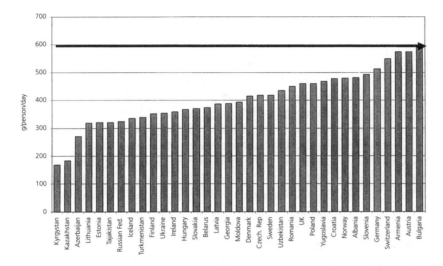

Fig. 9.4 Vegetable and fruit availability in the WHO European Region. Only France, the Netherlands, Spain, Bel-Luz, Malta, Portugal, Italy, Israel, Turkey, and Greece have more than 600 g/day/person of vegetables and fruit available (data not shown) to ensure consumption of the recommended 400 g/day/ person (assuming $\frac{1}{3}$ is wasted). (Source: FAOSTAT 1994.)

buy, should not be underestimated. Unfortunately much of the marketing aimed at young people is for sweets, snack items, convenience and fast foods, and very little is spent on promoting consumption of vegetables and fruits. International comparative surveys, such as *A spoonful of sugar, television advertising aimed at children*, carried out by Consumers International in 1996, confirm this. Concern was expressed about the negative effect of aggressive advertising of foods high in fat, sugar, and/or salt in contrast to very few adverts promoting vegetables and fruit. There was also concern about the marketing techniques, such as the use of promotional gifts, cartoon characters, and personalities as well as sponsorship, teleshopping, and premium-rate phone services targeting children. (Consumers International 1996). Their research showed that the highest level of food advertising was in Australia where, on average, there were 29 television adverts per hour: more than double that found in many European countries and up to 15 times more than in Sweden and Norway, countries with the least advertising.

Sweden and Norway do not permit any advertising on national television to be directed towards children under 12 years old, and no advertising at all is allowed during children's programmes. However, in 1997 the European Court ruled that Sweden could not block commercials broadcast from other EU member states. This ruling was made despite the view of most consumer organizations that international broadcasters should be obliged by law to observe the national advertising rules of the receiving state.

In Scotland, over £80 million was spent on advertising chocolates in 1991, compared with a meagre £1 million advertising vegetables. There is no doubt that it pays the food industry to advertise. Most probably as a result of advertising, sales of soft drinks have escalated in central and eastern Europe: between 1992 and 1996 sales increased by 112 per cent on average, and 200 per cent in Poland. The average consumption of soft drinks in CCEE is now higher than the average in EU countries and appears to be increasing.

Brand recognition is one of the main aims of companies' marketing strategies. In a 1994 survey carried out in China, a well-known US soft-drink manufacturer was recognized by two-thirds of the population, making it the second best-known brand name in China. Companies spend huge amounts on promoting their brand name, and of the 15 branded food products with the highest sales in the UK in 1996–97 (Table 9.2), six were soft drinks and three were chocolate brands. These nine brands were promoted with an advertising budget of around £60 million (US$90 million), compared to the budget of the Health Education Authority for promoting better diets of less than £1 million.

Since the collapse of communism, advertising is a new phenomenon in CCEE. Whereas western Europe is flooded by advertising on the media, newspapers, and special mailings, a survey published in the *Central European Economical Review* of the *Wall Street Journal Europe* showed that around half of the people in Hungary, Slovakia, the Czech Republic, and Poland said that they enjoyed receiving mailed adverts in 1997. The impact of advertising is great because not only do people enjoy receiving it, but in addition many also believe that advertised products are superior to those that are not advertised.

Table 9.2
The 15 top-selling food brands in the UK, 1996–7 (source: *Food Magazine* (1998) Vol. 42, pp. 14–15, Food Commission, London)

Brand	Sales (£ millions)	Advertising (£ millions)
Coca-Cola	542	26.0
Walkers crisps	385	7.0
Pepsi	180	8.6
Robinsons drinks	160	3.3
KitKat chocolate	140	4.7
Muller yogurt	135	5.0
Ribena	130	0.9
Flora	125	5.2
Mars Bar	120	1.4
Heinz soup	115	0.3
Anchor butter	115	5.3
Lucozade	105	7.0
Tango drink	100	6.6
Cadbury's chocolate	100	0.3
Kellog's Corn Flakes	95	11.7

If locally produced foods, such as vegetables and fruits, are not advertised, their future market potential could be threatened.

The lesson here is that marketing messages do influence purchasing behaviour and that marketing messages overwhelm health messages if the latter are not strongly promoted. Health messages and marketing messages both influence buying patterns. When health messages act alone, for example the encouragement to drink lower-fat milk, then the message seems to influence purchasers. In order to ensure that health takes higher priority, health messages, for example to promote fruit and vegetable consumption, need to be strengthened relative to the contrary marketing messages – either by increasing the budget for health education or by restricting the activities of the relevant commercial interests.

New food culture

Physical access to food has altered dramatically in developed countries in recent years. A diminishing proportion of people know how to grow food. Small shops in many cities have closed or have limited their product range to non-perishable, long shelf-life items. In the UK, the number of local food shops has fallen dramatically and 44 000 small shops, out of the 60 000 in 1950, had closed down by 1990. If this trend spreads to other countries, it could have a major negative impact on health.

Analysts predict an expansion of supermarkets and hypermarkets (very large complexes which contain supermarkets and are usually situated in outer-city areas surrounded by large car parks) in CCEE at a pace not seen before. Hungary had around 5000 super- and hypermarkets in 1997 and in Poland the number of hypermarkets was predicted to rise from only seven in 1995, to 70 in the year 2000. Major food retailers are dictating what foods should be produced. For example, supermarkets buy more than 70 per cent of the vegetables and fruit produced in the UK.

Alternative markets, such as local greengrocers, are disappearing because they cannot compete. For example, large retail stores have far stricter criteria than either the EU or governmental definitions of top-class vegetables and fruit. If growers cannot meet the rigorous standards demanded by super-markets for width, shape, and colour, the retailers go to other countries to buy fruit that conforms to their standards. One supermarket demands that Cox apples measure 60–90 mm across and be up to 30 per cent red. Another wants strawberries to be perfectly red and have a circumference of 22 mm, despite the fact that there is nothing wrong with a fruit or vegetable that is not symmetrical. The health value and taste is just the same, but nevertheless hundreds of tonnes of non-standard fruits and vegetables are destroyed, causing social, environmental, and economic havoc. Retailers claim they are responding to consumer demand.

Retailers have recently started to support the survival of local shops. In the

UK, for example, rural shops now have the right to buy supermarket own-brand products at favourable prices in order to re-sell them. This initiative comes after years of decline of the village shop, which is now extinct in 40 per cent of English parishes. If vulnerable groups do not have land or are unable to grow food, easy access to nearby shops or home delivery services at affordable prices is essential to ensure that healthy choices are not only possible but easy.

9.4.5 Food poverty

The diets of low-income groups are likely to be inadequate. In the UK such diets are characterized by low fruit, vegetable, and fish consumption. Nutrient intakes are consequently low in dietary fibre, antioxidant and other vitamins, folate, iron, and essential fatty acids (Dowler and Dobson 1997).

Information on the extent of food poverty in Europe is scarce. Using the EU definition of general poverty (less than 50 per cent of average income) it is evident that some 57 million individuals, including 13 million children, lived below the poverty line in 1993 in the EU's 12 member states (Lang 1998). The Eurostat survey found that some 37 per cent of poor households could not manage financially, 17 per cent could not afford meat or fish every second day, and one-third could not afford to have friends or family for a drink or a meal at least once per month. National disparities in the extent of poverty were substantial. The UK had the highest proportion of children in poverty (32 per cent) and Denmark the lowest (5 per cent).

The income gap between the rich and poor, both within and between countries in Europe, is increasing (Wilkinson 1996). Among European industrialized nations, the United Kingdom was exceptional in the pace and extent of the increase in inequality in the 1980s and by 1990 the level of inequality was almost back to the levels of 1930 (Leather 1996).

Lack of food associated with poverty can be estimating from the percentage of disposable income spent on food: in Romania the average figure is around 60 per cent, in Poland around 40 per cent, compared with the EU average of 22 per cent (OECD 1996).

Coping within a limited budget may mean that healthier, safer foods are not affordable. In Poland the prevalence of nutrient deficiencies is highest amongst the unemployed and low-income families with many children. It is not clear whether this phenomenon affects the rest of Europe, but unpublished data from DAFNE (Data Food Networking 1997) suggests that from around 20 per cent of the population of Greece to 70 per cent of the population of Ireland do not have access to sufficient vegetables and fruit.

In the European Region around 70 per cent of the population is suffering from physical and mental exhaustion as people cope with increasingly uncertain conditions related to very rapid economic and social change. This is especially true for the countries of the former Soviet Union, where the transition to a market economy has resulted in soaring consumer prices due to a reduction in subsidies while salaries have remained low. In addition, there is rising unemployment as a result of industrial restructuring and the new monetary polices have hit vulnerable groups in particular.

A system to identify and protect vulnerable groups against food poverty is needed in all countries. Many initiatives are related to the physiologically vulnerable, such as children, pregnant women, or the elderly. In addition, welfare safety nets, aimed at ensuring a minimum family income by setting minimum wages, pensions, and unemployment benefits, are considered necessary for economically vulnerable groups, such as the poor, those on low incomes, the unemployed, refugees or immigrants, and those with large or one-parent families.

9.5 Local production for local consumption

Subsistence and small-scale agriculture can provide one solution in circumstances of food shortages or income inadequacy. Local production has many advantages:

(1) Health benefits: improved physical and mental health and sense of well-being.

(2) Social benefits: leisure, community cohesion, and social inclusion.

(3) Environmental benefits: improved water supply and conservation, air quality, soil quality, carbon dioxide balance, biodiversity, and energy savings through local production.

(4) Direct economic benefits: income generation, local employment, development of small enterprises and production of vegetables for local consumption.

(5) Indirect economic benefits: education, recreation, waste management (reduced costs of waste disposal), use of under-used resources (rooftops, roadsides, water bodies), economic diversity/stability, changes in economic value of land, and possible multiplier effects such as attracting new businesses such as restaurants, local shops, and markets.

In central and eastern Europe large-scale agricultural output has decreased in recent years, but local food production and subsistence cultivation are growing rapidly. This survival strategy is traditionally resorted to during times of social stress, economic hardship, or war, in order to ensure food security and to supplement income. The phenomenon was observed in most countries during the Second World War, when Britain was urged to 'dig for victory', and more recently in Sarajevo during the war in Bosnia.

One of the reasons why families living in countries undergoing economic transition in central and eastern Europe are not suffering from lack of protein or energy, is because many produce a large percentage of their own food. In Russia, town dwellers produce 88 per cent of their potatoes, 43 per cent of their meat, 39 per cent of their milk, and 28 per cent of their eggs on urban household plots. This important share of production is generated on plots of 0.2–0.5 hectares, which together constitute only 4 per cent of the total amount of agricultural land in Russia.

The pattern of urban construction under the former communist regimes creates a unique opportunity to promote urban food and nutrition security. Because urban expansion was concentrated in planned high-rise mini-cities, there is a great deal more open land near centres than in North America or western Europe. There is considerable potential for expanding food production as energy and transport costs multiply under the new capitalist economic system. Such small horticulture businesses offer a number of advantages, including cost savings.

Paradoxically, times of economic hardship can be associated with health benefits. For example, in Norway during the Second World War there was a 20–30 per cent decrease in mortality of heart disease, which was probably related to a decrease in the proportion of dietary energy from saturated fat from around 22 per cent to 10 per cent (Johansson et al. 1996), with energy from total fat of only 24 per cent. Similarly, in Sarajevo during the war non-insulin-dependent diabetics lost around 12 kg and only 18 per cent were obese in 1995, compared with 60 per cent before the war. There were large improvements in blood glucose control (measured by haemoglobin A_{1c}) and blood pressure levels, and a 30 per cent reduction in prescribed medication (Kulenovic et al. 1996).

These health gains were achieved largely by increasing potato, vegetable, and fruit production and consumption, together with a reduction in the amount of processed and energy-dense foods in the food supply. Policy makers need to harness this information in order to develop local food policies (Box 9.2) and create environments where these approaches can flourish without being enforced by hardship, poverty, or war. One answer may be to reorientate cities to grow more of their own food locally and to capitalize on the assets of the growing number of people flooding into cities. Rural migrants initially come with food-production skills but, if not quickly harnessed, these vital life skills are soon lost. 'Local production for local consumption' provides an alternative to globalization and fits well into a sound environmental perspective ('Think global, act local').

9.6 Policy implications

Citizens have a vested interest in supporting the supply of safe food of good quality which is nutritionally healthy and produced in environmentally sustainable ways. For policy makers there are opportunities to promote public

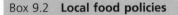

Box 9.2 **Local food policies**

1. create more opportunities for local employment;
2. stimulate local economic growth;
3. enhance social cohesion
4. improve the aesthetics of the environment;
5. increase opportunity for a more active life style;
6. improve mental and psychological health;
7. facilitate the recycling of carefully treated water and organic waste;
8. provide a closer link between consumers and producers;
9. enable environmental improvements; and
10. lead to more sustainable health, food, and environmental systems.

health. The challenge is to create the political awareness that investment for health makes good economic sense and is a prerequisite for human and economic development. Policies that make healthier choices easier choices are relatively inexpensive to implement in relation to the potential benefits, such as increased productivity, and thus government revenue, and reduced health inequalities. One approach is to build stronger health alliances with public interest groups working in the voluntary sector. In an EU-wide (Eurobarometer) survey carried out in 1996, consumer and environmental organizations were judged the most trustworthy sources of information by the public.

Some recommendations (targeted mainly at national policy) that emerge from the issues discussed in this chapter are listed below and then expanded:

(1) Nutrition recommendations and dietary guidelines are needed to assist individuals, institutions, and countries to move towards food policy targets.

(2) Health information systems should collect data on the food supply, population nutrition, food poverty, obesity, and physical inactivity.

(3) The health sector's effectiveness should be strengthened by increasing the knowledge of public-health specialists and developing closer collaboration with related professional groups, such as nutritionists and food safety experts.

(4) Health policy makers should strengthen alliances with consumers and the voluntary sector, in order to create a food system that is compatible with public health and a sustainable environment.

(5) The health sector of each country should participate actively in the work of international committees such as the Codex Alimentarius Commission

and EU committees, since the decisions made by these bodies are important determinants of health.

(6) Nutrition and health objectives should be incorporated into the new Common Agricultural Policy.

(7) Acquisition of food skills should be a component of national school curricula.

(8) National, regional, and local food and nutrition policies and strategies should be developed.

9.6.1 Nutrition recommendations and dietary guidelines

Guidelines are needed in Europe to assist individuals and policy makers, and to provide a basis for monitoring dietary change (Schmitt et al. 1998). For instance, the guideline for fruit and vegetable consumption is 400 g/person/ day or more (Box 9.3). Availability in Europe is very variable (Fig. 9.4), being less than 200 g/person/day in Krygyzstan and more than five times this amount (over 1 kg/person/day) in Greece.

Some dietary problems may best be tackled at national level. Prevention of iodine deficiency, which is especially common in young children and women, by universal salt iodisation, is one example. In the Nordic countries and the UK people get their iodine mostly from milk and milk products because iodine is added to cow fodder. In the Netherlands the salt in bread made by central bakeries is iodized. In Italy a campaign aims to eliminate iodine deficiency through the promotion of iodized salt, but at the same time aims to prevent hypertension by limiting salt intake to 6 g/day.

9.6.2 Information systems

Almost all countries need to improve their food and nutrition information gathering, and to integrate it with health data systems. Many western European countries have established surveillance systems that provide information on food consumption and nutritional status on a routine basis (Schmitt et al. 1998). Other countries have no information, some use secondary data or access nutrition information from national budget surveys. Some have information from special surveys sponsored through international co-operation. Obesity receives little attention within the health sector, and this probably reflects the lack of data on body weight and height. It illustrates the need for countries to collect anthropometric data as part of their health information system.

Although national nutrition surveys are not carried out on a regular basis in many countries, other strategies can be useful. The DAFNE project 1997 extracts nutrition-related data from household budget surveys. FAO food balance sheets provide data such as the percentage energy

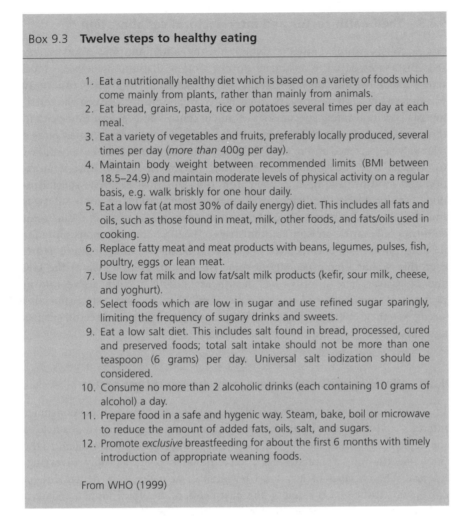

Box 9.3 **Twelve steps to healthy eating**

1. Eat a nutritionally healthy diet which is based on a variety of foods which come mainly from plants, rather than mainly from animals.
2. Eat bread, grains, pasta, rice or potatoes several times per day at each meal.
3. Eat a variety of vegetables and fruits, preferably locally produced, several times per day (*more than* 400g per day).
4. Maintain body weight between recommended limits (BMI between 18.5–24.9) and maintain moderate levels of physical activity on a regular basis, e.g. walk briskly for one hour daily.
5. Eat a low fat (at most 30% of daily energy) diet. This includes all fats and oils, such as those found in meat, milk, other foods, and fats/oils used in cooking.
6. Replace fatty meat and meat products with beans, legumes, pulses, fish, poultry, eggs or lean meat.
7. Use low fat milk and low fat/salt milk products (kefir, sour milk, cheese, and yoghurt).
8. Select foods which are low in sugar and use refined sugar sparingly, limiting the frequency of sugary drinks and sweets.
9. Eat a low salt diet. This includes salt found in bread, processed, cured and preserved foods; total salt intake should not be more than one teaspoon (6 grams) per day. Universal salt iodization should be considered.
10. Consume no more than 2 alcoholic drinks (each containing 10 grams of alcohol) a day.
11. Prepare food in a safe and hygenic way. Steam, bake, boil or microwave to reduce the amount of added fats, oils, salt, and sugars.
12. Promote *exclusive* breastfeeding for about the first 6 months with timely introduction of appropriate weaning foods.

From WHO (1999)

coming from carbohydrate, fat, protein, and alcohol, and the quantity of food commodities available nationally. These data are directly accessible at the FAO web-site (FAO statistical databases (FAOSTAT DATA): http:// apps.fao.org/cgi-bin/nph-dp.pl). Mortality data are available from the WHO 'Health for All' database which is accessible at the WHO web-site. (WHO web-site: http://www.who.ch/ and 'Health for All': http://www.who.dk/ mainframe.htm) These data allow comparison of mortality statistics between countries. It is hoped that in the future the EU will encourage existing and new member states to develop standard nutrition information systems (Schmitt et al. 1998). This would allow comparison of data on dietary intake, nutritional status, and diet-related behaviour in member states and so facilitate the development of health-promoting food and nutrition policies.

9.6.3 The health sector and inter-sectoral collaboration

Good collaboration between public health, nutrition, and food safety specialists is essential. Consumers do not usually distinguish between food safety and nutrition, they just want good wholesome food they can enjoy without anxiety. There appears to be more collaboration between the nutritionists and food safety specialists working in central and eastern Europe than those in western Europe. There may be several reasons for this. Nutrition is a relatively new science and in the CCEE its evolution seems to be closely linked to 'hygiene' and the sanitary epidemiology system. In eastern Europe nutrition and food hygiene have evolved from the same post graduate specialization, usually within medicine. In former socialist countries food safety is traditionally under ministries of health, whereas in some western European countries only nutrition is under ministries of health and the responsibility for food legislation and enforcement may be with ministries of agriculture. However, this is changing, especially in some EU member states such as the UK and Norway, where ministries of health are taking a more active role in protecting consumers and their health. Public-health specialists could also strengthen their collaboration with the main players in the food sector, such as agriculture, the food industry, and retailers.

9.6.4 Working with consumers and the voluntary sector

Links with voluntary sector and public-interest groups representing consumer interests could facilitate improvements in population nutrition. An obstacle to the implementation of food policies is the differing level of commitment to the public-health interest versus each stake-holder's own, possibly diverging, interest. The survival of any food business is, however, very dependent on consumer attitudes. Consumers, the customers of the food industry, have a right to be more involved in the food-policy process.

9.6.5 International committees

Most countries in the WHO European Region are already members of, or are lining up to join, either the WTO or the EU, or both. Their national food legislation will become harmonized with the international standards set either by Codex or EU directives. It is essential that health professionals, especially those working in public health, become more informed about international agreements on global food trade. Ministries of health should ensure that health professionals are always represented in the delegations attending the Codex Committee on Sanitary and Phytosanitary Measures (WHO 1997). Only if public-health specialists participate can they hope to influence future food policies in favour of health.

9.6.6 Common Agricultural Policy

About half of the EU budget is spent on agricultural support. In 1995 this amounted to a tax of some 39 billion ECU. There is much to be gained by including public-health criteria in the new CAP arrangements.

9.6.7 Food skills

As the availability of fast food and convenience foods proliferates, there is alarming evidence that the skills, knowledge, and culture surrounding food is being lost. A UK survey in 1993 showed that 93 per cent of children aged 7–15 years knew how to use a computer, but only 38 per cent could cook a jacket potato. The lack of food skills teaching in many national curricula contributes to the loss of these skills. Results from focus group interviews in Denmark showed that parents could not cook and thus could not pass on cooking skills to their children.

Food skills teaching in schools can provide an interesting, practical part of cross-curricular themes by, for example, combining the natural sciences and environmental studies. Food growing and preparation can be part of activities after school hours. Schools in Nordic countries are experimentally providing students with a piece of fruit or vegetable every day to encourage consumption and give children the opportunity to experience and enjoy eating fresh produce. In North Karelia, Finland, schools have special days when students collect berries or mushrooms for the school kitchen during winter.

9.6.8 Food-policy development

Some countries pay scant attention to the link between diet and non-communicable diseases, and instead give undue attention to the less widespread problems of protein and micronutrient deficiency. In public-health terms, this approach is neither optimal nor cost-effective. Further, there remains a tendency in some countries to prescribe special diets for a variety of disorders, despite the lack of evidence for their efficacy. Many individuals referred for dietary treatment have obesity, diabetes, high blood pressure, or heart disease. Such cases should be given advice based on the nutrition principles developed for the population: increasing consumption of vegetables and fruit, getting at least half of their energy from bread, pasta, and potatoes, and reducing intake of fattening energy-dense foods that provide few micronutrients. Dental caries is also widespread in many European countries and this is related to frequent, high intakes of sugars.

A comparative analysis of nutrition policies in WHO European Member States was made on the basis of country reports submitted at a Member State FAO/WHO consultation held in Warsaw in 1996. Albania, Israel, Kazakstan, Latvia, Romania, Slovakia, the Republic of Moldova, Ukraine, and Uzebekistan made no mention of the link between diet and non-communicable diseases in their country reports. In addition only one-third (12) of the 35 countries mentioned obesity as a problem despite the high prevalence in Europe (see Table 9.1).

Policies that support improved eating habits and more active living are needed. It is recommended that prevention efforts are focused on population-based public-health strategies. Such strategies need to go beyond traditional health education programmes and might involve economic incentives for sustainable production of food to meet health targets, regulation to protect local food production, better mass catering standards, and improved urban planning and transport policies.

9.7 Acknowledgements

We are grateful for the expert editorial assistance of Patricia Crowley.

References

Abel-Smith, B., Figueras, J., Holland, W., McKee, M. and Mossialos, E. (1995). *Choices in health policy – an agenda for the European Union*. Office for Official Publications of the European Communities, Luxembourg.

Anonymous (1997*a*). Predicting obesity in young adulthood from childhood and parental obesity. *N. Engl. J. Med.* **337**, 869–73.

Anonymous (1997*b*). *Food, nutrition and the prevention of cancer: a global perspective*. American Institute for Cancer Research, Washington.

Barker, D.J.P., Gluckman, P.D., Godfrey, K.M., Harding, J.E., Owens, J.A., and Robinson, J.S. (1993). Fetal nutrition and cardiovascular disease in adult life. *Lancet* **341**, 938–41.

Bobak, M., Brunner, E.J., Miller, N.J., Skodova, Z. and Marmot, M.G. (1998). Could antioxidants play a role in high rates of coronary heart disease in the Czech Republic? *Eur. J. Clin. Nutr.* **52**, 632–6.

Brunner, E.J. (1997). Stress and the biology of inequality. *BMJ* **314**, 1472–6.

Brunner, E.J., Juneja, M. and Marmot, M.G. (1998). Abdominal obesity and disease are linked to social position. *BMJ* **316**, 508–9.

Cannon, G. (1998). *Food and Health: the experts agree*. Consumers Association, London.

Consumers International (1996). *A spoonful of sugar*. Consumers International, London.

(DAFNE – Data Food Networking, Network for the Pan-European food data bank based on household budget surveys. Methodology for the exploitation of Household Budget Survey data and results on food availability in 5 European countries. cost action 99 EUR 17909 EN 1997)

Davey Smith, G., Hart, C., Blane, D., Gillis, C. and Hawthorne, V.M. (1997). Lifetime socioeconomic position and mortality: prospective observational study. *BMJ* **314**, 547–52.

Dowler, E.A. and Dobson, B.M. (1997). Symposium on 'Nutrition and poverty in industrialized countries'. *Proc. Nutr. Soc.* **56**, 51–62.

Economic Research Service (1997). *Russian food consumption: emerging demand for quality, Newly Independent States and Baltic update.* Agriculture and Trade Report, Economic Research Service WRS-97-S1, 28 March.

FAO (1997). *Codex Alimentarius* (2nd edition), Rome.

Howie, P.W., Forsyth, J.S., Ogston, S.A., Clark, A. and Florey, C.D. (1990). Protective effect of breastfeeding against infection. *BMJ* **300**, 11–6.

James, W.P.T., Nelson, M., Ralph, A. and Leather, S. (1997). Socioeconomic determinants of health: The contribution of nutrition to inequalities in health. *BMJ* **314**, 1545–9.

Johansson, L., Drevon, C.A. and Bjorneboe, G.E. (1996). The Norwegian diet during the last hundred years in relation to coronary heart disease. *Eur. J. Clin. Nutr.* **50**, 277–83.

Keys, A. (1970). Coronary heart disease in seven countries. *Circulation* **41** (Suppl.1), 1.

Kulenovic, I., Robertson, A., Grujic, M., Suljevic, E. and Smajkic, A. (1996). The impact of war on Sarajevans with non-insulin dependent diabetes mellitus. *Eur. J. Publ. Hlth* **6**, 252–6.

Lang, T. (1998). *Food and nutrition in the EU: its implications for public health.* EU Main Public Health Issues Project, pp. 1–50.

Larsson, B., Bengtsson, C., Bjorntorp, P., Lapidus, et al. (1992). Is abdominal body fat distribution a major explanation for the sex difference in the incidence of myocardial infarction? *Am. J. Epidemiol.* **135**, 266–73.

Leather, S. (1996). *The making of modern malnutrition: an overview of food poverty in the UK.* Caroline Walker Trust, London.

The North Karelia Project (1995). *20 year results and experiences.* Eds. Pushka, P., Tuomilehto, J., Nissinen, A., and Vartiaianen, E. The National Public Health Institute (KTL), Helsinki.

OECD (1996). *Purchasing power parities and real expenditure.* OECD, Paris.

Popkin, B.M., Adair, L., Akin, J.S., Black, R., Briscoe, J. and Flieger, W. (1990). Breastfeeding and diarrheal morbidity. *Paediatrics* **86**, 874–82.

Robertson, A., Fronczak, N., Jaganjac, N., Hailey, P., Copeland, P. and Duprat, M. (1995). Nutrition and immunization survey of Bosnian women and children during 1993. *Int. J. Epidemiol.* **24**, 1163–70.

Rose, G. (1992). *The strategy of preventive medicine.* Oxford University Press, Oxford.

Schmitt, A., Chambolle, M., Millstone, E., Brunner, E.J. and Lobstein, T.

(1998). Nutritional surveillance in Europe. ESTO/IPTS C-1097, pp. 173. VDI Technology Centre. Dusseldorf.

Steinberg, D. (1992). Antioxidants in the prevention of human atherosclerosis. *Circulation* **85**, 2338–44.

Taylor, A. (1998). Violations of the international code of marketing of breast milk substitues: prevalence in four countries. *BMJ* **316**, 1117–22.

Victora, C.G., Smith, P.G., Vaughan, J.P., et al. (1997). Evidence for the protection by breast-feeding against infant deaths from infectious diseases in Brazil. *Lancet* **350**, 319–22.

WHO (1990). *Diet, nutrition, and the prevention of chronic diseases.* Technical Report Series, no. 797. WHO, Geneva.

WHO (1999). CINDI Dietary Guidelines. WHO, Copenhagen.

WHO (1997). *Food Safety and Globalization of trade in food: a challenge to the public health sector,* WHO Geneva.

Wilkinson, R.G. (1996). *Unhealthy societies: the afflictions of inequality.* Routledge, London.

Wilson, A.C., Forsyth, J.S., Greene, S.A., Irvine, L., Hau, C. and Howie, P.W. (1998). Relation of infant diet to childhood health: seven year follow up of cohort of children in Dundee infant feeding study. *BMJ* **316**, 21–5.

10 Poverty, social exclusion, and minorities

Mary Shaw, Danny Dorling and George Davey Smith

10.1 Introduction

Poverty, the extent of relative deprivation, and the processes of social exclusion in a society have a major impact on the health of its population. All over Europe, in richer countries as well as poorer ones, those people who are worse off in socio-economic terms have worse health outcomes and higher death rates than those who are better off. Particular 'minority' ethnic groups are often in poor socio-economic positions within particular countries and hence often experience poor health, which can be exacerbated by the additional effects of prejudice and racism. The harm to health comes not only from material deprivation but also from the social and psychological problems resulting from living in relative poverty.

This chapter first presents a small sample of the vast body of available evidence that shows a clear relationship between poverty, deprivation, and health, and then discusses briefly why poverty affects health. Evidence of the increasing incidence of poverty and social exclusion in both western and eastern Europe, and the implications of this for health, are then presented. Following this, attention turns to the concept of 'social exclusion' in Europe and focuses on the evidence of the detrimental effect on health for particular 'minority' groups: the unemployed, refugees, poorer migrants, ethnic minorities, and the homeless. The chapter closes by offering short- and long-term policy suggestions for the reduction of health problems resulting from poverty, relative deprivation, and social exclusion.

10.2 Poverty and health

Whether we refer to mortality, morbidity, or self-reported health, and whichever indicator of socio-economic position we employ – income, class, housing tenure, deprivation, or education – we find that those who are worse off socio-economically have worse health. It is not only the case that the poorest in society have poor health, but a gradient of ill health and mortality spans all socio-economic strata. This gradient can be found across the industrialized world, although the strength of the relationship varies somewhat between different countries, for different age groups, by the health measures used, and for men and women (Kunst et al. 1995).

Recent evidence from Britain, where there is a long tradition of research into inequalities in health, shows that variations in life expectancy by social class continue to be found and are in fact widening. Table 10.1 shows that for men the life expectancy difference between social classes I and II (high) and IV and V (low) increased from 3.7 years in the late 1970s to 4.7 years a decade later; for women this gap has increased from 2.1 to 3.4 years (Drever and Whitehead 1997). Figures 10.1 and 10.2 display this data graphically and the steepening of the gradient is clearly visible. Occupational groups I and II include professionals, such as doctors and lawyers, as well as managerial occupations. Occupational groups IV and V include semi-skilled manual occupations, such as some coal miners and machine operators, and unskilled manual occupations, such as cleaners and labourers.

Similar findings of differences in mortality and life expectancy by social and occupational classes are reported for other European countries. For example, Kunst and Mackenbach (1992) compared mortality by occupational social class in six European countries (Denmark, England and Wales, Finland, France, Norway, and Sweden) and found that socio-economic gradients in mortality varied in each country and in different age groups, but that there were, none the less, gradients in each of these countries.

Kunst (1997) reports findings of socio-economic differences in mortality for a number of eastern and western European countries, in terms of occupational class and educational groups. Table 10.2 shows death rate ratios in the 1980s for males in manual versus non-manual occupational

Table 10.1
Life expectancy at age 15 by social class (using collapsed categories) for men and women (adapted from Drever and Whitehead 1997)

	Men			Women		
	1977–81	1982–86	1987–91	1977–81	1982–86	1987–91
Life expectancy Classes I+II	58.8	59.9	60.5	64.1	64.3	65.8
Difference in years between I+II and:						
III Non-manual	−1.9	−1.7	−0.7	0.0	0.0	−0.5
III Manual	−2.2	−2.5	−2.4	−1.9	−1.4	−2.6
IV+V	−3.7	−4.0	−4.7	−2.1	−1.5	−3.4

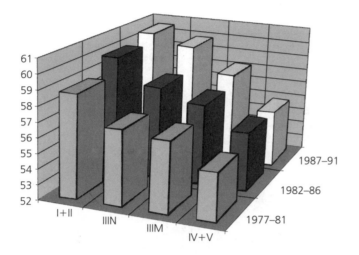

Fig. 10.1 Life expectancy at age 15 by social class (using collapsed categories) for men (from Drever and Whitehead 1997).

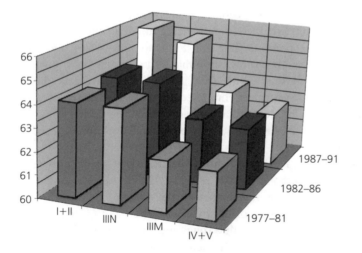

Fig. 10.2 Life expectancy at age 15 by social class (using collapsed categories) for women (from Drever and Whitehead 1997).

classes for various countries. Differences are particularly large for the former communist countries of the Czech Republic and Hungary, showing that socio-economic gradients in mortality are not the preserve of the capitalist countries of the West.

Table 10.2
Death rate ratios for males in manual versus non-manual occupational classes in the 1980s (adapted from Kunst 1997)

Country	Death rate ratio 30–44 years	45–59 years
Czech Republic	2.25	1.83
Denmark	1.53	1.33
England and Wales	1.46	1.44
Finland	1.76	1.53
France	*	1.71
Hungary	2.89	2.65
Ireland	1.43	1.38
Italy	1.35	1.35
Norway	1.65	1.34
Portugal	1.5	1.36
Spain	*	1.37
Sweden	1.66	1.41
Switzerland	1.45	1.35

* Data not reported for this age group.

In Britain, alternative socio-economic measures, such as housing tenure and access to a car, are increasingly being used as indicators of social position. Table 10.3 presents data for England and Wales, and shows a similar polarization to that shown in Table 10.1. Compared to owner occupiers, those who rent their home from a public or private landlord have increasingly higher death rates; compared to those who have access to one or more cars, those who do not have access to a car have increasingly higher death rates. Similar findings are reported when education is used as the social indicator.

Some researchers have looked more specifically at the health effects of relative deprivation, a concept that refers to the disadvantaged position of an individual, family, or group relative to the society to which they belong, and focuses on the condition of deprivation as well as the lack of resources (Townsend et al. 1988). Using the Townsend index of deprivation, a composite indicator for areas (which includes unemployment, percentage of households with no car, the extent of overcrowding, and housing tenure), Eames et al. (1993) found that higher deprivation was associated with higher rates of premature death in every region in England and Wales, although the association was stronger in some regions than others. There is also some evidence that living in a relatively deprived area can have a detrimental effect on an individual's health, even when the individual level of deprivation has been taken into account, i.e. that there is an area health effect over and above the effect of individual deprivation. This has been found in the USA (Haan et

Table 10.3
Direct age-standardized rate ratios for deaths under 65 by housing tenure and car access: 1971 and 1981 census cohorts (Longitudinal Study data) (adapted from Filakti and Fox 1995)

	Males		Females	
	1971–81	**1981–89**	**1971–81**	**1981–89**
Housing tenure				
Owner occupiers	1	1	1	1
Private renters	1.32	1.38	1.32	1.38
Social housing	1.35	1.62	1.42	1.44
Car access				
1+cars	1	1	1	1
No cars	1.44	1.57	1.40	1.56

al. 1987) and in British studies of both mortality and morbidity (Langford and Bentham 1996; Shouls et al. 1996; Davey Smith et al. 1998a).

Suicide rates, in particular, have been found to be associated with deprivation. For example, Gunnell et al. (1995) report that socio-economic deprivation is an indicator and possible determinant of psychiatric morbidity and suicide. Similarly, McLoone (1996) reports that the greatest rates of increase in suicide rates in Scotland between 1981 and 1993 were for deprived young people – their suicide rates being approximately twice those of young people in affluent areas.

10.2.1 Why poverty is bad for health: the material, social, and psychological consequences of living in poverty

An understanding of why those who live in conditions of poverty and relative deprivation have poorer health is necessary in order to begin effectively to redress the issue. A number of different explanations for this relationship have been suggested, including living and working conditions, limitations on resources, and the subsequent effect on social relationships. Individual life-style factors, such as smoking, alcohol consumption, exercise, and diet, have been suggested by some as the main underlying causes. However, while such factors may indeed form a part of the explanation for inequalities in health, they should not be considered the exclusive cause, nor viewed as being distinct from the socio-economic environment.

The majority of the evidence suggests that material conditions are the underlying root of ill health, which includes being the determining factor for health-related behaviours (Davey Smith et al. 1994). Poverty imposes constraints on the material conditions of everyday life – by limiting access to the fundamental building blocks of health such as adequate housing, good nutrition, and opportunities to participate in society (Black and Laughlin 1996). The concomitants of poverty are often poor nutrition; overcrowded, damp, and inadequately heated housing; increased risk of infections; and inability to maintain optimal hygiene practices (Davey Smith 1998). Poor housing, for example, can be damp, cold, and contain mould, conditions which are associated with wheezing, breathlessness, cough, phlegm, meningococcal infection, and respiratory diseases and asthma (Ineichen 1993). Poor housing conditions can also bring a risk of fire and accidents, and overcrowded housing not only increases the risk of infection but impacts upon mental health through factors such as high noise levels and lack of privacy.

Blackburn (1991) asserts that poverty affects health through not only nutrition and housing, but also in terms of the effect on mental health and caring for children. Income levels affect the way parents are able to care for their own and their children's health. As well as affecting other aspects of their lives – where they live, where their children go to school – living on a low income makes it difficult to exercise control over family health, and as a result the health needs of parents, particularly women, are often compromised for those of children. For example, Graham (1995) found that smoking rates in young women in manual households were related to the strains of caring responsibilities as well as to greater material disadvantages – it was a combination of the psychological and material difficulties of life that led to their greater smoking prevalence. By compromising their own health women thus felt better equipped to cope with the care of their children and families. It is thus necessary to understand how material restrictions operate through a number of processes – 'unhealthy' behaviours need to be understood in the context of the constraints on everyday life which accompany them.

It is important to recognize the processual nature of poverty, but also that it has a cumulative effect. A body of evidence is now emerging which shows that health outcomes in adulthood reflect the accumulating influence of poor socio-economic circumstances throughout life (Davey Smith et al. 1997). Adverse socio-economic conditions in early life can produce lasting increases in the risk of cardiovascular disease, respiratory disease, and some cancers late in life. Adverse socio-economic conditions in adulthood compound these earlier-life influences, resulting in health differentials in adulthood which reflect the social patterning of exposure acting across the life course (Davey Smith et al. 1998b). The particular influence of deprivation in childhood should focus attention on some current social policies which are leading to an increasing concentration of poverty in households with young children (Davey Smith 1998).

10.2.2 Increasing poverty, unemployment, and inequality

What we know about the relationship between poverty and health should be cause for great concern, given that the proportion of people living in relative poverty is increasing in many European countries. This is the case in western as well as eastern Europe.

The extent of poverty and relative deprivation has increased in European countries in the past two decades. Between 1980 and 1988 poverty rates increased in all European Community countries, with the exceptions of the Netherlands, Portugal, and Spain (Oppenheim and Harker 1996). The sharpest rises were seen in Italy, Germany, and the UK. In terms of income inequality, the UK, Sweden, Denmark, Norway, the Netherlands, and Belgium have all experienced increases over the time period 1967–92; the UK, Norway, the Netherlands, Belgium, and Germany all experienced increases in child poverty (Goodman et al 1997).

Vogel (1997) points to economic developments, underlying these increases in poverty and inequality, which can be seen across the European Union: mass unemployment, reductions in welfare transfer systems, and cuts in public services. Socio-demographic changes, ageing populations, increasing divorce rates, and increasing numbers of lone parents also contribute to the increased proportion of people living in poverty. Vogel reports a clear tendency towards growing poverty rates in 9 of the 12 European countries he considers (increased poverty in the Netherlands, Denmark, Belgium, Luxembourg, Spain, Ireland, UK, Greece, and Portugal).

Although there is wide variation in the unemployment rates of European countries and methodological problems of comparing rates (Green 1998), most countries have experienced mass unemployment in the past two decades. Approximately half of the unemployment rate consists of long-term unemployed (those unemployed for more than 12 months), and the youth unemployment rate is higher than the general rate (Vogel 1997). This growth in unemployment and insecure employment, as well as rises in the numbers on welfare, rising debts and arrears, increase in the number of lone parents, and increasing numbers of homeless people is referred to by Room (1991) as the 'new poverty' of the European Community. This is in addition to, and not replacing, older forms of poverty among the elderly, sick, and children.

Examining the case in Britain, where much data is available, in the post-war period there have been considerable improvements in terms of living standards, and this has been reflected in falling overall mortality rates. However, despite this overall growth in prosperity, there has also been an increase in poverty and inequality. The case of housing provides an example. Home ownership in Britain increased from 57 per cent in 1981 to 68 per cent in 1991 (Dorling 1995). The proportion of households with central heating increased from 37 per cent in 1972 to 83 per cent in 1992, the proportion of households with more than one car from 9 per cent in 1972 to 24 per cent in 1992

(Wadsworth 1996). However, the number of households in insecure housing tenures has also risen, reflected in increases in the number of mortgage repossessions and households in temporary accommodation – the number of which rose from over 10 000 in 1982 to over 67 000 in 1992 (Wadsworth 1996). The number of households applying to local authorities as homeless and the number of single homeless has also risen (Victor 1997). Thus in the context of increased overall prosperity, relative poverty is on the increase.

The situation regarding the distribution of wealth and income in Britain has been examined in detail in recent years by Hills (1995a,b, 1998). He reported (Hills 1995a) that income inequality grew between 1970 and 1990, and that while income inequality also grew in a number of other advanced industrialized countries, the rate of increase in Britain was faster than in any other country except New Zealand. The extent of inequality is such that the lowest-income groups have not benefited from economic growth, and since 1977 the proportion of the population with less than half the average income has more than trebled, from 7 per cent to 24 per cent. As a result of high unemployment and economic activity (such as early retirement and invalidity), more people became dependent on state benefits. Those particularly vulnerable to low income are pensioners, lone parents, households with no earners, and families with children.

At the same time as economic inequality has increased in Britain, so too has the gap between the death rates of the better off and the deprived (McLoone and Boddy 1994; Phillimore et al. 1994). For example, Raleigh and Kiri (1997) looked at life expectancy and deprivation in district health authorities in England and Wales between 1984 and 1994. Those areas with the greatest gains in prosperity had the greatest gains in life expectancy, whereas in deprived areas improvements in life expectancy were negligible. They report a difference in life expectancy of 6.7 years for men and 4.7 years for women between the most and least deprived areas.

Recently, Blane and Drever (1998) have calculated this widening gap of health in terms of years of potential life lost. While standardized mortality ratios have the advantage of taking into account the different age structures of the social class groups, they are heavily influenced by the number of deaths occurring in the oldest age category. However, the largest relative class differences in absolute mortality are at younger ages, and so it is also worth considering the relative number of years of productive life which are lost through premature mortality (Davey Smith et al. 1994). As Table 10.4 shows, the ratio of years of life lost for social class V as compared to social class I between the early 1970s and early 1990s rose from 2.1 to 3.3.

Thus increasing poverty and income inequality are mirrored by increasing health inequalities. A specific disease which traditionally has been associated with poverty, tuberculosis, is reported to be rising in eastern Europe. Raviglione et al. (1994) report increases in Romania, Armenia, Kyrgystan, Latvia, Lithuania, Moldova, and Turkmenistan and no further decline in

Table 10.4
Annual age-adjusted rate of years of potential life lost per 1000 population for all causes of death in men aged 20–64 in England and Wales for 1970–72, 1979–80 and 1982–83, and 1991–93 (standardized to population of England and Wales 1981) (from Blane and Drever 1998)

Social class	1970–2	1979–80, 1982–83	1991–93
I	48.7	36.5	28.0
II	51.9	42.2	31.6
III non-manual	65.0	53.9	45.7
III manual	66.0	58.0	50.5
IV	75.6	67.7	52.8
V	103.0	105.8	93.3
Ratio V: I	2.1	2.9	3.3

other countries. Recent rises in Britain have been linked with increased poverty, deprivation, and unemployment (Darbyshire 1995; Kumar et al. 1995).

Similar polarization can be seen on a larger scale. Shaw et al. (1998) have analysed changing all-cause standardized mortality ratios (SMRs) for deaths under the age of 65 for 160 regions of the European Union. Data were analysed at the NUTS 2 (Nomenclature of Statistical Territorial Units) level, which are generally provinces, *Regierungsbezike* (German regions), or groups of counties (for example, Herefordshire and Worcester and Warwickshire in the UK). Regions were amalgamated into population deciles according to their SMRs in 1990.

Table 10.5 indicates that while a number of the deciles had decreasing SMRs, including those that already had relatively low SMRs in 1990, deciles 5, 6, 7, and 10 have experienced increasing SMRs over the study period. Most notably, the SMR of the population decile with the highest death rates was 130.1 in 1990 but by 1994 the SMR of this population decile was 134.9. Thus the difference between the regions with the highest and the lowest SMRs is becoming greater. A cursory inspection of the geographical patterning of this polarization of mortality across Europe suggests that it reflects, to a large extent, the European geography of polarizing wealth and employment.

10.3   Central and Eastern Europe

Increases in inequalities in health can thus be interpreted as a result of increases in poverty and inequality, and this phenomenon can be seen in the former communist countries of eastern and central Europe. While overall

Table 10.5
SMRs (all cause, under 65) by population deciles, 1990 and 1994 (standardized to the European average) (from Shaw et al. 1998)

Decile	1	2	3	4	5	6	7	8	9	10
1990	75.0	85.1	90.6	94.6	97.4	100.6	105.1	109.0	116.3	130.1
1994	73.5	84.0	89.4	94.4	97.8	102.2	105.9	108.7	113.7	134.9
Change	−1.5	−1.1	−1.2	−0.2	+0.4	+1.6	+0.8	−0.3	−2.6	+4.8

death rates have been falling in western Europe, in eastern and central Europe mortality has been rising since the mid 1960s (Shloknikov et al. 1998). In the years since the collapse of communism, death rates have risen sharply. Between 1989 and 1994 life expectancy in Russia fell by 6.5 years for men and 3.5 years for women (Shloknikov et al. 1998); similar changes have been seen in other former Soviet countries (Dennis et al. 1993). By 1993, death rates had risen substantially in all of the former Warsaw Pact countries with the exception of Hungary (UNICEF 1993). These changes have not been spread evenly throughout the population, for example in Russia, death rates have risen fastest among those with lower levels of education (Shloknikov et al. 1998).

As well as increasing rates of tuberculosis, Davis (1993) notes that in eastern Europe morbidity as a result of diseases such as diphtheria, measles, whooping cough, and syphilis is also increasing; nutritional, infectious, and degenerative diseases have all become more widespread. In terms of mortality, a great proportion of the increase is due to male deaths from accidents and homicide, and many of these deaths are alcohol related (Ellman 1994; Leon et al. 1997). For example, Ellman states that for males aged 15–59, between 1987 and 1991, 77 per cent of the total increase in mortality was accounted for by accidents and homicide. These increases in morbidity and mortality are all occurring within the context of a ravaged healthcare system:

> Medical facilities are underfunded and afflicted by shortages of all categories of supplies . . . The quality of medical care in state facilities has almost certainly fallen. These negative trends have not been offset by the increase in sophisticated treatment in private facilities, which only a small minority can afford . . .
> *(Davis 1993, p. 34)*

Severe environmental pollution has also been suggested as a possible contributory factor (Feshbach and Friendly 1992). However, as increases in mortality rates have particularly affected certain groups – young men of working age in particular – it has been argued that this is unlikely to be a predominant cause of the overall increases (Watson 1995). Similarly, Hertzman (1995) argues that pockets of pollution tend to affect health at the local level and this effect is not enough to influence significantly national mortality rates.

Others point to behavioural changes as a major factor in these poorer health outcomes, particularly increased alcohol consumption. For example, Cockerham (1997) argues that life-style factors – alcohol consumption, smoking, poor diet, and lack of exercise – account for this increase in mortality. Bobak and Marmot (1996) also point to the role of unhealthy behaviours and life styles, arguing that smoking has probably had the largest impact; Leon et al. (1997) highlight alcohol consumption. However, these authors also emphasize that individual behaviours need to be understood in their broader social context, we must look to the far-reaching changes in socio-economic conditions for explanations as to why large groups of people behave as they do. Local considerations may also need to be borne in mind. For example, in a recent paper reporting mortality in a cohort of the Nova Huta steelworkers in Poland, Watson (1998) suggests the results need to be understood not only in the context of broader political and economic circum-stances, but also regarding the history and experience of employment at that particular steelworks. Similarly, Phillimore and Morris (1991) argue that in order to understand geographical patterns in mortality we need an under-standing of what constitutes a 'place', and this may include looking not only at levels of deprivation but also examining closely the social and economic histories of particular localities, such as the provision of housing and the pattern of deprivation over a number of decades.

An understanding of place-specific factors, cultures, and societies is also needed at the international level. In virtually all states of central and eastern Europe and the former Soviet Union political and economic changes have been accompanied by drastic reductions in production output and in real wages, and living standards have fallen (Davis 1993). As a consequence, many people now find themselves in a condition of sudden impoverishment (Cornia and Paniccia 1995) and there have been widening income inequalities. Many people now have two jobs and work very long hours in order to provide for themselves and their families. For example, Ellman (1994) reports that, in Russia in 1992, 37 per cent of the Russian population were below the poverty line (defined in this study as an income which would allow a level of food consumption adequate to maintain a normal body weight at an average level of activity), and 47 per cent of children below the age of 15 were living below the poverty line. These conditions have direct effects, such as on food con-sumption (due to both lack of availability and lack of purchasing power), and also lead to social stress (Shapiro 1995). Marriage rates have declined and crime rates soared. People have not only lost their incomes, but also a sense of pride, power, and participation, in relation to both work and national identity. Watson (1995) argues that it is likely that rising mortality rates in eastern European countries are not only associated with falling absolute standards of living for the majority of the population, but are also related to increased social and economic inequalities, a sense of hopelessness and disenfranchisement with the political process, and higher levels of insecurity and uncertainty, particularly in employment.

There are thus psychosocial implications (Davey Smith and Egger 1996) of social and economic stress, which may influence rates of murder, depression, suicide, and alcohol consumption. As Ellman says:

> . . . someone whose job is insecure and who may become unemployed (or who has actually become unemployed), who is living on a low and uncertain income (which may frequently not be paid when due) under conditions of very high inflation and very high crime, and whose access to meat, vegetables, fruit and medical care has sharply worsened, may die in a brawl, car crash or of alcohol poisoning.
> (Ellman 1994, p. 343)

Economic conditions thus have a knock-on effect. Increased poverty and the difficulties that accompany it affect health in terms of morbidity and mortality, and it is those who are worse off whose health suffers most. This is the case in established market economies as well as societies in the process of transition.

10.4 Social exclusion

In many areas the terminology of social exclusion is superseding poverty or deprivation in popularity. 'Poverty' emphasizes lack of economic resources, and the term 'relative deprivation' stresses the conditions of living. 'Social exclusion' refers not only to the economic hardship of relative economic poverty, but also incorporates the notion of the *process* of marginalization – how individuals come, through their lives, to be excluded and marginalized from various aspects of social and community life.

There is no European-wide definition of social exclusion, but it is generally considered to include a number of dimensions:

> Exclusion processes are dynamic and multidimensional in nature. They are linked not only to unemployment and/or to low income, but also to housing conditions, levels of education and opportunities, health, discrimination, citizenship and integration in the local community
> (European Social Policy White Paper (1994), cited in Oppenheim and Harker 1996, p. 156).

The term 'social exclusion' also relates to cultural aspects of exclusion and discrimination and refers to the relationship between the included and excluded, the meaning and identity of the excluded. Social exclusion is about multidimensional disadvantage – there is not one 'social exclusion' but many 'social exclusions' (Room 1995) and, as with social class and relative economic deprivation, there are degrees of exclusion. The term 'socially excluded' can refer to those who may be stigmatized and marginalized, such as people with HIV, who might not be considered in traditional analyses of economic deprivation. Those who are more socially included have greater access to resources, not only in economic terms but also resources which come from living within a society – such as educational opportunities, social networks, and support; those who are excluded are denied these (see Chapter 8). As Wilkinson says:

> To feel depressed, cheated, bitter, desperate, vulnerable, frightened, angry, worried about debts or job and housing insecurity; to feel devalued, useless, helpless, uncared for, hopeless, isolated, anxious and a failure: these feelings can dominate people's whole experience of life . . . The material environment is merely the indelible mark and constant reminder of the oppressive fact of one's failure, of the atrophy of any sense of having a place in a community, and of one's social exclusion and devaluation as a human being
> *(Wilkinson 1996, p. 215)*

The processes leading to social exclusion in Europe include economic change (increased unemployment and widespread job insecurity), demographic change (increased proportions of single households, lone parents, and elderly), changes to welfare regimes (cuts and withdrawal), and specific spatial processes of segregation and separation (stigmatization and marginalization of certain groups, often leading to spatial segregation of minorities) (White 1998).

White (1998) refers to four aspects of social exclusion (Fig. 10.3). First there is exclusion from civil society through legal constraint or regulation. This is particularly relevant to migrants, for example the children born to foreign immigrants (with no German ancestry) in Germany, who remain foreigners in legal terms. Secondly, there is the failure to supply social goods to a group with particular needs; for example, facilities for the disabled, language services, or accommodation for the homeless. Thirdly, there is exclusion from social production, not being able to be an active contributor to society; certain groups may be labelled as undesirable, unacceptable, or in need of control, for example gypsies and travellers. Finally, there is economic exclusion from normal social consumption – not having access to the normal perquisites, routines, and experiences of everyday life.

Social exclusion can refer to individuals, but it is not just individuals who manifest conditions of exclusion and accompanying stress and insecurity. Spatial concentration and segregation can mean that areas can become deprived, disadvantaged or stigmatized, this may affect all of those in the area, and affect their potential for mobility. For instance, living in an area where factories are closing and where there are no job vacancies increases an individual's chance of unemployment. An area which has high unemployment and high levels of deprivation is also likely to have poor schools – an individual's circumstances depend very much on his or her geographical setting.

The health-damaging and health-promoting features of local areas in Glasgow, Scotland's largest city, have recently been investigated in work by

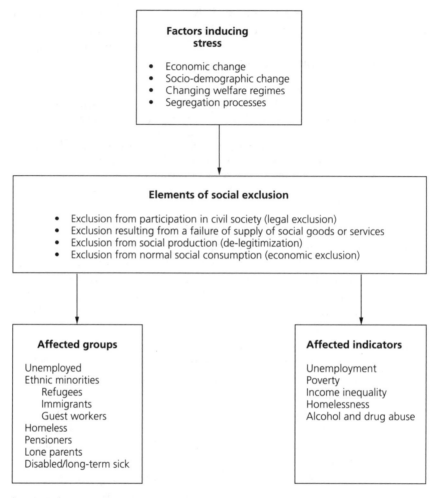

Fig. 10.3 The process and outcome of social exclusion in Europe (adapted from White 1998).

Sooman and MacIntyre (1995). They found that not only were there differences in self-reported health between local areas, with those in more advantaged areas reporting fewer health problems, but there was also an association between the respondents' perceptions of their local social and physical environment which could not be explained by social class differences. Important factors were local amenities and problems, area reputation, neighbourliness, fear of crime, and area satisfaction. These findings highlight that social exclusion is not just about individuals, but that there is also a spatial dimension.

10.4.1 The unemployed

The groups of people who are socially excluded and their characteristics vary from state to state. They can include the elderly, the disabled (especially disabled children), lone parents and their children, as well as those with certain health conditions (e.g. the mentally ill and the long-term sick). However, here we concentrate on the evidence showing that the unemployed, refugees, poorer migrants and ethnic minorities, and the homeless have adverse health outcomes. As noted above, unemployment has increased across the whole of Europe; relatively high unemployment rates seem to have become a permanent feature of developed economies at the end of the twentieth century. This unemployment tends to be concentrated in certain groups – there are growing numbers of long-term unemployed and youth unemployment is also widespread – increasing numbers of young people in Europe have never worked. Unemployment is essentially a spatial process, because people are limited in how far they can travel to work in a day; they rely on the supply of work in their local area and when this falls, unemployment rises. Unemployment in Europe is also concentrated disproportionately among immigrants. For example, in the mid 1990s in the Netherlands unemployment was 7 per cent for the Dutch themselves, but for non-Dutch workers it was 20 per cent, for those from Turkey and Morocco it was even higher (Pinder 1998).

The research showing that unemployment carries a risk of premature mortality is discussed in Chapter 5 of this volume. The effect operates over and above pre-existing health and social class position. According to Drever and Whitehead (1997), after adjusting for social class, the excess mortality for the unemployed is 25 per cent for men and 21 per cent for women. Nor is this increased mortality due solely to behavioural factors – data from the British Regional Heart Study have shown that differences in mortality between employed and unemployed men remain after adjustment for factors including smoking and alcohol consumption (Morris et al. 1994).

It is thus not just the economic hardship which accompanies unemployment which has repercussions for health, but the psychosocial condition of unemployment appears also have an effect. Consistent with this, job insecurity and the anticipation of job loss have been found to be associated with poorer health outcomes (Ferrie et al. 1995; Bartley et al. 1996; see also Chapter 6 on work).

10.4.2 Refugees, migrants, and ethnic minorities

Refugees and internationally displaced persons experience elevated risks of mortality in the period following their migration. For people fleeing from countries which have recently experienced conflict in Europe (the former Yugoslavia, Georgia, Azerbaijan, Chechnia and Kosovo), this includes not only war-related injuries but also communicable diseases, neonatal problems, and nutritional deficiencies (Toole and Waldman 1997). The stresses accompanying this process – past traumatic experiences, the loss of family and friends and disruption of social support networks, and problems of settling in a new environment – will also have an impact upon a number of dimensions of physical and mental health (see Chapter 8 on Social Support).

People also migrate in order to find work, unemployment being a spatial phenomenon. Some migrants and guest workers will experience similar problems to those of refugees (although perhaps to a lesser degree). There is a range of evidence that poorer migrants and ethnic minorities have different health outcomes to those of the general population of the society in which they are living. In terms of all-cause mortality, Drever and Whitehead (1997) report raised rates for most ethnic groups in Britain (Table 10.6).

Table 10.6 shows that migrants from the Indian subcontinent, East, West and southern Africa, as well as from Scotland and Ireland, have significantly higher SMRs than the average population in England and Wales, and that this is the case even after social class is taken into account. Only those who were born in the Caribbean have lower SMRs. This is likely to be explained by a healthy migrant effect, with only the healthiest from the Caribbean migrating to Britain (Marmot et al. 1984), or may possibly be due to the fact that many migrants return to the Caribbean shortly before their death and thus have not been included in these mortality data.

This elevated mortality has also been found to extend to the children of migrants. Harding and Balarajan (1996) found that the mortality of second-generation Irish migrants living in England and Wales was significantly higher for most causes of death than that of all men and women, and this was only partially explained by socio-economic variables (social class, car access, and housing tenure). In the Netherlands, the mortality rate of Turkish and Moroccan children under 15 is 23 times higher than that for Dutch children – the main causes of death responsible for this elevated rate being perinatal death (including congenital malformations), accidents (including drowning), and infectious diseases (Schulpen 1996).

There is also evidence in terms of particular health outcomes. Evidence

Table 10.6
SMRs, by country of birth, for men aged 20–64, all causes
(England and Wales 1991–93) (from Drever and Whitehead 1997)

	All countries	Caribbean	West/ South Africa	East Africa	Indian sub-continent	Scotland	Ireland (all parts)
SMR	100	89	126	123	107	129	135
SMR adjusted for social class	100	82	135	137	117	132	129

from Australia suggests that migrant workers may be more prone to work-related accidents, as Corvalan et al. (1994) found that language and duration of stay were related to occupation-related fatalities. In Canada, the stress of resettlement after migration has been linked to higher suicide rates (Trovato 1992).

Etienne et al. (1994) report that tuberculosis is higher in immigrants in Belgium; Elender et al. (1998) showed the same in England and Wales, although they note that this can be accounted for by overcrowded living conditions and poverty. Circumstances in country of origin may also play a role. In Sweden, there is evidence of elevated morbidity in labour migrants and refugees (Sundquist 1995). This research found that migrants were more likely to live in rented housing and have low material standards of living, they were also more likely not to feel secure in everyday life and to have poor leisure opportunities – being an immigrant was a risk factor for poor health of equal significance to life-style risk factors.

Nazroo (1998) also highlights the importance of social position in deter-mining the health of migrants. He asserts that much of the variation in health by ethnicity can be explained by standards of living. The health of ethnic minorities may also be influenced by geographical concentration in certain areas, as well as the experience of harassment and discrimination. Nazroo warns:

> The ethnic classifications we use do not reflect unchangeable and natural divisions within groups. Also ethnicity does not exist in isolation, it is within a social context that ethnicity achieves its significance, and part of that social context is the ways in which those seen as members of ethnic minority groups are racialised. Indeed, one of the most important purposes for undertaking work on ethnicity and health is to extend our understanding of the nature and extent of the social disadvantage faced by ethnic minority groups. Not only is health part of the disadvantage, it is also a consequence.
> *(Nazroo 1998, p. 8)*

Methodological issues also need to be considered when looking at the health of migrant workers. Egger et al. (1990) report on health inequalities by occupational class in Switzerland, suggesting that class differences may be understated as large numbers of migrant workers (mostly from Yugoslavia, Italy, Spain, and Portugal), concentrated in partly skilled and unskilled manual occupations, are not routinely included in official statistics. Even within particular occupational groups there is evidence that migrant workers experience worse conditions, and hence demonstrate unfavourable health out-comes, compared to the indigenous Swiss population.

10.4.3 The homeless

Even in developed societies with relatively high gross domestic product (GDP) and highly developed welfare systems, we see the problem of homelessness.

While there are many methodological problems with the definition and enumeration of homelessness (Pleace and Quilgars 1996), there has undoubtedly been a general upward trend in the number of homeless people living in many European countries.

In the former German Democratic Republic (GDR), while there are problems with enumeration of the homeless (by no means unique to that state), there are strong indications that this phenomenon is growing – from 26 000 at the beginning of the 1970s to 100 000 in 1989 (Rossler and Salize 1994). There is also evidence that homelessness is rising in the Netherlands (Schnabel 1992), where the homeless tend to be concentrated in city centres. Brandt and Munk-Jorgensen (1996) point out that in Denmark, a rich country with a relatively good social welfare system, homelessness can none the less be found. While few of these people sleep rough on the streets, they can be defined as homeless in that they lack their own home – they live in institutions, sleep on friends' floors, or in lodging houses – by this definition 0.3–0.4 per cent of Denmark's population are homeless. Since the late 1970s this number has been growing, and the homeless are becoming younger.

Fernandez (1996) points out that in Ireland, as in the UK, there has been a reduction in the state provision of housing, and homelessness is a growing problem. In the mid 1990s there were believed to be 5000 homeless (out of a population of 3.5 million) in addition to over 7000 travellers and nearly 30 000 approved applicants on housing lists, with over 30 000 child dependants. Factors which have contributed to this are high unemployment and long-term unemployment, a halt in emigration (due to worldwide economic trends), lack of availability of low-cost rented accommodation, and progressive disinvestment in local authority housing.

There is a great deal of evidence that the homeless have poor health outcomes, and this can be seen in terms of a range of both physical and mental health problems. A comprehensive study of the health problems of homeless people in Britain (Bines 1994) found that people using hostels, living in bed and breakfast accommodation, and those sleeping rough were not only more likely to have health problems than the general population, but were also more likely to have multiple health problems. Health data were collected from 1280 people living in hostels and bed and breakfast accommodation and 507 people sleeping rough and using day centres and soup runs. These were compared to data from the first wave of the British Household Panel Survey (BHPS), which is a representative sample of 10 264 individuals from over 5000 households (Buck et al. 1994). Bines calculated standardized *morbidity* ratios which take into account the age and sex structure of each group. This is a more accurate comparison than merely reporting rates of ill health, as the homeless group is, on average, much younger than the general population and so should 'expect' good health. The standardized morbidity ratios are presented in Table 10.7. As with standardized mortality ratios, the rate of the general population is set at 100. A number higher than 100 means that the

Table 10.7
Standardized morbidity ratios (SMorbRs) for reported health problems for hostel users and rough sleepers compared to the general population (from Bines 1994)

Health problem	Hostels and B&Bs	Sleeping rough	
		Day centres	Soup runs
Musculoskeletal problems	153	185	221
Wounds, skin ulcers, or other skin complaints	105	189	298
Chronic chest or other breathing problems	183	259	365
Fits or loss of consciousness	651	2109	1892
Frequent headaches	264	338	365

SmorbRs for the general population (from the BHPS) are 100.
B&B, bed and breakfast.

group is more likely than the general population to experience that particular health problem.

We can see from this table that the homeless have higher rates of morbidity than the general population. Those in hostels have rates higher than the general population (whose rates are set equal to 100) and those sleeping rough have even higher rates. For example, those living in hostels and bed and breakfast accommodation have an SMorbR of 183 for 'chronic chest or other breathing problems' – meaning they are nearly twice as likely to report suffering from this health problem. Those using soup runs are almost four times as likely to report this problem, with an SMorbR of 365. Rates are highest, however, for 'fits or loss of consciousness', a result which is likely to be related to the high levels of drug and alcohol use amongst these groups, in conjunction with the deprivations of living on the streets.

Other studies have found that tuberculosis is also more common and rising amongst the homeless in England and Wales (Ramsden et al. 1988). Darbyshire (1995) links recent increases in tuberculosis in England and Wales with poverty, unemployment, and homelessness. Kumar et al. (1995) found that nearly one-quarter of the 642 shelter users examined had abnormal chest radiographs and 5 per cent had active tuberculosis.

A recent Office of Population Censuses and Surveys survey of psychiatric morbidity amongst homeless people included hostel residents, residents of private-sector leased accommodation (used as a substitute for bed and break-fast accommodation by local authorities), adults staying in nightshelters, and people sleeping rough (Gill et al. 1996). The results (Table 10.8) show high rates of physical and mental illness, and many individuals reporting both.

Table 10.8 also indicates high rates of alcohol and drug dependence, with

Table 10.8

Selected results of the OPCS survey of psychiatric morbidity (% self-reported items) (adapted from Gill et al. 1996)

	Sample size*	Physical illness only	Physical and mental illness	Mental illness only	Alcohol dependence	Drug dependence	GP registration
Hostels	530	36	6	6	16	11	92
PSLA	268	33	2	3	3	7	95
Nightshelters	187	26	9	12	44	29	71
Sleeping rough	181	39	14	7	50	24	58

* Not all respondents completed all parts of the questionnaire.
PSLA, private-sector leased accommodation.

half of the rough sleepers alcohol dependent, and one-quarter drug dependent. This compares to rates for the general population of about 5 per cent and 2 per cent, respectively (Meltzer et al. 1995). This can lead to cirrhosis, overdoses, and accidents. Injecting drug use also brings problems such as thrombosis, abscesses, and infected injecting sites. When needles are shared, there is also the risk of HIV infection.

Another health issue associated with homelessness is suicide (Baker 1997). Suicide and suicidal feelings are likely to occur at all stages of homelessness: fear of losing one's home, sudden and unprepared moves, having no settled home, seeking accommodation, waiting for a home, and settling into a new home (in some ways similar to the challenges faced by migrants). As Baker notes, various emotions are associated with homelessness:

> . . . a sense of isolation and loneliness, feeling worthless, a failure and uncared for, lacking hope for the future, feeling trapped and powerless to change things, despised, rejected and marginalised by society, feeling frustrated, betrayed and misunderstood.
>
> *(Baker 1997, p. 24)*

Keyes and Kennedy (1992) found that homeless people were 34 times more likely to kill themselves than the general population; similarly, Grenier (1997) reports that they are 35 times more likely to do so. Craig et al. (1996) found that one-third of young homeless people had attempted suicide and that self-harm (for example, cutting or burning) is also common.

Violence from others is also an everyday threat faced by those without a home, especially homeless women and those sleeping on the streets. North et al. (1996), in a study of the use of accident and emergency departments by homeless people, found that their accidental injuries were four times as likely to be the result of assault as those of housed people. Keyes and Kennedy (1992) found that homeless people were 150 times more likely to be fatally assaulted and eight times more likely to die in an accident than the general population.

The homeless have also been found to have much higher overall mortality rates than the housed population. In the USA, Hwang et al. (1997) report the average age of death of homeless people in Boston to be 47 years. A study in Georgia reports an average age of death of 46 years; 42 per cent of deaths were from injuries, mostly accidental, nearly half of which were related to acute or chronic effects of alcohol (Hanzlick and Parrish 1993). However, due to problems with estimating the denominator – the number of homeless people in each age group – it is difficult to compare death rates with those of the general population. In Britain, a study of deaths of rough sleepers found the average age of death to be 42 (Grenier 1997) – this has been found to translate to a standardized mortality ratio of over 2500 (Shaw and Dorling 1998). The street homeless are 25 times more likely to die in any given period than the people who walk past them on the streets.

The direction of the relationship between health and homelessness, and particularly mental health, is unclear – the health problems of some homeless people may predate their homelessness (Pleace and Quilgars 1996). For example, Bines' study (1994) found that between 12 per cent and 20 per cent of homeless people had previously stayed in a psychiatric institution. However, between 9 per cent and 21 per cent had been in a young offenders' institution, and 15–24 per cent had been in a children's home; over half had been resident in some kind of institution before becoming homeless. Moreover, while some health problems may precede homelessness, it is certainly the case that the daily conditions of homelessness, both material and psychosocial, compound existing health problems, cause additional problems (such as problems with feet and respiratory illness), and make access to healthcare more problematic (Fisher and Collins 1993; Pleace and Quilgars 1996). The increasing homelessness in many European countries is thus likely to lead to elevated rates of morbidity and mortality for the people concerned.

10.5 Conclusion and implications for policy

There is a well-established link between poverty and poor health – those who are socially excluded, such as the unemployed, refugees and other poorer migrants, and the homeless, experience worse or very worse health outcomes than the general population. In the context of increasing poverty, inequality, and social exclusion in Europe, health inequalities are also polarizing.

In the long term, the way to address the poor health of the socially excluded is to pursue economic policies that lead to greater economic equality. A redistribution in wealth will have the greatest influence on improving the health of those who are worse off. There is also evidence that societies that are more economically equal and socially cohesive have lower overall mortality than those that are more unequal (Wilkinson 1996).

However, in the short term, and in the light of the fact that poverty and social exclusion are currently increasing rather than decreasing, a number of specific actions can be taken to improve the health of the socially excluded. As social exclusion is dynamic and multidimensional, so should be the policies to combat it and its effects. Policies include:

(1) Legislation to protect the rights of minority and migrant groups, particularly concerning citizenship and employment rights, anti-discrimination, and protection of those seeking asylum.

(2) Income support/welfare regimes to provide an adequate standard of living for the unemployed. Adequate minimum wages to protect those on low incomes.

(3) Policies should focus on reducing the proportion of children born into and living in poverty (which will have short-term as well as long-term effects on health).

(4) Policies should aim to reduce inequalities in income and wealth within populations, for example, through progressive taxation of income and inherited wealth.

(5) Policies to ensure access to educational, training, and employment opportunities, especially for those such as the long-term unemployed.

(6) Barriers to access to health and social services should be removed, which will involve understanding where and why such barriers exist.

(7) Adequate follow-up support is needed for those leaving institutional care.

(8) Housing policies should aim to provide enough affordable housing of reasonable standard.

(9) Employment policies should aim to preserve and create jobs.

(10) Improving the health of migrants requires attention to the unfavourable socio-economic position of many migrant groups and also particular difficulties of access to health, and other care services.

Policies such as these, which are focused on the many dimensions of social exclusion and which aim to reduce inequality in a society, will have an effect on health. As Blane and co-workers say:

> A society which nurtures people's skills and abilities throughout the population, which provides economic opportunities for all, and fosters a cohesive and integrated social environment, would do more for health than curative medical services are able to.
> *(Blane et al. 1996, p. 12)*

References

Baker, L. (1997). *Homelessness and suicide.* Shelter, London.

Bartley, M., Montgomery, S., Cook, D. and Wadsworth, M. (1996). Health and work insecurity in young men. In: *Health and social organization: towards a health policy for the 21st century* (ed. D. Blane, E. Brunner, and R. Wilkinson). Routledge, London.

Bines, W. (1994). *The health of single homeless people.* Centre for Housing Policy, University of York, York.

Black, D. and Laughlin, S. (1996). Poverty and health: the old alliance needs new partners. *Benefits* Sept./Oct., 5–9.

Blackburn, C. (1991). *Poverty and health: working with families.* Open University Press, Buckingham.

Blane, D. and Drever, F. (1998). Inequality among men in standardised years of potential life lost, 1970–93. *BMJ* **317**, 255.

Blane, D., Brunner, E. and Wilkinson, R. (1996). The evolution of public health policy: an Anglocentric view of the last fifty years. In: *Health and social organization: towards a health policy for the 21st century* (ed. D. Blane, E. Brunner, and R. Wilkinson). Routledge, London.

Bobak, M. and Marmot, M. (1996). East–West mortality divide and its potential explanations: proposed research agenda. *BMJ* **312**, 421–5.

Brandt, P. and Munk-Jorgensen, P. (1996). Homelessness in Denmark. In: *Homelessness and mental health* (ed. D. Bhugra). Cambridge University Press, Cambridge.

Buck N., Gershuny J., Rose D. and Scott, J. (ed.) (1994). *Changing households. The British Household Panel Survey 1990–1992*. ESRC Centre for Micro-Social Change, Colchester.

Cockerham, W.C. (1997). Life expectancy in Russia and Eastern Europe: a lifestyle explanation. *J. Hlth Soc. Behav.* **38**, 117–30.

Cornia, A.G. and Paniccia, R. (1995). The demographic impact of sudden impoverishment: Eastern Europe during the 1989–94 transition. In: *UNICEF Innocenti Occasional Papers*, Economic Policy Studies, No. 49. UNICEF, Florence.

Corvalan, C.F., Driscoll, T.R. and Harrison, J.E. (1994). Role of migrant factors in work-related fatalities in Australia. *Scand. J. Work, Environ. Hlth* **20**, (5), 364–70.

Craig, T.K.J., et al. (1996). *Off to a bad start*. Mental Health Foundation, London.

Darbyshire, J.H. (1995). Tuberculosis: old reasons for a new increase? *BMJ* **310**, 954–5.

Davey Smith, G. (1998). Poverty across the lifecourse and health. *Radical Statistics* **68**, 15–29.

Davey Smith, G. and Egger, M. (1996). Commentary: understanding it all – health, meta-theories, and mortality trends. *BMJ* **313**, 1584–5.

Davey Smith, G., Blane, D. and Bartley, M. (1994). Explanations for socio-economic differences in mortality: evidence from Britain and elsewhere. *Eur. J. Publ. Hlth* **4** (2), 131–44.

Davey Smith, G., Hart, C., Blane, D., Gillis, C. and Hawthorne, V. (1997). Lifetime socioeconomic position and mortality: prospective observational study. *BMJ* 314, 547–52.

Davey Smith, G., Hart, C., Watt, G., Hole, D. and Hawthorne, V. (1998*a*). Individual social class, area-based deprivation, cardiovascular disease risk factors, and mortality: The Renfrew and Paisley study. *J. Epidemiol. Commun. Hlth*, **52**, 399–405.

Davey Smith, G., Hart, C., Blane, D. and Hole, D. (1998*b*). Adverse socio-economic conditions in childhood and cause-specific adult mortality: prospective longitudinal study. *BMJ* **316**, 1631–5.

Davis, C.M. (1993). *Eastern Europe and the former USSR: an overview*. RFE/RL Research Report, Vol.2, No. 40, 8 October.

Dennis, B.H., Zhukovsky, G.S., Shestov, D.B., et al. (1993). The association of education with coronary heart disease mortality in the USSR. Lipid Research Clinics Study. *Int. J. Epidemiol.* **22**, 420–7.

Dorling, D. (1995). *A new social atlas of Britain*. Wiley, Chichester.

Drever, F. and Whitehead, M. (1997). *Health inequalities: decennial supplement*. ONS, The Stationery Office, London.

Eames, M., Ben-Shlomo, Y. and Marmot, M.G. (1993). Social deprivation and premature mortality: regional comparison across England. *BMJ* **307**, 1097–102.

Egger, M., Minder, C.E. and Davey Smith, G. (1990). Health inequalities and migrant workers in Switzerland. *Lancet* Sept. 29, 816.

Elender, F., Bentham, G. and Langford, I. (1998). Tuberculosis mortality in England and Wales during 1982–1992: its association with poverty, ethnicity and AIDS. *Soc. Sci. Med.* **46** (6), 673–81.

Ellman, M. (1994). The increase in death and disease under 'katastroika'. *Camb. J. Econ.* **18**, 329–55.

Etienne, T.J., Spiliopoulos, A. and Megevand, R. (1994). Surgery for lung tuberculosis and related lesions: change in clinical presentation as a consequence of migration of population. *Acta Chir. Belg.* **94** (2), 101–4.

Fernandez, J. (1996). Homelessness: an Irish perspective. In: *Homelessness and mental health* (ed. D. Bhugra). Cambridge University Press, Cambridge.

Ferrie, J., Shipley M.J., Marmot, M.G., Stansfeld, S. and Davey Smith, G. (1995). Health effects of anticipation of job change and non-employment: longitudinal data from the Whitehall II study. *BMJ* **311**, 1264–9.

Feshbach, M. and Friendly, A. (1992). *Ecocide in the USSR*. Basic Books, New York.

Filakti, H. and Fox, J. (1995). Differences in mortality by housing tenure and by car access from the OPCS Longitudinal Study. *Popn Trends* **81**, 27–30.

Fisher, K. and Collins, J. (1993). Access to health care. In: *Homelessness, health care and welfare provision* (ed. K. Fisher and J. Collins). Routledge, London.

Gill, B., Meltzer, H., Hinds, K. and Petticrew, M. (1996). *Psychiatric morbidity among homeless people*. OPCS Surveys of Psychiatric Morbidity in Great Britain. HMSO, London.

Goodman, A., Johnson, P. and Webb, S. (1997). *Inequality in the UK*. Oxford University Press, Oxford.

Graham, H. (1995). Cigarette smoking: a light on gender and class inequality in Britain? *J. Soc. Policy* **24** (4), 509–27.

Green, A. (1998). Problems of measuring participation in the Labour Market. In: *Statistics in society* (ed. D. Dorling and S. Simpson). Arnold, London.

Grenier, P. (1997). *Still dying for a home: an update of Crisis' 1992 investigation into the links between homelessness, health and mortality*. Crisis, London.

Gunnell, D.J., Peters, T.J., Kammerling, R.M. and Brooks, J. (1995). Relation between parasuicide, suicide, psychiatric admissions, and socioeconomic deprivation. *BMJ* **311**, 226–30.

Haan, M., Kaplan, G. and Camacho, T. (1987). Poverty and health: prospective evidence from the Alameda County Study. *Am. J. Epidemiol.* **125** (6), 989–98.

Hanzlick, R. and Parrish, R.G. (1993). Death among the homeless in Fulton County, GA, 1988–90. *Publ. Hlth Rep.* **108**, 488–91.

Harding, S. and Balarajan, R. (1996). Patterns of mortality in second generation Irish living in England and Wales: longitudinal study. *BMJ* **312**, 1389–92.

Hertzman, C. (1995). *Environment and health in central and eastern Europe.* World Bank, Washington DC.

Hills, J. (1995*a*). *Joseph Rowntree Foundation inquiry into income and wealth,* Vol. I. Joseph Rowntree Foundation, York.

Hills, J. (1995*b*). *Joseph Rowntree Foundation inquiry into income and wealth,* Vol. II. Joseph Rowntree Foundation, York.

Hills, J. (1998). *Income and wealth: the latest evidence.* Joseph Rowntree Foundation, York.

Hwang, S.W., Orav, E.J., O'Connell, J.J., Lebow, J.M. and Brennan, T.A. (1997). Causes of death in homeless adults in Boston. *Ann. Int. Med.* **126**, 625–8.

Ineichen, B. (1993). *Homes and health: how housing and health interact.* Chapman and Hall, London.

Keyes, S. and Kennedy, M. (1992). *Sick to death of homelessness.* Crisis, London.

Kumar, D., Citron, K.M., Leese, J. and Watson, J.M. (1995). Tuberculosis among the homeless at a temporary shelter in London: report of a chest X ray screening programme. *J. Epidemiol. Commun. Hlth* **49**, 629–33.

Kunst, A. (1997). Cross-national comparison of socio-economic differences in mortality. Ph.D. Thesis, Erasmus University, Rotterdam.

Kunst, A.E. and Mackenbach, J.P. (1992). *An international comparison of socio-economic inequalities in mortality.* Erasmus University, Rotterdam.

Kunst, A.E., Guerts, J.J.M. and van der Berg, J. (1995). International variation in socioeconomic inequalities in self reported health. *J. Epidemiol. Commun. Hlth* **49**, 117–23.

Langford, I.H. and Bentham, G. (1996). Regional variations in mortality rates in England and Wales: an analysis using multilevel modelling. *Soc. Sci. Med.* **42** (6), 897–908.

Leon, D.A., Chenet, L., Shloknikov, V.M., et al. (1997). Huge variation in Russian mortality rates 1984–1994: artefact or alcohol or what? *Lancet* **350**, 383–8.

McLoone, P. (1996). Suicide and deprivation in Scotland. *BMJ* **312**, 543–4.

McLoone, P. and Boddy, F.A. (1994). Deprivation and mortality in Scotland, 1981 and 1991. *BMJ* **309**, 1465–70.

Marmot, M.G., Adelstein, A.M. and Bulusu, L. (1984). *Immigrant mortality in England and Wales, 1970–78: causes of death by country of birth*. Studies on medical and population subjects, No. 47. HMSO, London.

Meltzer, H., Gill, B., Petticrew, M. and Hinds, K. (1995). *The prevalence of psychiatric morbidity among adults living in private households*. HMSO, London.

Morris, J.K., Cook, D.G. and Shaper, A.G. (1994). Loss of employment and mortality. *BMJ* **308**, 1135–9.

Nazroo, J. (1998). The racialisation of ethnic inequalities in health. In: *Statistics in society*, (ed. D. Dorling and S. Simpson). Arnold, London.

North, C., Moore, H. and Owens, C. (1996). *Go home and rest? The use of an accident and emergency department by homeless people*. Shelter, London.

Oppenheim, C. and Harker, L. (1996). *Poverty: the facts*. Child Poverty Action Group, London.

Phillimore, P.K. and Morris, D. (1991). Discrepant legacies: premature mortality in two industrial towns. *Soc. Sci. Med.* **33** (2), 139–52.

Phillimore, P., Beattie, A. and Townsend, P. (1994). Widening inequality of health in northern England, 1981–1991. *BMJ* **308**, 1125–8.

Pinder, D. (1998). New Europe or New Europes? East–West development dynamics in the twentieth century. In: *The New Europe: economy, society and environment* (ed. D. Pinder). Wiley, Chichester.

Pleace, N. and Quilgars, D. (1996). *Health and homelessness in London: a review*. King's Fund, London.

Raleigh, V.S. and Kiri, V.A. (1997). Life expectancy in England: variations and trends by gender, health authority, and level of deprivation. *J. Epidemiol. Commun. Hlth* **51** (6), 649–58.

Ramsden, S.S., Baur S. and el Kabir, D.J. (1988). Tuberculosis among the central London homeless. *J. R. Coll. Gen. Pract.* **22**, 16–17.

Raviglione, M.C., Rieder, H.L., Styblo, K., Khomenko, A.G., Esteves,K. and Kochi, A. (1994). Tuberculosis trends in eastern Europe and the former USSR. *Tubercle and Lung Dis.* **75** (6), 400–16.

Room, G. (1991). *New poverty in the European Community*. Macmillan, Oxford.

Room, G. (1995). Conclusions. In: *Beyond the threshold: the measurement and analysis of social exclusion* (ed. G. Room). The Policy Press, Bristol.

Rossler, W. and Salize, H.J (1996). Longitudinal statistics of mental health care in Germany. *Soc. Psychiatry Psychiat. Epidemiol.* **29**, 112–18.

Schnabel, P. (1992). Down and out; social marginality and homelessness. *Int. J. Soc. Psychiat.* **38** (1), 59–67.

Schulpen, T.W. (1996). Migration and child health: the Dutch experience. *Europ. J. Pediat.* **155** (5), 351–6.

Shapiro, J. (1995). The Russian mortality crisis and its causes. In: *Russian economic reform at risk* (ed. A. Aslund). Pinter, London.

Shaw, M. and Dorling, D. (1998). Mortality among street youth in the UK. *Lancet* **352**, 743.

Shaw, M., Orford, S., Brimblecombe, N. and Dorling, D. (1998). *Widening inequality in mortality between 160 regions of 15 European countries in the early 1990s.* Proceedings of the 8th International Symposium in Medical Geography, Baltimore, USA, 13–17 July, pp. 371–90.

Shloknikov, V.M., Leon, D.A., Adamets, S., Andreev, E. and Deev, A. (1998). Educational level and adult mortality in Russia: an analysis of routine data 1979 to 1994. *Soc. Sci. Med.*, in press.

Shouls, S., Congdon, P. and Curtis, S. (1996). Modelling inequality in reported long term illness in the UK: combining individual and area characteristics. *J. Epidemiol. Commun. Hlth* **50**, 366–76.

Sooman, A. and MacIntyre, S. (1995). Health and perceptions of the local environment in socially contrasting neighbourhoods in Glasgow. *Hlth Place* **1**, 15–26.

Sundquist, J. (1995). Living conditions and health: a population-based study of labour migrants and Latin American refugees in Sweden and those who were repatriated. *Scand. J. Primary Hlth Care* **13** (2), 128–34.

Toole, M.J. and Waldman, R.J. (1997). The public health aspects of complex emergencies and refugee situations. *Ann. Rev. Publ. Hlth* **18**, 283–312.

Townsend, P., Phillimore, P. and Beattie, A. (1988). *Health and deprivation: inequality in the north.* Croom Helm, London.

Trovato, F. (1992). Violent and accidental mortality among four immigrant groups in Canada. *Soc. Biol.* **39** (1), 82–101.

UNICEF (1993). *Central and eastern Europe in transition: public policy and social conditions.* Regional Monitoring Report No. 1. International Child Development Centre, Florence.

Victor, C.R. (1997). The health of homeless people in Britain: A review. *Eur. J. Publ. Hlth* **7**, 398–404.

Vogel, J. (1997). *Living conditions and inequality in the European Union 1997.* Eurostat Working Papers. University of Umea, Stockholm.

Wadsworth, M. (1996). Family and education as determinants of health. In: *Health and social organization: towards a health policy for the 21st century* (ed. D. Blane, E. Brunner and R. Wilkinson). Routledge, London.

Watson, P. (1995). Explaining rising mortality among men in Eastern Europe. *Soc. Sci. Med.* **41** (7), 923–34.

Watson. P. (1998). Health differences in Eastern Europe: preliminary findings from the Nowa Huta study. *Soc. Sci. Med.* **46**, 549–58.

White, P. (1998). Urban life and social stress. In: *The New Europe: economy, society and environment* (ed. D. Pinder). Wiley, Chichester:

Wilkinson, R.G. (1996). *Unhealthy societies: the afflictions of inequality.* Routledge, London.

Acknowledgements

All the authors have been funded by the Economic and Social Research Council's Health Variations Programme.

11 Social patterning of individual health behaviours: the case of cigarette smoking

Martin J. Jarvis and Jane Wardle

11.1 Introduction

Poverty is linked intimately to a variety of behaviours that impact on health. As illustrated in Table 11.1, poor people in a country such as the UK are less likely than those who are well off to eat a good diet, more likely to have a sedentary life style, more likely to be obese, and more likely to be regularly drunk. These associations may be due to a variety of factors, including poverty itself, as well as poorer access to education and information, rather than reflecting a single invariant cause, and not all of these associations may be found in all societies. Nevertheless, their consistency is impressive. Nowhere are the links between deprivation and health behaviours stronger than in the case of drug use, both legal and illegal. Alcohol abuse is frequently a marker for acute social break-down and, through accidents and violence induced by drunkenness, has a significant impact on death rates (Makela et al. 1997). Binge drinking, which is more common in deprived groups in the population, may lead directly to sudden cardiac death (Kauhanen et al. 1997). Drug users are differentially represented in groups with disturbed family backgrounds, low self-esteem, and impaired psychological functioning. The costs to society through drug-related crime and social disruption are immense. Cigarette smoking stands out as somewhat different: the acute effects of nicotine do not lead directly to disturbed behaviour, crime, or violence, but cigarette smoking imposes the greatest costs of all in terms of premature death. It, too, shows a strong association with indicators of social disadvantage.

Smoking, drinking, and drug use are individual behaviours which involve an element of personal choice. It is perhaps for this reason that they have frequently been seen not in a broad social context but as a matter of individual responsibility: if smokers wish to avoid the adverse effects of tobacco on their health, it is for them to change their behaviour and quit. If they don't, they have brought ill health on themselves and it is no-one

Table 11.1
Distribution of some health behaviours by level of socio-economic
deprivation (from Colhoun and Prescott-Clarke: Health Survey for England 1994)

| | Level of socio-economic deprivation | | | |
	0 least deprived	1	2	3+ most deprived
Men				
% eat fruit less often than weekly	6.3	9.7	15.2	21.3
% sedentary life style	14.3	14.5	21.0	28.9
% body mass index > 30	13.3	13.4	13.8	17.0
% drunk at least once per week	7.0	13.2	16.1	15.9
Women				
% eat fruit less often than weekly	4.2	6.9	10.7	14.1
% sedentary life style	14.5	17.3	24.6	31.5
% body mass index > 30	14.9	16.0	21.0	25.2
% drunk at least once per week	3.0	5.9	7.6	8.1

else's fault. Persistence in unhealthy behaviours is sometimes seen simply as fecklessness rather than as a response to social circumstances. This victim-blaming approach is unhelpful, in that it fails to address underlying questions of why disadvantaged people are drawn to these behaviours and the nature of the social and individual influences that maintain them. It has also been signally unsuccessful in leading to the development of effective interventions to achieve behaviour change in disadvantaged groups.

This chapter will focus on cigarette smoking, as the individual health behaviour with the single largest impact on health inequalities. As a legal, widespread, and, until recently at least, little stigmatized behaviour, there is a wealth of detailed data available documenting its natural history, social patterning, and impact on health. Drawing on data from the UK, a country where the smoking epidemic is now mature, we consider first the nature and extent of the association of smoking with indicators of disadvantage, and trends in rates of current and ex-smoking by deprivation. We then briefly give estimates of the contribution of smoking to death rates in different social groups, before attempting to address the question of why poor people are more likely to smoke and why they find it harder to give up. The final section outlines possible policy options to reduce smoking-induced inequalities.

11.2   Rates of cigarette smoking by material and cultural disadvantage

The gradient in cigarette smoking prevalence by occupational class is well known, as is also the high rate of smoking in lone parents (Marsh and McKay

1994), the unemployed (Lee et al 1991) and the mentally ill (Hughes et al. 1986). But these links by no means fully characterize the extent of smoking's association with disadvantage. Table 11.2, which draws on several years' data from the General Household Survey (Bennett et al. 1996), documents how a whole range of circumstances independently predict current cigarette smoking. Thus the odds of being a smoker are significantly increased in those in lower occupational class groups, those living in rented housing, without access to a car, who are unemployed, and in crowded accommodation. Above and beyond this there is a substantial gradient by educational level, and an increased risk in those who are divorced or separated or lone parents. With the exception of lone parenthood, which is uncommon in men and appears not to carry a risk of smoking for them, the magnitude of the associations is very similar in men and women. These independent associations imply extreme differences in smoking prevalence between groups with different constellations of circumstances. For example, by comparison with professional owner-occupiers with degree-level education and owning a car, the predicted odds of smoking for unemployed, unskilled manual workers living in rented, crowded accommodation and with no car are 17.8, corresponding to smoking prevalences in these groups of about 15 per cent and 75 per cent, respectively. It should be noted that these variables do not provide an exhaustive list of factors influencing smoking prevalence, as other work shows that smoking is more common in people suffering from mental illness or who are heavy drinkers or who are homeless. Indeed, groups who have an extreme clustering of deprivation indicators, such as prisoners in gaol and homeless people sleeping rough, have been observed to have rates of smoking prevalence of 80–90 per cent (Bridgwood and Malbon 1995; Gill et al. 1996).

The factors that predict smoking include material circumstances, cultural deprivation, and indicators of stressful marital, personal, and household circumstances. This illustrates what might be proposed as a general law of Western industrialized society; namely, that any marker of disadvantage that can be envisaged and measured, whether personal, material, or cultural, is likely to have an independent association with cigarette smoking. Of course, this may not be true of all societies, such as, for example, Asian countries where there is an overriding cultural prohibition on women's smoking, and in particular may not be true of developing societies in which cigarette smoking is associated with images of glamour and Western prosperity, rather than disadvantage and poverty.

11.3 Trends in cigarette smoking prevalence and rates of cessation by deprivation

Cigarette smoking prevalence has been on a declining trend in Britain for over 20 years, reducing overall from 53 per cent in 1973 to 29 per cent in 1996 in

Table 11.2 Predictors of current cigarette smoking among men and women (General Household Survey 1988–96)

	Men		Women		All	
	OR	95%CI	OR	95%CI	OR	95%CI
Social class						
I	1.00		1.00		1.00	
II	1.37	1.20–1.56	1.47	1.29–1.68	1.41	1.28–1.54
III NM	1.18	1.04–1.35	1.46	1.28–1.66	1.31	1.20–1.44
III M	1.65	1.45–1.88	1.86	1.63–2.12	1.74	1.59–1.90
IV	1.58	1.38–1.82	1.74	1.52–1.99	1.63	1.49–1.80
V	1.59	1.35–1.88	1.88	1.60–2.21	1.71	1.52–1.91
Rented tenure	1.88	1.78–1.99	1.85	1.75–1.95	1.87	1.80–1.95
No car	1.43	1.33–1.53	1.33	1.25–1.41	1.38	1.32–1.45
Unemployed	1.59	1.46–1.74	1.43	1.28–1.58	1.53	1.44–1.64
Crowding	1.25	1.15–1.35	1.10	1.01–1.19	1.17	1.10–1.23
Education						
Degree level	1.00		1.00		1.00	
Higher < degree	1.51	1.34–1.71	1.84	1.58–2.12	1.63	1.48–1.79
A level	1.62	1.44–1.82	1.62	1.40–1.87	1.61	1.47–1.76
O level	1.95	1.74–2.18	2.02	1.78–2.30	1.94	1.78–2.10
CSE grade	2.03	1.79–2.39	2.50	2.18–2.86	2.22	2.07–2.43
No qualification	2.49	2.23–2.78	3.10	2.72–3.53	2.73	2.52–2.97
Lone parent	0.90	0.73–1.10	1.49	1.36–1.64	1.33	1.22–1.44
Divorced or separated	1.73	1.56–1.92	1.38	1.26–1.51	1.53	1.43–1.64

OR, odds ratio.

men, and from 42 per cent to 28 per cent in women. But over this same period there has been a substantial widening of the gulf in prevalence between social groups. Figure 11.1a shows trends by a composite index of deprivation which incorporates several of the variables in Table 11.2. Respondents are assigned a score of 1 for each of the following: manual occupational class, rented housing, no car, unemployed, and living in crowded conditions (one or more persons per room). The resulting index, with scores ranging from 0 among the affluent to 5 among the most deprived, is similar to the indices employed by Townsend (Townsend et al. 1988) and by Carstairs (Carstairs and Morris 1989), but is applied to individuals rather than to areas. In both 1973 and 1996, for both men and women, there was an approximately linear increase in cigarette smoking with increasing deprivation. Among the most affluent, smoking rates more than halved over the years, reaching a figure of 17 per cent in 1996. Among the most deprived, on the other hand, 70 per cent or more were smokers in 1973, and that still remained the case some 23 years later.

Figure 11.1b shows rates of smoking cessation by deprivation in 1973 and 1996 (Jarvis 1997). Mirroring the observations on prevalence, it indicates that while rates of cessation more than doubled in affluent people, from 25 per cent to 55 per cent, among the poorest groups there was little or no change, with 10 per cent or less of ever-regular smokers giving up.

11.4 Contribution of smoking to differences in death rates by social group

It has long been acknowledged that smoking has a major bearing on observed differences in death rates by social class. One in two of those who smoke are ultimately killed by the habit if they persist and do not give up (Doll et al. 1994; Thun et al. 1995) and, in view of higher prevalence and lower rates of cessation, it would be anticipated that smoking-related disease would bear more heavily on poorer groups. Poorer diet and factors such as earlier age of starting to smoke (leading to longer duration of smoking at any given age) and higher levels of smoke intake in poorer smokers (see below) would act to amplify smoking risks.

Unsurprisingly, observed rates of death from smoking-related diseases show a gradient that parallels the gradient in smoking prevalence. Standardized mortality ratios in unskilled male workers are three times higher than in professionals for heart disease, five times higher for lung cancer, six times higher for emphysema, and 14 times higher for chronic airways obstruction (Drever and Whitehead 1997). Similar but somewhat smaller variations are seen in women. As would be expected from the preceding discussion, alternative indicators of socio-economic status, such as housing tenure or access to

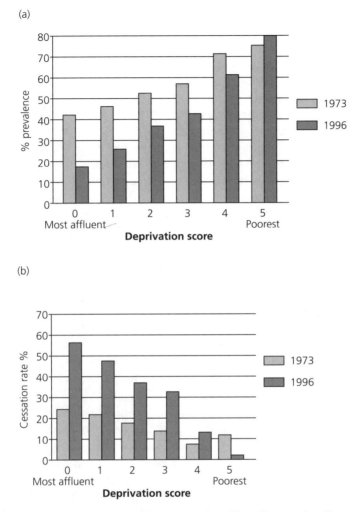

Fig. 11.1 Deprivation in Great Britain and (a) cigarette smoking; (b) smoking cessation. (General Household Survey data 1973 and 1996; from Jarvis 1997.)

a car, are additionally predictive of death rates (Goldblatt 1990; Smith and Harding 1997).

Recently the indirect methods developed by Peto and Lopez (Peto et al. 1992, 1994) to estimate deaths from smoking in different countries have been applied to deaths by socio-economic status within countries (Jarvis et al. 1999). For men aged 35–69 in England and Wales, estimates have been made of the proportion of deaths attributable to smoking by social class for the years since 1970. In 1970–72 among men in social class I and II the overall risk of dying in middle age was 36 per cent, and just over one-third of these deaths (13 per cent) were estimated to be attributable to smoking. By 1996 the overall risk of dying had declined to 21 per cent, and tobacco-attributable deaths were 4 per cent. Thus the reduction in deaths attributable to tobacco was responsible for over half of the overall reduction in risk of death. Men in social class V, by contrast, had an overall risk in 1970–72 of dying in middle age of 47 per cent, and over half of this (25 per cent) was accounted for by tobacco. By 1996 the risk had declined only modestly to 43 per cent and the estimated smoking attributable element to 19 per cent.

Of course, the accuracy of these estimates depends on the adequacy of the data and of the assumptions underlying their calculation. The overall number of deaths attributed to tobacco is subject to considerable uncertainty, due to fairly approximate assumptions. For example, only half of the apparent excess of vascular deaths observed in smokers is attributed to tobacco. This somewhat arbitrary proportion, intended to be conservative, may either underestimate true smoking effects, or not be conservative enough. However, for the method to give seriously misleading results for differences in the proportions of deaths attributable to smoking in different social class groups, there would have to be major bias introduced in the calculations across different classes. It is difficult to see that any major bias could be present which would invalidate the estimates.

These findings carry a number of implications. First, the observed widening in overall risk of death between men in social classes I and II and V that has been observed over the past 25 years largely reflects changes in tobacco-attributable mortality. Deaths caused by tobacco have dropped far more steeply in social class I and II than in social class V, paralleling changes in smoking prevalence and cessation in these groups. Men in social class V have not experienced an absolute increase in risk of death: the widening of health inequalities that has occurred has been due to their failure to share to the same extent in the major overall reduction in risk of death consequent upon smoking cessation. This implies that further reductions in smoking prevalence, unless they are concentrated in poorer groups, may only serve to widen inequalities in death rates still further. The 1996 data indicate that around two-thirds of the observed difference in risk of death across social class groups in middle age is caused by tobacco.

11.5 Why do poor people smoke?

The discussion so far has shown that disadvantaged groups in society are disproportionately likely to smoke and least likely to give up cigarettes. As a consequence, the burden of smoking-related disease also falls disproportionately on these groups. Those who can least afford to smoke, smoke the most and suffer most from it. That nicotine is a powerful drug of addiction no doubt has much to do with this state of affairs, but we need to move beyond this to ask why it is that the poor are particularly drawn to this drug. The association could be mediated by higher rates of smoking initiation, stronger perceived rewarding effects (either positive or negative) leading to higher levels of dependence, or to greater difficulties in cessation through lower motivation, higher dependence, or fewer available coping resources. These influences are not mutually exclusive, and it could be that a variety of factors operates at each stage of the smoker's career to accentuate the link with disadvantage.

A particularly important distinction to be drawn is between ever becoming a regular cigarette smoker and persisting with the habit. Among those who take up smoking but give up before their early 30s, there is no detectable increase in risk of premature death in comparison with never smokers (Doll et al. 1994). As shown in Fig. 11.2, there exists a gradient between ever-regular cigarette smoking and deprivation in both men and women, but among those aged 35–64 the gradient with current smoking is far steeper. Thus although poor people are somewhat more likely to become smokers, the strongest association is with persisting smoking. What we need to explain above all is not so much why poor people start smoking, but why they do not give it up.

11.5.1 Disadvantage and smoking uptake

A gradient in uptake of smoking by level of deprivation is not hard to explain. Children growing up in poverty experience social environments outside the home where most adults are smokers, and the vast majority, 80 per cent or more, will live in households where one or both parents smoke. Thus cigarette smoking is modelled as normal adult behaviour and cigarettes are readily available to experiment with. But in addition to this there is evidence that smoking is a measure of social trajectory, with prevalence being more closely related to people's social destination than to their circumstances of origin (Glendinning et al. 1994). In the national cohort of all the babies born in one week in 1958, who have been followed up at regular intervals ever since (Ferri 1993), cigarette smoking at age 16 increased from 24 per cent among those from the most affluent homes to 48 per cent among the most deprived. But the gradient at age 16 was much sharper (80 per cent among the most deprived) when cohort members were characterized by deprivation measured 7 years later at age 23 by their own achieved social position rather than by the characteristics of the parental household. This implies that factors conferring an increased risk of smoking at age 16 (such as poorer school achievement and lower levels of self-esteem) also have a bearing on subsequent downward social mobility.

11.5.2 Motivation to give up smoking

A superficially attractive hypothesis to explain poor people's lower likelihood of quitting smoking is that they are less well informed and concerned about

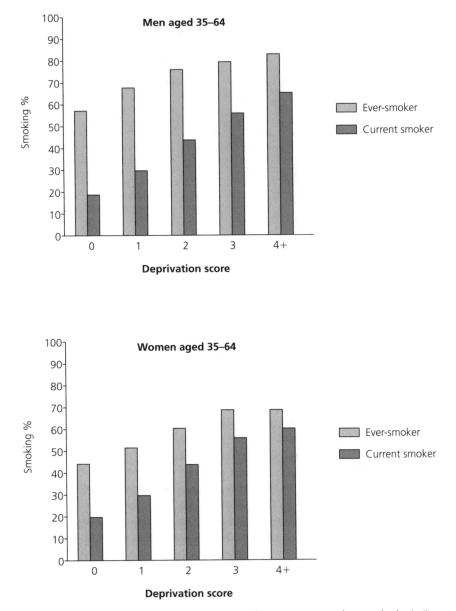

Fig. 11.2 Rates of current and ever-regular cigarette smoking among men and women by deprivation. (General Household Survey data 1988–96.)

effects on health, leading to a lower probability of attempts at quitting. On this view, the problem is that the health education message simply isn't getting through. Motivation to quit is not an easy construct to measure reliably, as it can fluctuate greatly over time and in different situations (raised in the doctor's surgery, for example, but much lower when drinking in the pub with friends). At present we are not able to do much better than ask people the question how much they want to give up smoking altogether. Responses to this have been shown to have some validity by predicting future quit attempts. In the General Household Survey, levels of expressed motivation to quit are essentially flat across deprivation categories, just over two-thirds of cigarette smokers in each group saying that they want to give up. To the extent, therefore, that this measure can be taken at face value, there is no evidence that disadvantaged groups are any less likely than the more affluent to want to give up.

11.5.3 Nicotine dependence and deprivation

By contrast with the lack of variation in motivation to quit by disadvantage, there is strong emerging evidence that level of nicotine dependence increases systematically with deprivation. This is evident both from questionnaire indicators of dependence in the General Household Survey (e.g. time to first cigarette of the day; and perceived difficulty of going for a whole day without smoking) and from quantitative measures of smoke intake. Figure 11.3 shows levels of plasma cotinine (a measure of total nicotine intake) among smokers in the Health Survey for England (Bennett et al. 1995). Increasingly high levels of nicotine intake are seen with increasing deprivation, with average intake being close to 50 per cent higher in the most deprived than in the most affluent smokers. Poor people achieve their higher intakes both by choosing to

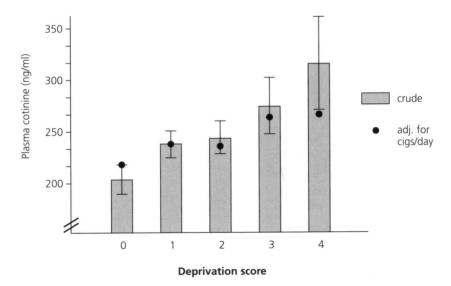

Fig. 11.3 Plasma cotinine by deprivation in adult smokers (Health Survey for England data 1993).

smoke more cigarettes and by smoking each cigarette more intensively. There are indications that this may turn out to be a phenomenon of wide generality, as similar observations have been made in the USA, comparing black with white smokers (Wagenknecht et al. 1990; English et al.1994; Caraballo et al. 1998; Perez-Stable et al. 1998) and a gradient in intake by level of education has been observed in Czech smokers (M. Bobak, personal communication). Since nicotine dependence is an important determinant of ease of quitting, these findings suggest one reason for lower rates of cessation in those who are disadvantaged. Since smoking-related disease bears a dose response relation to intake, they have implications for a higher risk of disease in poor than in affluent smokers. They also raise the question of just why it should be that poor smokers seek higher nicotine doses.

11.5.4 Functional aspects of nicotine use: positive and negative rewards

Nicotine has a number of positively rewarding effects which could serve as the basis for cigarette use. Although euphoriant effects are not as prominent as with many drugs, they are reported for at least some cigarettes by smokers (Pomerleau and Pomerleau 1992) and could achieve a greater valence for people whose lives are generally deficient in rewards. It is difficult to think of evidence which would strongly support this hypothesis, but equally it should not be ruled out.

An alternative functional view of smoking is that it is self-medication. Cigarette smoking is seen as a means of regulating mood, of managing stress, and of coping with all the hassles and strain resulting from material deprivation (Graham 1987; Smith and Morris 1994). This account corresponds with smokers' self-reports of calming effects from cigarettes and with poor women's observation that smoking is the one thing they do for themselves, that gives them space from the difficult task of caring for children in poverty (Graham 1994). It also recalls soldiers' demands for cigarettes in the First World War to help them cope with the rigours of the trenches.

Attractive though the self-medication view of smoking is, it faces several major objections. The most serious of these is the nature of nicotine as a drug. Pharmacologically nicotine is a stimulant, similar to drugs such as amphetamine. Sedative or anxiolytic effects, if they exist, are very hard to find either in animal models or in humans. Smoking is closely associated with adverse mood states, but there is no evidence that it ameliorates them other than through withdrawal relief (Anda et al. 1990; Schoenborn and Horm 1993). Smokers' self-reports of calming effects from cigarettes could refer to relief of nicotine withdrawal by smoking. Onset of withdrawal symptoms is rapid and certainly occurs with overnight abstinence during sleep, and may, in a more subtle way, begin within an hour or two of the last cigarette. Stress modulation over the course of the day suggests that mood-elevating effects of cigarettes are attributable to relief of adverse mood from incipient withdrawal rather than to any absolute benefits (Parrott 1995). Studies of the process of smoking cessation have found that successful quitting leads to lower, rather than to higher, levels of perceived stress, consistent with the idea that smoking may actually be a stressor rather than relieve stress (Cohen and Lichtenstein 1990).

11.5.5 Giving up smoking could be particularly difficult for poor people

If it is difficult to find unequivocal reasons why smoking should be more rewarding for the poor and disadvantaged, there are a number of identifiable factors which would tend to make it harder for them to give up. Even if poor people are as likely to make an attempt at quitting, higher levels of nicotine dependence would place a barrier between the attempt and success. Poor people's generally smokier environment and their much greater likelihood of having a smoking partner would further reduce their chances of succeeding (Jarvis 1997). It is important to appreciate how hard it is for smokers to give up. Estimates of the chances of succeeding for at least a year in a serious unaided quit attempt are no better than about 1 in 100 (Cohen et al. 1989; Jarvis 1997). When preparing themselves for an attempt at giving up smoking, smokers need to take a medium- to long-term view and be prepared to tolerate the discomfort of nicotine withdrawal and cravings for several weeks at least before things start to get easier. If this is difficult for everybody, it may be especially difficult for those whose lives are stressful and full of hassles to forego the certainty of short-term craving relief and elimination of withdrawal for longer-term gains in disposable income, health, and well-being. The logic of addiction, if not of economics, may win out and dictate buying the next pack of cigarettes.

11.6 Implications for policies to promote cessation

Two general kinds of approach can be identified which might reduce the association of smoking with disadvantage. Improvements in housing, education, and employment would target the underlying social conditions which foster high levels of smoking. There is little doubt that substantial progress in this direction would greatly facilitate reductions in smoking, as well as contributing to the wider adoption of other desirable health behaviours, such as an improved diet. But such change is not easy to achieve, and most government policy has sought instead to target the downstream factors which more proximally determine smoking behaviour.

The policies to reduce smoking that have been followed over the past decade or more have been successful in reducing overall prevalence, but have had the paradoxical effect of increasing health inequalities. The main planks of policy have been interventions designed to increase people's motivation to quit: price, restrictions on smoking in public places, and health education campaigns. Addressing dependence has received less attention. While price increases are effective in reducing consumption, there is some uncertainty about their impact on the poor, for whom tobacco expenditure amounts to a high proportion of disposable income (Marsh and McKay 1994). Some economists have argued that poor smokers respond equally as much, or more, to price as do affluent smokers (Townsend et al. 1994), while others are less certain. The very low rates of cessation seen in disadvantaged groups are inconsistent with the idea that for them price is an effective means of promoting cessation. Price increases may influence poor people to switch to cheaper and higher yielding brands (Jarvis 1998), to roll their own cigarettes, and to cut down on the number of cigarettes they smoke, rather than to quit altogether. Because of the phenomenon of nicotine compensation, lowering cigarette consumption is unlikely to confer any benefit in lowering risk of smoking-related disease.

The key factor amenable to intervention would appear to be nicotine dependence, and new policy initiatives need to take seriously the issue of delivering dependence treatments of proven efficacy to the groups most needing to quit. Nicotine replacement therapy (NRT) has been shown to be an effective and cost-effective aid to cessation (Buck et al. 1997; Cromwell et al. 1997), approximately doubling success rates from both brief and intensive treatments (Silagy et al. 1997) and with evidence that its success is maintained in real world settings (Shiffman et al. 1998). NRT specifically targets the dependence problem. Making NRT reimbursable would have the effect of delivering treatment free to the groups most needing help. Recent evidence from the USA has shown clearly that full reimbursement for smoking cessation treatments offers the greatest public health benefit by maximizing rates of quitting in the target population (Curry et al. 1998).

If the potential return from promoting cessation in the poor is seen as questionable, an alternative, or complementary, approach would be to take new initiatives in the area of product modification to make smoking less harmful. The advent of novel forms of nicotine delivery, as in NRT and some innovative products from the tobacco industry (Sutherland et al. 1993), is focusing attention on harm reduction as a potentially important new arm of policy (Warner et al. 1997). There is compelling evidence that people smoke for nicotine, but much of the burden of smoking-related disease is attributable to other smoke components, particularly the tar fraction. Smoking cigarettes has been likened to injecting drugs through a dirty syringe. The potential benefit of shifting the market toward safer forms of nicotine delivery is illustrated by the case of Sweden, a country that has the lowest male rate of cigarette smoking in Europe (below 20 per cent) and also the lowest rate of lung cancer. But its rate of tobacco dependence is not low, as 20 per cent of adult males use moist oral snuff, a non-combustible form of nicotine delivery which carries considerably less risk than cigarettes (Bolinder 1997).

The risk is that an intensification of current smoking control policies without fresh thinking may well succeed in further reducing prevalence, but only at the cost of still wider health inequalities.

References

Anda, R.F., Williamson, D.F., Escobedo, L.G., Mast, E.E., Giovino, G.A. and Remington, P.L. (1990). Depression and the dynamics of smoking: A national perspective. *JAMA* **264** (12), 1541–5.

Bennett, N., Dodd, T., Flatley, J., Freeth, S. and Bolling, K. (1995). *Health Survey for England 1993*. HMSO, London.

Bennett, N., Jarvis, L., Rowlands, O., Singleton, N. and Haselden, L. (1996). *Living in Britain: Results from the 1994 General Household Survey*. HMSO, London.

Bolinder, G. (1997). Smokeless tobacco a less harmful alternative? In: *The tobacco epidemic* (ed. C.T. Bolliger and K.O. Fagerstrom). Progress Respiratory Research, Vol. 28, pp. 199–212. Karger, Basel.

Bridgwood, A. and Malbon, G. (1995). *Survey of the physical health of prisoners*. HMSO, London.

Buck, D., Godfrey, C., Parrott, S. and Raw, M. (1997). *Cost effectiveness of smoking cessation interventions*. Centre for Health Economics.

Caraballo, R.S., Giovino, G.A., Pechacek, T.F., *et al.* (1998). Racial and ethnic differences in serum cotinine levels of cigarette smokers. *JAMA* **280**, 135–9.

Carstairs, V. and Morris, R. (1989). Deprivation and mortality: An alternative to social class? *Commun. Med.* **11** (3), 210–19.

Cohen, S. and Lichtenstein, E. (1990). Perceived stress, quitting smoking, and smoking relapse. *Hlth Psychol.* **9** (4), 466–78.

Cohen, S., Lichtenstein, E., Prochaska, J.O., et al. (1989). Debunking myths about self-quitting. Evidence from 10 prospective studies of persons who attempt to quit smoking by themselves. *Am. Psychol.* **44** (11), 1355–65.

Colhoun, H., Prescott-Clarke, P. (Eds) (1996). *Health Survey for England 1994*. HMSO, London.

Cromwell, J., Bartosch, W.J., Fiore, M.C., Hasselblad, V. and Baker, T. (1997). Cost-effectiveness of the clinical practice recommendations in the AHCPR guideline for smoking cessation. *JAMA* **278**, 1759–66.

Curry, S., Grothaus, L.C., McAfee, T. and Pabiniak, C. (1998). Use and cost effectiveness of smoking-cessation services under four insurance plans in a health maintenance organization. *N. Engl. J. Med.* **339**, 673–9.

Doll, R., Peto, R., Wheatley, K., Gray, R. and Sutherland, I. (1994). Mortality in relation to smoking: 40 years' observations on male British doctors. *BMJ* **309** (6959), 901–11.

Drever, F. and Whitehead, M. (ed.) (1997). *Health inequalities*. The Stationery Office, London.

English, P.B., Eskenazi, B. and Christianson, R.E. (1994). Black–White differences in serum cotinine levels among pregnant women and subsequent effects on infant birthweight. *Am. J. Publ. Hlth*, **84** (9), 1439–43.

Ferri, E. (ed.) (1993). *Life at 33: the fifth follow-up of the National Child Development Study*. National Children's Bureau, London.

Gill, B., Meltzer, H., Hinds, K. and Pettigrew, M. (1996). *Psychiatric morbidity among homeless people*, Vol. 7. HMSO, London.

Glendinning, A., Shucksmith, J. and Hendry, L. (1994). Social class and adolescent smoking behaviour. *Soc. Sci. Med.* **38**, 1449–60.

Goldblatt, P. (ed.) (1990). *Longitudinal study: mortality and social organization*. HMSO, London.

Graham, H. (1987). Women's smoking and family health. *Soc. Sci. Med.* **25** (1), 47–56.

Graham, H. (1994). Gender and class as dimensions of smoking-behavior in Britain – insights from a survey of mothers. *Soc. Sci. Med.* **38** (5), 691–8.

Hughes, J.R., Hatsukami, D.K., Mitchell, J.E. and Dahlgren, L.A. (1986). Prevalence of smoking among psychiatric outpatients. *Am. J. Psychiat.* **143** (8), 993–7.

Jarvis, M.J. (1997). Patterns and predictors of unaided smoking cessation in the general population. In: *The tobacco epidemic* (ed. C.T. Bolliger and K.O. Fagerstrom). Progress in Respiratory Research, Vol. 28, pp. 151–64. Karger, Basel.

Jarvis, M.J. (1998). Supermarket cigarettes: the brands that dare not speak their name. *BMJ* **316**, 929–31.

Jarvis, M.J., Boreham, J., Bunting, Lopez, A.D. and Peto, R. (1999). In preparation.

Kauhanen, J., Kaplan, G.A., Goldberg, D.E. and Salonen, J.T. (1997). Beer binging and mortality: Results from the Kuopio ischaemic heart disease risk factor study, a prospective population based study. *BMJ* **315** (7112), 846–51.

Lee, A.J., Crombie, I.K., Smith, W.C.S. and Tunstall-Pedoe, H.D. (1991). Cigarette smoking and employment status. *Soc. Sci. Med.* **33**, 1309–12.

Makela, P., Valkonen, T. and Martelin, T. (1997). Contribution of deaths related to alcohol use of socioeconomic variation in mortality: register based follow up study. *BMJ* **315** (7102), 211–16.

Marsh, A. and McKay, S. (1994). *Poor smokers*. Policy Studies Institute, London.

Parrott, A.C. (1995). Stress modulation over the day in cigarette smokers. *Addiction* **90** (2), 233–44.

Perez-Stable, E.J., Herrera, B., Jacob, P. and Benowitz, N.L. (1998). Nicotine metabolism and intake in black and white smokers. *JAMA* **280**, 152–6.

Peto, R., Lopez, A.D., Boreham, J., Thun, M. and Heath, C. Jr (1992). Mortality from tobacco in developed countries: Indirect estimation from national vital statistics. *Lancet* **339** (8804), 1268–78.

Peto, R., Lopez, A.D., Boreham, J., Thun, M. and Heath, C. (1994). *Mortality from smoking in developed countries 1950–2000: indirect estimates from national vital statistics.* Oxford University Press, Oxford.

Pomerleau, C.S. and Pomerleau, O.F. (1992). Euphoriant effects of nicotine in smokers. *Psychopharmacology* **108** (4), 460–5.

Schoenborn, C.A. and Horm, J. (1993). *Negative moods as correlates of smoking and heavier drinking: implications for health promotion.* National Center for Health Statistics, Hyattsville, Maryland.

Shiffman, S., Gitchell, J., Pinney, J.M., Burton, S.L., Kemper, K.E. and Lara, E.A. (1998). Public health benefit of over-the-counter nicotine medications. *Tobacco Control*, **6**, 306–10.

Silagy, C., Mant, D., Fowler, G. and Lancaster, T. (1997). The effect of nicotine replacement therapy on smoking cessation. In: *The tobacco addiction module of the Cochrane Database of Systematic Reviews* (ed. T. Lancaster, C. Silagy and D. Fullerton). The Cochrane Collaboration, Oxford.

Smith, G.D. and Morris, J. (1994). Increasing inequalities in the health of the nation. *BMJ* **309** (6967), 1453–4.

Smith, J. and Harding, S. (1997). Mortality of women and men using alternative social classifications. In: *Health inequalities: decennial supplement* (ed. F. Drever and M. Whitehead). The Stationery Office, London.

Sutherland, G., Russell, M.A.H., Stapleton, J.A. and Feyerabend, C. (1993). Glycerol particle cigarettes: a less harmful option for chronic smokers. *Thorax* **48** (4), 385–7.

Thun, M.J., Day-Lally, C.A., Calle, E.E., Flanders, W.D. and Heath, C.W. (1995). Excess mortality among cigarette smokers: changes in a 20-year interval. *Am. J. Publ. Hlth* **85** (9), 1223–30.

Townsend, J., Roderick, P. and Cooper, J. (1994). Cigarette smoking by socio-economic group, sex, and age: Effects of price, income, and health publicity. *BMJ* **309** (6959), 923–7.

Townsend, P., Phillimore, P. and Beattie, A. (1988). *Health and deprivation: inequality and the North.* Croom Helm, London.

Wagenknecht, L.E., Cutter, G.R., Haley, N.J., et al. (1990). Racial differences in serum cotinine levels among smokers in the Coronary Artery Risk Development in (Young) Adults Study. *Am. J. Publ. Hlth* **80** (9), 1053–6.

Warner, K.E., Slade, J. and Sweanor, D.T. (1997). The emerging market for long-term nicotine maintenance. *JAMA* **278**, 1087–92.

Acknowledgements

Dr Jarvis and Professor Wardle are funded by the Imperial Cancer Research Fund.

12 Putting the picture together: prosperity, redistribution, health, and welfare

Richard G. Wilkinson

12.1 Introduction

Given the strong statistical associations between people's material circumstances and their health, it may seem that the soundest approach to improving public health would be to increase everyone's prosperity by maximizing economic growth rates while ensuring that some degree of 'trickle-down' spreads the health benefits to the poor. Indeed, a possible dilemma facing public-health policy in the context of the social gradient in health is that redistributive policies may appear to achieve no more than a redistribution of a finite quantity of health-producing goods and services from the rich to the poor. Perhaps health gains for some would be cancelled out by health losses for others. And if levels of unemployment and educational opportunities are regarded as fixed, it is possible that programmes designed to improve the opportunities of disadvantaged individuals may seem to do little more than redistribute the scarce opportunities among the disadvantaged.

While this last point rightly underlines the need for structural policies aimed at decreasing unemployment levels and increasing the number of educational opportunities, the health implications of economic growth and of redistribution are more surprising. The well-known problems of drawing inferences from ecological data and assuming they tell us about causal processes at the individual level (the ecological fallacy) are matched by the problems of making inferences the other way round – from individual-level data to societal policies (the individualistic fallacy). Part of the association between people's material circumstances and their health appears to be not so much a direct relationship between exposure to unhealthy material circumstances, as a relationship between relative income, or social position, and health. If what matters causally is socio-economic status rather than increased levels of consumption *per se*, then it may be wrong to assume that societal improvements in income or educational standards will improve health as

256

much as the individual associations with either income or education seem to suggest.

What, then, is the solution if projects designed to improve individual job and educational prospects are flawed because they do not change the sum total of disadvantage, and societal policies to improve overall incomes and educational standards may mistake the effects of social position for an effect of absolute material standards? Fortunately, there is a solution. Evidence from a number of sources suggests that in more egalitarian societies, where differences in incomes and in social status are smaller, the average health standards of the population may be substantially improved. But as well as more egalitarian societies having a smaller burden of relative deprivation pressing down on health standards, they also seem to be more socially cohesive. Complementing the picture of better health among more egalitarian populations is evidence that, at least among the rich developed countries, health is indeed related to relative rather than absolute income, and that, as a consequence, health may not be strongly related to economic growth. This chapter will summarize some of this evidence and offer some tentative explanations before returning to the policy implications.

12.2 Relative income

The main *material* and behavioural determinants of health – diet, absolute poverty, unemployment, exercise, drug abuse, housing, etc. – tend to be more widely recognized than the contribution to ill health from psychosocial sources. But research suggests increasingly that many of the socio-economic determinants of health have their effects through psychosocial pathways. Important parts of the picture have been discussed by Eric Brunner and Michael Marmot in their chapter on the biology of stress (Chapter 2), by Michael Marmot, Johannes Siegrist, Tores Thoerell, and Amanda Feeney in their discussion of the workplace (Chapter 6), and by Stephen Stansfield on social support and social cohesion (Chapter 8). Here I will first describe some indications of the overall importance to population health of the kinds of psychosocial pathways they describe, and then suggest how key psychosocial risk factors, such as social affiliations, early emotional development, and social status, are related to each other.

There are two important pieces of ecological (or macro-) level evidence which suggest that psychosocial pathways may exert a more powerful influence on health in the developed world than do pathways involving direct exposure to material hazards. Both suggest that correlations between income and health should be interpreted primarily as correlations between health and relative – rather than absolute – income or material standards. The implication is that what is important is not what your absolute level of material prosperity is, but how it compares, or where it places you, in relation to others in society. Interestingly, this accords well with the original basis on which the British Registrar General ranked occupations according to their 'general social standing' in order to show the social gradient in death rates.

Relationships between the average income and average health of developed countries are much weaker than the relationships found when using grouped data on income and health differences within them. Thus the USA has a gross domestic product per capita (GDPpc) which is well over twice as high as that of Greece, yet life expectancy is higher in Greece than in the USA. Among the developed countries this is not an exception to a more general relationship. The cross-sectional correlation between life expectancy among the 23 richest member countries of the Organization for Economic Co-operation and Development (OECD) (the rich market democracies) and GDPpc (converted at purchasing power parities) is very weak (in 1993, $r = 0.08$). Although we tend to assume that the gradual increase in life expectancy is a direct reflection of increasing prosperity, in fact the association even between long-term economic growth rates per capita and changes in life expectancy is also weak: the correlation coefficient between the percentage increase in GDPpc and the increase in life expectancy among the same group of rich countries over the period 1970–93 was only 0.30. (Although life expectancy rises with economic development in developing countries, this relationship almost disappears among the developed countries. Among them, continued increases in life expectancy have little relation to economic growth (Wilkinson 1996).) This contrasts sharply with the very close relationships between income and mortality rates found using grouped data *within* countries, where correlations as strong as 0.8 or 0.9 are not uncommon. Indeed, mortality rates for small areas or occupations are usually almost perfectly rank ordered by income within countries. This is, of course, an expression of the relationship between a wide variety of measures of socio-economic status and health within countries – known as 'health inequalities' or the 'social gradient' in health – which has featured so prominently in earlier chapters.

Dealing as we are with whole nations, the much weaker or non-existent income health relationships between countries cannot be attributed to sampling error; nor is it attributable to differences in national cultures. For instance, among the 50 states in the USA, where cultural differences are smaller and people shop at many of the same chain stores selling the same range of goods throughout the country, the correlation between median state income and mortality is only 0.28, and even this weak relation disappears when it is controlled for income inequality ($r = 0.06$) (Kaplan et al. 1996).

This suggests that income is related to health not so much through its role as a determinant of material living standards, but rather as a marker for social status. Where (as within countries) income differences map onto differences in social status, they are closely related to health. Where (as between countries) they have no significance for social status, they are not closely related to health. The implication is that the bulk of the relation between income and health, at least in the developed countries, is a relation between health and relative income or socio-economic status. Health appears to be related less to people's absolute material living standards than to their position in society, as expressed by their income.

This interpretation finds strong support in the association between a society's income distribution and population health. More egalitarian societies, that is societies with smaller differences in income between rich and poor, tend to have better health and increased longevity. There have been numerous reports of an association between income distribution and measures of health (Kawachi et al. 1999a). As well as evidence from international comparisons, studies within countries also suggest that more egalitarian areas tend to have better health. Thus, although mortality in US states is not related to median state income (Kaplan et al. 1996), it has been shown to be closely related to measures of income inequality within those states (Kennedy et al. 1996) – and to income inequality among the 282 Standard Metropolitan Areas of the USA (Lynch et al. 1998). Indeed, the relation between income distribution and health now seems safe: alongside the 20 or so reports of an association between measures of income inequality and population health, there are only two reports (using the same data set) suggesting that the relation is weak or non-existent.

There has been some discussion as to whether the relation of income distribution to health is simply a reflection of a tendency for the health of the poor to be more sensitive to changes in income than the rich, and could be accounted for by the relationships between individual incomes and health. There have now been a number of studies which have looked at the effects of different degrees of income inequality after controlling for individual incomes. All but one concluded that greater income equality has a beneficial effect on health even after taking individual incomes into account (Kennedy et al. 1998a; Soobader and LeClere 1998; Diez-Roux et al. 1999). The methods of the one study which produced results at odds with the others (Fiscella and Franks 1997) have been criticized (Kennedy et al. 1998a; Diez-Roux et al. 1999). However, the distinction between the health effects of individual income and the societal effects of income inequality is more important for those who believe that it coincides with the distinction between the effects of individual absolute income (as a determinant of material living standards), and the effects of societal social processes related to inequality. In the light of the preceding discussion, it seems more likely that the distinction is the less fundamental one between the psychosocial effects of individual relative income – or social position – and the societal effects of inequality. As we shall see, both are likely to involve similar pathways to do with issues of social status and social relations. The distinction may therefore be less important than first thought.

Having seen that among populations where there are greater income differences, implying greater disparities of socio-economic status and a correspondingly greater burden of relative deprivation, health tends to be less good, we shall now go on to outline two powerful routes through which relative income and income inequality are likely to affect health. One is through the direct psychosocial effects of low social status; and the other is through the poorer quality of social relations found in more hierarchical societies.

12.3   Inequality and psychosocial welfare

The strongest evidence that there are psychosocial health effects attributable directly to low social status itself comes from work on the physiological effects of social status among non-human primates. Work on baboons in the wild and on macaques in captivity indicates important psychosocial pathways linking the chronic anxiety of subordinate social status to raised basal cortisol levels and attenuated responses to acute stress, increased atherosclerosis, worse HDL : LDL ratios, central obesity, depression, and poorer immune function (Sapolsky 1993; Shively and Clarkson 1994; Sapolsky et al. 1997; Shively et al. 1997). The effects of chronic anxiety and the consequent rise in basal cortisol levels appear to be so far-reaching that they have been likened to a process of more rapid ageing (Sapolsky 1994). Many of the physiological risk factors which are also associated with social status among humans (see Brunner and Marmot, Chapter 2 this volume) seem, among non-human primates, to be directly attributable to the psychosocial effects of subordinate social status itself. In experiments on captive animals (Shively and Clarkson 1994; Shively et al. 1997) it is possible to manipulate social status by moving animals between cages with different groups, while at the same time controlling diet and the environment. This means that there is almost no way of explaining the physiological correlates of social status except to say that they are the direct result of subordinate social status. Important biological effects of social status differences remain among the monkeys even after the effects of factors like poor housing and diet, smoking and job insecurity have been excluded. (That is not to suggest that the excluded factors do not have an important influence on the health of people exposed to them: the evidence shows quite clearly that they do. What it does mean is that there is also a substantial direct psycho-social effect of social status on health.)

Not only are the common physiological correlates of social status in humans unlikely to derive from totally different sources in species which are so closely related to us genetically, but there are a number of suggestions in the psychological literature that issues to do with shame, inferiority, sub-ordination, people being put down and not respected, etc. are extremely important – if largely unrecognized – sources of recurrent anxiety resulting from hierarchy. The possible centrality of shame, fears of incompetence and inferiority in relation to people in superior positions needs to be emphasized for two reasons. First, because a central part of the research task is to identify the most potent sources of recurrent anxiety related to low social status and, secondly, because these issues go beyond health: the same psychosocial processes may also contribute to a number of other social problems associated with relative deprivation.

Crucially important here is the evidence that the social environment becomes less supportive and more conflictual where income differences are bigger. Both Kaplan et al. (1996) and Kennedy et al. (1998b) have shown close relationships between homicide and income inequality. We also have the benefit of a meta-analysis of some 34 papers, based on data comparing countries as well as areas within countries, which suggests that this is a robust relationship (Hsieh and Pugh 1993). Kawachi et al. (1997) have shown that the proportion of people who feel they can trust others declines sharply where income differences are bigger. Also closely related to income inequality are the differences in the average hostility scores for 10 US cities, which were measured by Williams et al. (1995): the wider the income differences, the greater are the hostility scores. These measures of the social environment were all closely related to mortality as well as to income inequality: correlations were commonly as high as 0.7 or higher.

In his study of people's engagement in community life in the regions of Italy, Putnam (1993) notes that income inequality is strongly related to his index of 'civic community' and says (referring here more to an egalitarian social ethos rather than to income distribution) that 'Equality is an essential feature of the civic community' (p. 105). I have also pointed to qualitative evidence suggesting that societies which were unusually egalitarian and unusually healthy were also unusually cohesive (Wilkinson 1996). The examples I discussed included Britain during the two world wars, post-war Japan, Roseto in Pennsylvania (Bruhn and Wolf 1979), and eastern Europe during the 1970s and 1980s. The more recent quantitative evidence (above) which includes a path analysis (Kawachi et al. 1997), strongly suggests that the pathway is from income distribution, through the quality of social relations, to health.

As Stephen Stansfeld shows (Chapter 8), it is now well established that the quality of people's social relations seems to have a powerful influence on their health. Several studies have reported death rates two or three times as high among people with low levels of social integration compared to people with high levels (House et al. 1988; Berkman 1995). In valiant attempts to avoid psychosocial explanations, some people have suggested that the health benefits of friendship may result primarily from the gains that come from practical material support, overlooking the fact that the most common things which friends share or give each other are cigarettes, alcoholic drinks, and the proverbial 'cup of sugar' borrowed from neighbours – not to mention AIDS. Hardly a recipe for good health! Much more plausible is that it is the psychosocial effect of the social relation itself which is important to health. Once more confirming the psychosocial pathway, studies of non-human primates have now shown that animals with fewer social affiliations have the familiar pattern of reduced basal cortisol levels and attenuated stress responses associated with chronic anxiety (Sapolsky et al. 1997).

Here it is conceptually helpful to see that friendship and social hierarchy are linked as opposite types of social relation: they may be thought of as opposite sides of the same coin. Friendship is about mutuality, reciprocity, and the recognition that the needs of friends are needs for us. In contrast, hierarchy, dominance, and subordination is a pecking order based on power, coercion, and access to resources regardless of the needs of others. Putnam refers to them as horizontal and vertical relations. He contrasts the horizontal relations between equals which are conducive to civic community with the vertical patron/client relations which predominate in the areas where community life is weaker. In studies of animal social behaviour it is also clear that horizontal affiliations (based largely on grooming) not only confer obligations of mutual aid and reciprocity, but are used to improve or defend positions in the vertical dominance hierarchy.

The incompatibility of friendship and inequality has often been noted. Indeed, Plato (*The Laws*, p. 229) remarked 'How correct the old saying is, that equality leads to friendship! It's right enough and it rings true'. In this context it is interesting to note that the current Cambridge Scale for ranking occupations in hierarchical order, uses information on friendships as a measure of social distance (Prandy 1990). It is based on data from a sample of the population who are asked details of their own occupations and those of six friends. Occupations with many friendships between them are regarded as being at a similar social level, whereas those with few friendships between them are assumed to be separated by a large social distance. So great is the friction between inequality and friendship that research has been undertaken to see 'how individuals maintain or repair a close social bond when a perceived difference in status . . . has disrupted a close relationship' (Harris 1997).

If increased income inequality is closely accompanied by a weakening of social bonds, the combination of the two can hardly fail to have a potent effect on health. Partly because of the large proportion of the population exposed to these risks, low social status and poor social relations are probably two of the most powerful risk factors influencing population health.

Reading between the lines of the evidence, we can see that a crucial source of chronic anxiety, related both to social hierarchy and inversely to friendship, is likely to centre on feelings aroused by social comparisons to do with confidence, insecurity, and fears of inadequacy. Social hierarchy induces worries about possible incompetence and inadequacy, feelings of insecurity, and fears inferiority. In contrast, the experience of friendship is primarily about the sense of being accepted and appreciated, and of having a positive, confidence-boosting, self-image reflected back. The importance of social comparisons in inducing stress has been demonstrated in research which involves exposing people to experimentally induced stressors. Having to do a difficult and demanding task in isolation does not in itself seem enough to raise cortisol levels. But cortisol levels do rise when the same tasks are performed in a situation where failure is experimentally induced and people's results are publicly compared with others at frequent intervals (Pruessner et al. 1999).

A third pointer (in addition to the health impact of social status and friendship) which seems to confirm the centrality of these basic issues of confidence and insecurity comes from the effects of early childhood emotional development on health. Because of the inherent methodological difficulties of collecting data during early life and relating it to disease in adulthood, there is still a serious shortage of evidence on the relationship between the emotional environment in early childhood and poor health in later life. However, all the pointers are there. Using retrospective data, Lundberg (1993) found that 'family dissension' in childhood was associated with a 52 per cent increase in mortality risk among Swedish adults 30–75 years old, and was a more important determinant of health in later life than economic hardship. Similarly, Montgomery et al. (1997) found that domestic conflict in early childhood predicted slow growth and unemployment in adulthood. In addition, lack of secure attachment in early life, domestic conflict, and family instability have been shown to be related to the behavioural, developmental, psychosocial, and physiological markers suggesting that the early emotional environment is strongly related to adult disease. Wadsworth discusses some of the links in Chapter 3 (see also Wadsworth 1984).

In a review paper, Fonagy (1998) says that domestic conflict and poor early attachment lead to a lower IQ and less good educational achievement, anti-social behaviour, depression, and aggression. Power et al. (1991) reported that in the National Child Development Study the best predictors of health in early adulthood were teachers' assessments of the behaviour of children when they were 16 years old. A review by Hertzman and Wiens (1996), which shows that various psychosocial interventions in early childhood can be effective in preventing or overcoming these difficulties, also confirms the importance of emotional development.

There is now strong evidence, mainly from animal studies, that the psychosocial effects of early emotional trauma are partly mediated by the activation of the hypothalamic–pituitary–adrenal axis and raised basal cortisol levels. Experiments on several species have shown that early handling, maternal licking in infancy, and good mothering results in lower cortisol levels through-out life (Meaney et al. 1988; Suomi 1991; Liu et al. 1997; Fonagy 1998).

The emerging picture seems to combine two large bodies of apparently separate sociological and psychological literature. The mass of sociological literature on social stratification and social class contrasts sharply with the minor importance accorded to these issues in the psychological literature. Yet, for its part, psychology has an enormous literature on the importance of early childhood which is not matched in sociology. From our point of view these sociological and psychological literatures are closely related. The basic confidence or insecurity which comes from emotional experience in early childhood affects people's vulnerability to the insecurity induced by low social status in the social hierarchy. The social hierarchy seems to present itself to us as if it were a hierarchy of human adequacy, from the most superior, successful, and capable, at the top, to the most incapable at the bottom. Indeed, that people with low social status take that as an indication of their own incompetence and lack of ability was the central message of Sennett and Cobb's (1973) *The hidden injuries of class*. While the nature of society and the extent of inequality are likely to be the primary determinants of the proportion of the population made to feel inferior, the security or insecurity of people's early attachments is likely to determine which individuals are most likely to succumb to status insecurities.

The health risks associated with low social status, lack of social ties, and early emotional insecurity may then all point to the same source of anxiety at the heart of social life. Thomas Scheff, working on the emotional complex involving a sense of inferiority, shame, and embarrassment which he calls the '*deference–emotion system*' (Scheff 1988), notes that 'there has been a continuing suggestion in the literature that shame is *the* primary social emotion, generated by the virtually constant monitoring of the self in relation to others' (p. 397). Similarly, Goffman (1967) argued that embarrassment played a prominent role in every social encounter; Gilbert and McGuire (1998) have suggested that 'shame' is distantly related to an evolved 'submission' response of subordinate animals to superiors in the social hierarchy; and Darwin (1872) devoted a whole chapter to blushing (and its relation to shame), which he said 'depends in all cases on . . . a sensitive regard for the opinion, more particularly the depreciation of others'. In Scheff et al.'s (1989) words:

> shame involves painful feelings that are not identified as shame by the person experiencing them. Rather they are labelled with a wide variety of terms that serve to disguise the experience of shame: having low self-esteem, feeling foolish, stupid, ridiculous, inadequate, defective, incompetent, awkward, exposed, vulnerable, insecure, helpless. Our culture provides a great many such codewords. Lewis (1971) classifies all these terms as shame markers, because they occurred only in a context [which] always involved a perception of self as negatively evaluated, by either self or other – the basic context for shame.
>
> *(Scheff et al. 1989, p. 181)*

> In these instances, the negative evaluation of self appears to cause so much pain that it interferes with the fluent production of thought or speech, even though the pain is mislabelled.
>
> *(Scheff et al. 1989, p. 182)*

The scene in TV soaps in which the boss and his wife come to dinner with the junior executive who is thereby reduced to a clumsy, gibbering idiot, unable to put a foot or a word right, is the comic representation of this process.

What is at stake is the sense of pride and need for self-confirmation on the one hand, and shame, humiliation, and rejection on the other. It is the unacknowledged or repressed nature of shame which 'explains how shame might be ubiquitous, yet usually escape notice' (Scheff et al. 1989, p. 183). So important are these processes in social life that it has been suggested that shame is the key to social conformity. The results of a number of social psychology experiments on people's tendency to conform (rather than sticking out from a group) are best explained in terms of their desire to avoid embarrassment, of being thought different, inadequate, or stupid: 'unacknowledged shame plays a central role in causing subjects to yield to group influence, even when it contradicts their own direct perceptions' (Scheff et al. 1989).

These processes, triggered by invidious social comparisons, seem the most plausible source of the chronic stress related to low social status, to lack of friendship, and to poor emotional attachment early in life – all of which have been shown to lead to raised basal cortisol levels and attenuated responses to experimental stressors. Although few studies have investigated the role of cortisol in health differences in human populations, the first to have done so provides strong evidence of its importance (Kristenson et al. 1998)

12.4   A culture of inequality

Given the close relationship between income inequality and both homicide and violent crime (Hsieh and Pugh 1993; Kaplan et al. 1996; Kennedy et al. 1998*b*), it is important to note that Scheff et al. (1989) also suggest that unacknowledged shame 'leads to anger, disrespectful communication and a spiral of exchanges between the parties [which] results in anger and further hostile communication' – the 'shame rage spiral'. 'As humiliation increases, rage and hostility increase proportionally to defend against loss of self-esteem . . . hostility can be viewed as an attempt to ward off feelings of humiliation (shame) generated by inept, ineffectual moves, a sense of incompetence, insults, and a lack of power to defend against insults' (Scheff et al. 1989, p. 188). The close accord between this and literature on violence and disrespect suggests an explanation for the link between violence and greater inequality. Gilligan (1996), who was a prison psychiatrist for 25 years, said: 'I have yet to see a serious act of violence that was not provoked by the experience of feeling shamed and humiliated, disrespected and ridiculed, and that did not represent the attempt to prevent or undo this "loss of face" – no matter how severe the punishment' (Gilligan 1996, p. 110). A paper examining the common links between inequality, health, and violence argued that as greater inequality cuts more people off from other sources of status, we become increasingly sensitive to status issues, ready to defend ourselves against being looked down on, thought incompetent, treated as inferior, and disrespected (Wilkinson et al. 1998).

The indications are that there is a culture of inequality which is less supportive, more aggressive, and usually more macho or 'laddish'. Not only is this suggested by the relation we have seen between income inequality and various measures of the social environment, but it is also suggested by the causes of death which are most closely related to differences in inequality. Although not accounting for the largest number of excess deaths in more unequal places, the death rates which usually show the biggest percentage differences between more and less egalitarian places seem to include violence, accidents, and alcohol-related deaths (McIsaac et al. 1997; Walberg et al. 1998). Because deaths from these causes affect men (particularly young men) more than women, greater income inequality is often associated with bigger differences between male and female mortality rates (Kawachi et al. 1999b; Wilkinson et al. 1999a).

The stresses of hierarchy and the effects of more hierarchical relations, of institutional structures of power and subordination, are passed downwards. The violence associated with wider income differences is not principally between rich and poor; it is most pronounced in the inner cities and among the poor themselves. People subordinated by their social or institutional superiors and threatened with humiliation, attempt to regain their sense of control and restore their self-esteem by asserting authority and control over those below them. At intermediate levels in the hierarchy this can be done through institutional sources of authority rather than through personal physical violence. But at the bottom, where people lack other ways of regaining their self-respect, the tendency is to try to regain it by asserting superiority over whatever minorities are most vulnerable. Hence the well-known pattern for discrimination and scapegoating of minorities to increase in times of high unemployment and economic hardship. Kennedy et al. (1997) have shown that there is more racial discrimination in those US states where income differences are bigger.

That men who have been humiliated are more likely to try to regain a sense of themselves by taking it out on women is likely to account for the connection between income inequality and the status of women (Kawachi et al. 1998). Gloria Anzaldua, who grew up where the word 'macho' gained its modern meaning, gives a graphic description of how machismo is predicated on hierarchy and leads to the oppression of women:

> For men like my father, being 'macho' meant being strong enough to protect and support my mother and us, yet being able to show love. Today's macho has doubts about his ability to feed and protect his family. His 'machismo' is an adaptation to oppression and poverty and low self-esteem. It is the result of hierarchical male dominance. The Anglo, feeling inadequate and inferior and powerless, displaces or transfers these feelings to the Chicano by shaming him. In the Gringo world, the Chicano suffers from excessive humility and self-effacement, shame of self and self-deprecation.
>
> The loss of a sense of dignity and respect in the macho breeds a false machismo which leads him to put down women and even to brutalize them.

> Coexisting with his sexist behavior is a love of the mother which takes
> precedence over that of all others. Devoted son, macho pig. To wash down
> the shame of his acts, of his very being, and to handle the brute in the mirror,
> he takes to the bottle, the snort, the needle and the fist.
> *(Anzaldua 1987, p. 83)*

Much the same processes are likely to lie behind the association between
greater inequality and more racial discrimination in the United States
(Kennedy et al. 1997).

In a different cultural context, but where some of the same forces operate,
James (1995) has reviewed evidence showing that greater inequality and
relative poverty increase the stresses on family life, so leading to more
domestic violence and to more children growing up to become violent adults.

12.5 Conclusions

Returning to the issues raised at the beginning of this chapter about the policy
conundrum round the dangers of both ecological and individualistic fallacies,
the solution involves tackling the structural determinants of the social
environment. This does not mean relying on economic growth, which, even
with 'trickle down', improves everyone's material prosperity in parallel while
leaving social relations unchanged. Nor does it mean pursuing policies that
simply affect which individuals suffer various forms of disadvantage without
affecting the total burden of disadvantage in the population. Instead, policies
need to aim at reducing the overall burden of disadvantage – tackling the
structural sources of inequality through policies on employment, incomes,
and education. (In Britain disparities in the educational achievements of
16-year-olds have been increasing.) In order to decrease socio-economic
inequality, we need to reduce both the proportion of the population who
fall behind, and the distance they fall behind, on each of these core criteria.

The admittedly speculative picture which has been suggested here is that
greater income inequality is one of the major influences on the proportion of
the population who find themselves in situations that deny them a sense of
dignity, situations that increase the insecurity they feel about their personal
worth and competence, and that carry connotations of inferiority in which
few can feel respected, valued, and confident. Instead of offsetting some of
this damage, friendships and social networks atrophy as people feel increasingly vulnerable to the way they are seen by others. Working through the kind
of deference–emotion system described by Scheff, people become more
vulnerable to feelings of shame and more likely to use violence to gain respect.
As well as increased violence, accidents, and alcohol-related deaths, these
feelings are plausibly one of the most powerful and recurrent sources of the
chronic stress that increases people's vulnerability to a wide range of infectious and cardiovascular diseases. This provides the most plausible model we

have of why low social status, weak social networks, and poor early attachment should be related not only to worse health but also to raised basal
cortisol levels and attenuated cortisol responses to experimental stressors.
The biological processes set in train by chronic anxiety appear to provide a
plausible candidate for the hypothesized 'general vulnerability factor' which
could explain why so many causes of death become more common further
down the social hierarchy (Marmot et al. 1984). Because they act cumulatively, they are also compatible with the additive effects of lifetime exposure to
adverse circumstances described by David Blane in Chapter 4.

The importance to health of the social environment and psychosocial
welfare does not, however, mean that we can ignore the material inequalities
which are its foundations. The strength of the statistical relationships suggest
that something between one-third and two-thirds of the differences in
measures of the social environment, in mortality and in violence may be
attributable to the extent of income inequality alone. Nor is improvement a
matter of reaching some utopian state of perfect equality. On the contrary,
rather than pointing to something unattainable, the statistical analyses show
the importance of the differences in inequality which currently exist between
developed market democracies or among the 50 states of the United States.

There are, of course, many other important sources of the relationship
between socio-economic circumstances and health. Diet, housing, job control,
exercise, social support, smoking, unemployment, job insecurity, and many
others all play a role. However, many of these risk factors will be influenced by
– or work through – a number of different processes. For instance, unemployment, low income, substantial income reductions (McDonough et al. 1997),
and lack of educational qualifications can all be experienced as a threat to
pride and dignity, and are potentially shaming. Income inequality is
important partly because it is indicative of a number of these different contributions to the scale of disadvantage in a society. But even apparently
independent risk factors, such as smoking and obesity, may not be completely
unaffected by this axis: there is some evidence to suggest that self-esteem and
a sense of control may make it easier to keep to resolutions about giving up
smoking (Action on Smoking and Health 1993; Marsh and McKay 1994.)
The same might be true of those who, despite their best intentions, continue to
'eat for comfort'. This might explain why behavioural risk factors such as
body mass index, smoking, and sedentarism appear to be related to the extent
of inequality (Diez-Roux et al. 1999).

There are numerous complimentary policy approaches to the issues
discussed in the earlier chapters of this book, and effective measures will
probably mean bringing several of them together. Take obesity as an example:

(1) A necessary but not sufficient condition for effective policy is a public
    awareness of its health risks and an understanding of the contribution of
    diet and exercise. That knowledge is probably fairly widespread already.

(2) On top of that is the need to tackle the food industry, which promotes, particularly to children, refined foods containing concentrated fats and sugars. (See Chapter 9.)

(3) The problem of low incomes: refined foods undoubtedly provide cheap calories, and diets that conform to nutritional recommendations usually cost more. This is an important part of the reason why more harmful diets are so much more common among poorer people.

(4) The amount of exercise people take is influenced not only by individual choice, but also by a society's transport policies – as Mark McCarthy explains in Chapter 7.

(5) It looks as if there is a direct contribution to central obesity and the 'metabolic syndrome' from chronic stress (Shively and Clarkson 1988; Brunner et al. 1997). (See Chapter 2.)

(6) There is little doubt that the tendency to eat (or drink) 'for comfort' will be stronger among those whose circumstances do not provide them with the social sources of that comfort. People who feel depressed and trapped, who lack the resources and opportunities that allow them to experience a sense of control over their circumstances, will find it hardest to make (and keep to) resolutions to take more exercise and go without comfort foods: that is easiest when you feel on top of things and life is going well.

Greater equality is likely to make a contribution to the third, fifth, and sixth of these approaches to reducing obesity. If a more egalitarian ethos also contributes to people's willingness to fund and use public transport, it will also contribute to the fourth. Examples of other health problems would have shown a similarly wide range of policy approaches, including ways in which a reduction in relative deprivation and in the hierarchical differentiation of the population would lead to improvements.

In a nutshell, then, the health importance of greater income equality, and of the improved social environment that comes with it, is that it enhances the population's psychosocial welfare. By improving social functioning, it increases the effectiveness of a wide range of public health and social policy initiatives – including the reduction in cardiovascular risk factors (Diez-Roux et al. 1999). Without tackling material inequalities, progress is likely to be slower and the quality of life poorer.

But it is not just health that is related to the extent of relative deprivation. We have already seen the links with violence and a less supportive social environment; equally strong is the association between deprivation and poorer educational performance of schoolchildren (Blane et al. 1996), and of course a number of other social problems are also recognized to be more common in deprived areas. It seems likely that the powerful psychosocial effects of relative deprivation and low social status can explain why a variety of social problems share roots in relative poverty. The implication is that there may be multiple benefits to policies that address the underlying causes.

Finally, if a range of health and other social problems are related to relative income rather than absolute living standards, and income inequality is associated, as we have seen, with ill health, violence, and a poorer social environment, it suggests that part of the almost universal desire for higher incomes may be a desire for improved social status. This has been suggested by several economists including Frank (1999) and Schor (1998), both of whom argue that consumption is competitive and fuelled by a concern to maintain or improve social status. Indeed, their views are reminiscent of Adam Smith's when he said:

> What is the end of avarice and ambition, of the pursuit of wealth, of power and pre-eminence? Is it to supply the necessities of nature? The wages of the meanest labourer can supply them . . . what are the advantages which we would propose to gain by that great purpose of human life which we call bettering our condition? To be observed, to be attended to, to be taken notice of with sympathy, complacency, and approbation, are all the advantages which we can propose to derive from it.
>
> *(Adam Smith,* Theory of the moral sentiments. *Book i, ch. ii.1, p. 50)*

Schor describes how American 'aspirational' incomes increased during the 1980s when income differences were widening. She says that in 1980 people used to aspire to life styles pegged to about 20 per cent above their prevailing standard of living, but then 'A shift took place in that comparative process – everyone, especially the entire middle class – began to compare themselves with the top 20 per cent of the income distribution', drastically widening the aspiration gap. She describes how a Roper poll in 1986 asked people 'How much money would you need to make all your dreams come true?' and found a mean reply of US$50 000. By 1994, that 'dream-fulfilling' level had doubled to US$102 000, and those earning US$50 000 or more felt they would need US$200 000. As a result, Americans spent higher fractions of their income, their savings declined, and they took on record levels of debt. She also presents data showing that the more television people watch, the less money they save, and the more they spend.

These trends are what one might expect if status differences are important in fuelling consumption. The implication is that it may not be legitimate to assume that individual desires for higher incomes can be summed into a societal demand for economic growth. Because it does nothing about relative social status, economic growth may be less important to welfare in the developed world than is often supposed. This means that if we are to move towards environmentally sustainable levels of consumption, it may be necessary to reduce the status differences which drive the competitive element in consumption. But, as Schor says, 'We live with high levels of psychological denial about the connection between our buying habits and the social statements they make'.

References

Action on Smoking and Health (1993). *Her share of misfortune.* ASH, London.

Anzaldua, G. (1987). *Borderlands.* Aunt Lute Books, San Francisco.

Berkman, L.F. (1995). The role of social relations in health promotion. *Psychosom. Res.* **57**, 245–54.

Blane, D., White, I. and Morris, J. (1996). Education, social circumstances and mortality. In: *Health and social organization*, (ed. D. Blane, E. Brunner and R. Wilkinson). Routledge, London.

Bruhn, J.G. and Wolf, S. (1979). *The Roseto Story.* Norman. University of Oklahoma Press.

Brunner, E.J., Marmot, M.G., Nanchahal, K., et al. (1997). Social inequality in coronary risk: central obesity and the metabolic syndrome. Evidence from the Whitehall II study. *Diabetologia* **40** (11), 1341–9.

Darwin, C. (1872). *The expression of emotion in men and animals.* John Murray, London.

Diez-Roux, A.V., Link. B. and Northridge, M.E. (1999). A multilevel analysis of income inequality and cardiovascular disease risk factors. *Soc. Sci. Med.* in press.

Fiscella, K. and Franks, P. (1997). Poverty or income inequality as predictors of mortality: longitudinal cohort study. *BMJ* **314**, 1724–8.

Fonagy, P. (1998). *Early influences on development and social inequalities: an attachment theory perspective.* Paper presented at the Kansas Conference on Health and its Social Determinants, Wichita, in press.

Frank, R.H. (1999). Luxury Fever. Free Press, New York.

Gilbert, P., McGuire, M.T. (1998). Shame, status, and social roles: psycho-biology and evolution. In: *Shame: interpersonal behavior, psychopathology, and culture.* Edited by Gilbert P. and Andrews B. Oxford University Press N.Y.

Gilligan, J. (1996). *Violence: our deadly epidemic and its causes.* G.P. Putnam.

Goffman, E. (1967). *Interaction ritual.* Anchor Doubleday, Garden City N.Y.

Harris, S.R. (1997). Status inequality and close relationships: an integrative typology of bond-saving strategies. *Symbolic Interaction* **20** (1), 1–20.

Hertzman, C. and Wiens, M. (1996). Child development and long-term out-comes: a population health perspective and summary of successful interventions. *Soc. Sci. Med.* **43**, 1083–95.

House, J.S., Landis, K.R. and Umberson, D. (1988). Social relationships and health. *Science* **241**, 540–5.

Hsieh, C.C. and Pugh, M.D. (1993). Poverty, income inequality, and violent crime: a meta-analysis of recent aggregate data studies. *Criminal Justice Rev.* **18**, 182–202.

James, O. (1995). *Juvenile violence in a winner–looser culture.* Free Association Books.

Kaplan, G.A., Pamuk, E., Lynch, J.W., Cohen, R.D. and Balfour, J.L. (1996). Inequality in income and mortality in the United States: analysis of mortality and potential pathways. *BMJ* **312**, 999–1003.

Kawachi, I., Kennedy, B.P., Lochner, K. and Prothrow-Stith, D. (1997). Social capital, income inequality and mortality. *Am. J. Publ. Hlth* **87**, 1491–8.

Kawachi, I., Kennedy, B.P., Gupta, V. and Prothrow-Stith, D. (1999b). Women's status and the health of women: a view from the States. *Soc. Sci. Med.,* in press.

Kawachi, I., Kennedy, B. and Wilkinson, R.G. (ed.) (1999a). *Income inequality and health: a reader.* New Press, New York, in press.

Kennedy, B.P., Kawachi, I. and Prothrow-Stith, D. (1996). Income distribution and mortality: cross sectional ecological study of the Robin Hood index in the United States. *BMJ* **312**, 1004–7. (See also Kennedy, B.P., Kawachi, I. and Prothrow-Stith, D. (1996). Important correction. *BMJ* **312**, 1194.)

Kennedy, B.P., Kawachi, I., Lochner, K., Jones, C.P. and Prothrow-Stith, D. (1997). (Dis)respect and black mortality. *Ethnic. Dis.* **7**, 207–14.

Kennedy, B.P., Kawachi, I., Glass, R., and Prothrow-Stith, D. (1998a). Income distribution, socioeconomic status, and self-rated health: a US multi-level analysis. *BMJ* **317**, 917–921.

Kennedy, B., Kawachi, I., Prothrow-Stith, D., Lochner, K. and Gibbs, B. (1998b). Social capital, income inequality, and firearm violent crime. *Soc. Sci. Med.* **47**, 7–17.

Kristenson, M., Orth-Gomer, K., Kucinskiene, Z., et al. (1998). Attenuated cortisol response to a standardised stress test in Lithuanian versus Swedish men: the LiVicordia Study. *Int. J. Behav. Med.* **5** (1), 17–30.

Liu, D., Diorio, J., Tannenbaum, B., et al. (1997). Maternal care, hippocampal glucocorticoid receptors, and hypothalamic–pituitary–adrenal responses to stress. *Science* **277**, 1659–62.

Lundberg, O. (1993). The impact of childhood living conditions on illness and mortality in adulthood. *Soc. Sci. Med.* **36**, 1047–52.

Lynch, J., Kaplan, G.A., Pamuk, E.R., et al. (1998). Income inequality and mortality in metropolitan areas of the United States. *Am. J. Publ. Hlth* **88**, 1074–80.

McDonough, P., Duncan, G.J., Williams, D. and House, J. (1997). Income dynamics and adult mortality in the U.S. 1972–89. *Am. J. Publ. Hlth* **87**, 1476–83.

McIsaac, S.J., Wilkinson, R.G. (1997). Income distribution and cause-specific mortality. *European Journal of Public Health,* **7**, 45–53.

Marmot, M.G., Shipley, M.J. and Rose, G. (1984). Inequalities in death – specific explanations of a general pattern? *Lancet* 5 May, 1003–6.

Marsh, A. and McKay, S. (1994). *Poor smokers.* Policy Studies Institute.

Meaney, M.J., Aitken, D.H., van Berkel, C., Bhatnagar, S. and Sapolsky, R.M. (1988). Effect of neonatal handling on age-related impairments associated with the hippocampus. *Science* **239**, 766–8.

Montgomery, S.M., Bartley, M.J. and Wilkinson, R.G. (1997). Family conflict and slow growth. *Arch. Dis. Child.* **77**, 326–30.

Plato (1970). *The Laws* (Translated by T.J. Saunders). Penguin, Harmondsworth.

Power, C., Manor, O., Fox, J. (1991) *Health and class: the early years.* Chapman and Hall, London.

Prandy, K. (1990). The revised Cambridge scale of occupations. *Sociology* **24** (4), 629–55.

Pruessner, J.C., Hellhammer, D.H. and Kirschbaum, C. (1999). Low self-esteem, induced failure and the adrenocortical stress response. *Personality and Individual Differences.* In press.

Putnam, R.D., Leonardi, R., Nanetti, R.Y. (1993). *Making democracy work: civic traditions in modern Italy.* Princeton U.P.

Sapolsky, R.M. (1993). Endocrinology alfresco: psychoendocrine studies of wild baboons. *Recent Prog. Horm. Res.* **48**, 437–68.

Sapolsky, R.M. (1998). *Why zebras don't get ulcers. A guide to stress, stress-related disease and coping.* Second edition, W.H. Freeman, New York.

Sapolsky, R.M., Alberts, S.C. and Altmann, J. (1997). Hypercortisolism associated with social subordinance or social isolation among wild baboons. *Arch. Gen. Psychiat.* **54** (12), 1137–43.

Scheff, T.J. (1988). Shame and conformity: the deference-emotion system. *American Sociological Review* **53**, 395–406.

Scheff, T.J., Retzinger, S.M., Ryan, M.T. (1989). Crime, violence, and self-esteem: review and proposals. In: *The social importance of self-esteem.* Edited by Mecca AM, Smelser NJ, Vasconcellos J. University of California Press, Berkeley.

Schor, J. (1998). *The overspent American: when buying becomes you.* Basic Books.

Sennett, R. and Cobb, J. (1973). *The hidden injuries of class.* Knopf, New York.

Shively, C.A. and Clarkson, T.B. (1988). Regional obesity and coronary artery atherosclerosis in females: a non-human primate model. *Acta Med. Scand. Suppl.* **723**, 71–8.

Shively, C.A. and Clarkson, T.B. (1994). Social status and coronary artery atherosclerosis in female monkeys. *Art. Thromb.* **14**, 721–6.

Shively, C.A., Laird, K.L. and Anton, R.F. (1997). The behavior and physiology of social stress and depression in female cynomolgus monkeys. *Biol. Psychiat.* **41**, 871–82.

Soobader, M.-J. and LeClere, F.B. (1999). Aggregation and the measurement of income inequality: effects on morbidity. *Soc. Sci. Med.* in press.

Suomi, S.J. (1991). Early stress and adult emotional reactivity in rhesus monkeys. In: *The childhood environment and adult disease* (ed. Ciba Foundation), pp. 171–186. John Wiley & Sons, Chichester.

Wadsworth, M.E.J. (1984). Early stress and associations with adult health, behaviour and parenting. In: *Stress and disability in childhood* (ed. N.R. Butler and B.D. Corner). Wright, Bristol.

Walberg, P., McKee, M., Shkolnikov, V., Chenet, L. and Leon, D.A. (1998). Economic change, crime, and mortality crisis in Russia: regional analysis. *BMJ* **317**, 312–18.

Wilkinson, R.G. (1996). *Unhealthy societies: the afflictions of inequality.* Routledge, London.

Wilkinson, R.G., Kawachi, I., Kennedy, B. (1998). Mortality, the social environment, crime and violence. *Sociology of Health and Illness* **20**, 578–97.

Wilkinson, R.G., Kennedy, B. and Kawachi, I. (1999a). Women's status and men's health in a culture of inequality.

Williams, R.B., Feaganes, J. and Barefoot, J.C. (1995). Hostility and death rates in 10 US cities *Psychosom. Med.* **57** (1), 94.

Acknowledgements

Professor Wilkinson's research is supported by a grant from the Medical Research Council.

Epilogue

Agis D. Tsouros and Jill L. Farrington

Introduction

There is no shortage of scientific information on the effects and the importance of a wide range of socio-environmental influences on peoples health. And yet, public health and health promotion action is often limited to addressing illnesses and lifestyle excesses trapped in a model that equates health to the absence of disease and nothing more. In the last ten years a host of global summits and international conferences have come to the same conclusion: there is no lack of technical knowledge, there is a lack of effective communication of scientific evidence to decision-makers and a lack of adequate political commitment to promoting healthy public policy which would enhance health and sustainable development.

Reaching out to decision-makers and promoting awareness, debate and action are the key goals of WHO's Social Determinants Campaign. The campaign was launched in June 1998 by the WHO Regional Office for Europe's Centre for Urban Health and the extensive Europe wide Healthy Cities network represents a principal vehicle of the Campaign. The purpose of this Epilogue is to describe the scope and purpose of the campaign and to give an overview of the Healthy Cities project, explaining its significance as a key mechanism for linking research to action.

The new policy context

The world is changing fast. Decisions are made differently. Politics are played differently. Since the adoption of WHO's strategy *Health for All*[1] in the early 1980s, there have been many changes which directly or indirectly affect the health policy making process. These relate both to changes in the policy environment, and to accumulating evidence concerning the determinants of health and their interrelationship with socio-economic development. New actors have

---

1 Health for All, health strategy for Europe was agreed by European States in 1984. The renewed European strategy Health 21 was agreed in 1998.

emerged and continue to emerge. Health promotion programmes are increasingly more strategic in their orientation; they employ a wider array of policy instruments, draw on the contributions of a greater number of partners from different sectors and allow more active community participation. Action at the local level is being recognized as an essential dimension in national and sub-national health development policies. This is paralleled by decentralization trends and strengthening of the leadership role local governments can play in health and sustainable development. Extensive networking between cities has developed into a formidable platform for innovation and change across Europe.

The health of a city's people is strongly determined by physical, social, economic, political, and cultural factors in the urban environment, including the processes of social aggregation, migration, modernization and industrialization, and the circumstances of urban living. Cities today present extreme disparities of wealth and environmental stress. It is almost invariably the case that the poorest and most disadvantaged populations experience the worst living and working conditions; the rich almost invariably live upstream, upwind, and uphill. Environmental degradation and pollution, unhealthy town planning, inadequate housing and overcrowding and lack of social systems are associated with stress and mental disorders, illness and deaths, violence and accidents, drug and alcohol abuse, desperation and helplessness.

There is no doubt that the urban context combines in high concentration, interaction and intensity the most challenging issues of modern public health. We know that these issues can only be tackled within a framework of integrated health development strategies and policies that address inequalities, social determinants of health, sustainable development, community empowerment, and accountability for health.

A series of global summits from Rio in 1992[2] (sustainable development and Agenda 21) to Istanbul in 1996[3] (human settlements and urbanization) generated an enormous momentum and interest for change amongst national, local governments, and activists alike. There is a remarkable convergence in the content of the strategy *Health for All*, the strategies that emerged from all the recent global summits and the policies of all major international bodies[4]. Change however requires political will, leadership, adequate capacity for management and implementation, strategic thinking and openness to innovation and institutional reform.

---

2 The United Nations Conference on Environment and Development was held in Rio de Janeiro, Brazil in June 1992.
3 The Second United Nations Conference on Human Settlements (Habitat II) was held in Istanbul in June 1996.
4 WHO Regional Office for Europe (1997) *Sustainable development and health: concepts, principles and framework for action for European cities and towns.* European Sustainable Development and Health Series: 1. ISBN 92–890–1281–1. Available from WHO Healthy Cities website.

The Healthy Cities Project

The WHO Healthy Cities Project (HCP) is a long-term international develop-ment project that seeks to put health on the agenda of decision-makers in cities and to build a strong lobby for public health at the local level. Healthy Cities is about changing the ways in which individuals, communities, private and volun-tary organizations, and local governments think about, understand, and make decisions about health. Ultimately, Healthy Cities is about enhancing the phy-sical, mental, social, and environmental well-being of the people who live and work in the cities. A fundamental principle of the Healthy Cities is the recogni-tion that a city can play a key role in promoting and maintaining the health of its citizens and a unique capacity to mobilize action for sustainable development.

The key words that run through the Healthy Cities project are: commitment to health development, healthy public policy, integration, leadership and management of change, partnerships for health, solidarity, international cooperation, and empowerment. Project implementation is achieved through a strategy that involves four elements of action: cross-party political support to the *Health for All*, Agenda 21[5] and Healthy Cities principles; commitment to developing and implementing a comprehensive city health development strategy; establishment of capacity to manage change and to facilitate institu-tional reform; and investment in local partnerships of health and interna-tional cooperation and networking.

Over the past ten years the WHO's Healthy Cities Project has developed into a major public health movement at local level, involving networks of over 1000 cities and towns throughout more than 27 countries of Europe. The strategic structures and systems consist of a system of interactive city net-works devoted to action and innovation supported by the newly established WHO European Centre for Urban Health. Embarking on its third phase in 1998, the Centre has outlined its strategic plan for the next five years (1998–2002)[6], in which a priority action area will be a focusing of attention and work on equity, social determinants of health and poverty, with the Healthy Cities networks representing its main political and implementation arm.

At the International Healthy Cities Conference held in Athens in June 1998, which marked a decade of Healthy Cities action, Mayors from over 100 European cities signed the *Athens Declaration for Healthy Cities*[7].

---

5 Earth Summit-Agenda 21. The United Nations Programme of Action from Rio. New York, United Nations, 1993.
6 WHO Regional Office for Europe Centre for Urban Health *Strategic plan: Urban Health/ HealthyCities Programme (1998–2002)*. June 1998. See also Healthy Cities Phase III (1998–2002) criteria. Available from the WHO Healthy Cities website (http:// www.who.dk/healthy-cities/).
7 Available from WHO Healthy Cities website (http://www.who.dk/healthy-cities/).

Through this, they pledged their commitment to improving the health of their citizens, guided by the key principles of equity, sustainability, inter-sectoral co-operation, and solidarity. They also stressed the importance of local level action as an essential component of any national or sub-national strategy or programme aimed at health and sustainable development and tackling the determinants of health. The Members of the WHO Regional Committee of the European Region issued a Resolution in September 1998 in support of the Healthy Cities movement as a principal vehicle for promoting health for all based policies in the European Region.

The scope and purpose of the Social Determinants Campaign

Recognizing the health impact of economic and social policies and conditions could have far reaching implications for the way society makes decisions about development, and it could challenge the values and principles on which institutions are built and progress is measured. The good news is that decision-makers at all levels increasingly recognize the need to invest in health and sustainable development. To do this they need clear facts as much as they need strategic guidance and policy tools. Nobody expects science to be black or white, but it must be accessible, creating opportunities for debate and informed decision-making.

At the WHO Regional Office for Europe, the Centre for Urban Health, in close partnership with the Communication and Public Affairs Unit and new European Health Communication Network, have embarked on a campaign to promote awareness, debate and action on the social determinants of health. The campaign aims at reaching the widest possible audiences of public health advocates and professionals, community activists, and decision-makers. The campaign will develop and employ materials that are attractive and easy to read and translate. A principal vehicle for the promotion of the campaign throughtout the European region will be the WHO Healthy Cities project. The timing of this effort is excellent, as it coincides with the launching of the renewed strategy health for all for the 21st century, the launching of Phase III (1998–2002) of the Healthy Cities project and the increasing commitment of a large number of cities to local Agenda 21.

The backbone of the Campaign is the provision of up-to-date information on the key areas of social determinants, in a clear and authoritative form. This was achieved through close partnership between WHO and the International Centre for Health and Society at University College London and led to the publication of the booklet *Social Determinants of Health: The Solid Facts*[8] which was launched in June 1998 and which provided the basis for this book, *The Social Determinants of Health*. This booklet identifies ten major social determinants of health in the form of ten messages and it provides the research in support of these messages. The booklet also contains specific policy proposals for both local and national governments. It aims to clarify the scientific findings and make them accessible to everyone, creating opportunities for debate and informed decision-making. The booklet has already proven enormously popular with policy makers and activists, both within and beyond Europe. It is being translated in several languages and used to promote awareness and debate amongst public health professional groups, politicians, communit activists and academic staff, both at local and national levels. Healthy Cities networks throughout Europe are committed to promoting sensitisation and action for the social determinants of health.

Conclusions

A call to address the social determinants of health should rest on clear evidence, and reach decision-makers and public health professionals in a format which is easily accessible and with a mechanism which facilitates implementation. Healthy Cities is an effective, well developed and well established mechanism for reaching and engaging local goverments. Thus, the WHO Social Determinants campaign is not limited to information dissemination but also has direct access to a large target policy-making audience that can provide the testing and implementation ground of the social determinants evidence provided in this book and the booklet.

---

8   WHO Regional Office for Europe (1998) Social Determinants of Health. The Solid Facts. ISBN 92–890–1287–0. Available from the WHO Healthy Cities website http:// www.who.dk/healthy-cities/

Index

Social determinants of health

The solid facts

Edited by Richard Wilkinson, Visiting Professor at the International Centre for Health and Society, UCL and Professor of Social Epidemiology at the Trafford Centre for Medical Research, University of Sussex and Michael Marmot, Professor of Epidemiology and Director of the International Centre for Health and Society, UCL

Policy and action for health need to be geared towards addressing the social determinants of health in order to attack the causes of ill health before they can lead to problems. This is a challenging task for both decision-makers and public health actors and advocates. The scientific evidence on social determinants is strong but is discussed mainly by researchers. This booklet is part of a WHO Regional Office for Europe campaign to present the evidence on social determinants in a clear and understandable form. The booklet identifies the broad implications for policy in ten selected areas. The campaign is meant to broaden awareness, stimulate debate and promote action.

Contents: Foreword; Preface; Introduction; The social gradient; Stress; Early life; Social exclusion; Work; Unemployment; Social support; Addiction; Food; Transport.

This booklet is available by post from:

Centre for Urban Health
World Health Organization
Regional Office for Europe
Scherfigsvej 8,
DK-2100 Copenhagen
Denmark
Telephone: +45 39 17 12 24
Fax: +45 39 17 18 60
E-mail: eip@who.dk

An electronic version of the booklet is available to download from:

http://www.who.dk/healthy-cities/determ.htm